The Whole Emergency Medicine Catalog

MICHAEL S. JASTREMSKI, M.D.

Associate Professor and Director
Critical Care and Emergency Medicine

RICHARD M. CANTOR, M.D.

Assistant Professor
Critical Care and Emergency Medicine and Pediatrics

CARIN M. OLSON, M.D.

Assistant Professor
Critical Care and Emergency Medicine

RODNEY W. SMITH, M.D.

Assistant Professor
Critical Care and Emergency Medicine

GARY J. TYNDALL, M.D.

Assistant Professor
Critical Care and Emergency Medicine

"All of the Department of Critical Care and Emergency Medicine
State University of New York
Upstate Medical Center
Syracuse, New York"

1985

W. B. SAUNDERS COMPANY

Philadelphia □ London □ Toronto □ Mexico City □ Rio de Janeiro □ Sydney □ Tokyo □ Hong Kong

W.B. Saunders Company: West Washington Square
Philadelphia, PA 19105

Library of Congress Cataloging in Publication Data
Main entry under title:

The Whole emergency medicine catalog.

    1. Emergency medicine—Handbooks, manuals, etc. I. Jastremski,
Michael S. [DNLM: 1. Emergency Medicine—methods. W 628]

RC86.7.W48   1985   616'.025   84–14106
ISBN 0–7216–1175–3

The Whole Emergency Medicine Catalog   ISBN   0–7216–1175–3

Last digit is the print number: 9   8   7   6   5   4   3   2   1

To our friend and colleague Eoin Aberdeen, whose compassionate approach to patient care and ever questioning mind continue to be an example and an inspiration for us.

"The secret of continuing medical education
is to learn to educate one's self."

HAROLD JEGHERS

If you wish to suggest an article for the second volume (a helpful hint, practical advice, or whatever), please cut out this page and send it to the first-named author with the information and your name and address. Credit will be given to you if the item is used.

To: Michael S. Jastremski, M.D.
      Critical Care and Emergency Medicine
      State University of New York
      Upstate Medical Center
      750 East Adams Street
      Syracuse, New York 13210

I wish to suggest the following article for the 2nd Volume of THE WHOLE EMERGENCY MEDICINE CATALOG:

(Name) _____

_____

_____

PREFACE

We decided to write a *Whole Emergency Medicine Catalog* because its predecessors in Pediatrics and Internal Medicine have been so useful to us in the Emergency Department. The other whole catalogs are among the most dog-eared books on the bookshelf of our Emergency Department when they can be found, since they are also among the books that often seem to mysteriously disappear. We hope that this volume will be of even more use to the emergency physician.

This book is not intended to be an all-inclusive textbook or procedure manual. In fact, we have tried to avoid information that is readily available in existing textbooks. It is intended to be a collection of useful, practical information, gleaned from many sources, that is usually not available when you need it the most. We think the book will be of the most use to you if you spend some time browsing through it to become familiar with its contents. Then, when you need a particular bit of information you will know where to find it. The references are not all-inclusive but should provide you with entry into the medical literature for that particular topic.

Since we believe that learning (and teaching) should be fun, we have tried to present the information in this style. Sprinkled among the facts, you will find various tidbits that interested us and hopefully will interest you.

We would appreciate any thoughts you might have about this volume or a second volume. We would be delighted to include contributions from our readers in a second volume. Please enjoy our book.

MICHAEL S. JASTREMSKI, M.D.
RICHARD M. CANTOR, M.D.
CARIN M. OLSON, M.D.
RODNEY W. SMITH, M.D.
GARY J. TYNDALL, M.D.

ACKNOWLEDGMENTS

We are deeply indebted to the many innovative and creative people whose work is quoted or referred to in this volume. They are the real authors of this book, and we are delighted to be able to share their wisdom with you. The humorous or philosophical quotes that are sprinkled semirandomly throughout the book come from many sources. Particular thanks should go to Robert Matz, M.D., who has collected and published several extensive listings of medical quotes in the New York State Journal of Medicine and to Marshall B. Segal, M.D., J.D., for his succinct observations on medical-legal issues that we found tacked to a bulletin board in the hospital. Some of the quotes were found in the International Dictionary of Thoughts edited by John Bradley, Leo Daniels, and Thomas Jones (published by J.W. Ferguson Publishing Company, Chicago).

Jack Hanley, formerly of W.B. Saunders, was instrumental in getting the book started, and John Dyson of W.B. Saunders patiently but firmly made sure that we finished it.

Susie Chilcoat, Clare Bohlig, and Darliene Dodds provided invaluable assistance with the many drafts and redrafts of the manuscript.

And finally, special thanks to our students, who asked the questions (and sometimes provided the answers) that led us to seek out the information included in this book.

CONTENTS

1   APPROACH TO THE PATIENT 1

2   RESUSCITATION................................. 34

3   TRAUMA 89

4   ENVIRONMENTAL HAZARDS AND POISONS 121

5   ORTHOPEDICS 176

6   SURGERY AND ITS SUBSPECIALTIES 197

7   MEDICINE 237

8   PEDIATRICS....................................278

9   LABORATORY...................................336

10   PSYCHIATRY...................................354

11   PROCEDURES 362

12   POTPOURRI...................................376

     INDEX 407

1

APPROACH TO THE PATIENT

WHAT IS AN EMERGENCY? 3

THE CODE 4

OUR APOLOGIES 5

AIR TRANSPORT OF THE CRITICALLY ILL 6

URINE TEMPERATURE: A CLUE TO EARLY DIAGNOSIS OF
FACTITIOUS FEVER 12

EMERGENCY AIR AMBULANCE 12

SURVEILLANCE: THE EMERGENCY PHYSICIAN'S ROLE IN
ORGAN DONATION 13

USE ALL YOUR SENSES 16

A BAREFOOT DOCTOR 18

TATTOOS 20

CAUSES OF GAS IN SOFT TISSUES .22

THE QUAKER AND THE NEWS DEALER — A FABLE 22

COST CONSCIOUSNESS QUIZ 23

STEROID SENSIBILITY 24

NOTES ON NARCOTICS 26

THE PATIENT WHO WALKS OUT 28

THE "EYE OF HORUS" 29

PRESCRIPTION CHECK LIST 30

PRESCRIBING LIQUIDS 32

FACTS OF HOSPITAL LIFE 32

TOP TEN UPDATE 33

WHAT IS AN EMERGENCY?

*The Patient's Rule: Its not a matter of life or death,
its more important than that.*

Anonymous

e·mer·gen·cy (i mûr jen sē) n., pl. - cies. A sudden, urgent, usually unforeseen occurrence or occasion requiring immediate action.[3]
emergo - mergere - mersi - mersum...v.t. to raise; emergi...v.i. to
emerge.[2]

Bona fide emergencies are "services performed in a hospital
emergency room that are necessary to prevent the death or serious
impairment of the health of the individual".[1]

"An unforeseen condition of a pathophysiological or psychological nature develops, which a prudent layperson, possessing an
average knowledge of health and medicine, would judge to require
urgent and unscheduled medical attention most likely available, after
consideration of possible alternatives, in a hospital emergency department. This would include:

1. Any condition resulting in admission of the patient to a
hospital or nursing home within 24 hours
2. Evaluation or repair of acute (less than 72 hours) trauma
3. Relief of acute or severe pain
4. Investigation or relief of acute infection
5. Protection of public health
6. Obstetrical crises or labor
7. Hemorrhage or threat of hemorrhage
8. Shock or impending shock
9. Investigation and management of suspected abuse or neglect
of person which, if not interrupted, could result in temporary or permanent physical or psychological harm
10. Congenital defects or abnormalities in a newborn infant, best
managed by prompt intervention
11. Decompensation or threat of decompensation of vital functions, such as sensorium, respiration, circulation, excretion, mobility,
and sensory organs
12. Management of a patient suspected to be suffering from a
mental illness and posing an apparent danger to the safety of himself
or herself or others
13. Any sudden or serious symptoms that might indicate a condition that constitutes a threat to the patient's physical or psychological
well-being requiring immediate medical attention to prevent possible
deterioration, disability, or death."[1]

The first dictionary definition emphasizes the unpredictability of
events, and the need for rapid treatment. The Latin root expresses the
developing nature of problems and the need for expectant management. The Health Care Financing Administration states that an

emergency, without intervention, must lead to poor health or death. The American College of Emergency Physicians (ACEP) definition acknowledges that patients or their advocates, in taking the initiative to seek care, decide what needs immediate attention. It is only after a thorough investigation that the true nature and potential consequences of the problems are known.

References:

1. Anthony KJ. ACEP board reviews definition of bona fide emergencies. ACEP News 1982; *1*(9):1 and 4. (Reproduced with permission of the author and publisher.)

2. Traupman JC. The New Collegiate Latin and English Dictionary. New York: Bantam Books, 1966: 98.

3. Urdang L, Flexner SB, eds. The Random House Dictionary of the English Language, College Edition. New York: Random House, 1968: 432.

> "The challenge for medical education today is to train physicians who not only share an understanding of the biology of disease and a mastery of the most advanced technology, but also retain a sense of compassion and understanding and a sensitivity to the patient as a person."
>
> FRANK H.T. RHODES

THE CODE

Preamble

The medical profession has long subscribed to a body of ethical standards developed primarily for the benefit of the patient. As a member of this profession, a physician must recognize responsibility not only to patients but also to society, to other health professionals, and to self. The following principles adopted by the American Medical Association are not laws but standards of conduct that define the essentials of honorable behavior for the physician:

A physician shall be dedicated to providing competent medical service with compassion and respect for human dignity.

A physician shall deal honestly with patients and colleagues and strive to expose those physicians deficient in character or competence, or who engage in fraud or deception.

A physician shall respect the law and also recognize a responsibility to seek changes in those requirements which are contrary to the best interest of the patient.

A physician shall respect the rights of patients, of colleagues, and of other health professionals, and shall safeguard patients' confidences within the constraints of the law.

A physician shall continue to study, apply, and advance scientific knowledge; make relevant information available to patients, colleagues, and the public; obtain consultation and use the talents of other health professionals when indicated.

A physician shall, in the provision of appropriate patient care, except in emergencies, be free to choose whom to serve, with whom to associate, and the environment in which to provide medical services.

A physician shall recognize a responsibility to participate in activities contributing to an improved community.

> *"Listen to the patient—he is telling you what is wrong."*
>
> Matz

OUR APOLOGIES

Throughout this text, a patient as well as a physician is often referred to as "he". We are aware that approximately half our patients are female, and we are also aware that a good many (and many good) physicians are female. However, the use of pronouns for both sexes ("he or she", "him or her", "his or her") is exceedingly awkward. And so, until a suitable genderless pronoun is found for the third-person singular, we are forced to resort to the traditional masculine form.

> *"When one's alright, he's prone to spite*
> *The doctor's peaceful mission;*
> *But when he is sick, it's loud and quick*
> *He bawls for a physician."*
>
> Eugene Field

AIR TRANSPORT OF THE CRITICALLY ILL

In 1870, 160 wounded soldiers, surrounded by Prussian troops, were lifted out of Paris by hot-air balloons and for the first time, patients were transported by air.

Although transfer of critically ill patients, particularly by air, is not always necessary or desirable, it may be the only way for those individuals to receive specialized medical services. The problems involved with flight at high altitude therefore must be recognized and remedied by the medical attendant.

Unpressurized aircraft do not fly above 20,000 feet. Private jets may fly at 40,000 feet, and commercial airliners may fly at 45,000 feet. While pressurized, most aircraft maintain a pressure difference between the cabin and the atmosphere of 7.5 to 8.7 psi. The cabin pressure is less than atmospheric pressure (at sea level) when the aircraft is flying above 22,500 feet.

Pressure Changes with Altitude[1]

ALTITUDE OF AIRCRAFT (ft)	ATMOSPHERIC PRESSURE (psi)	(mmHg)	CABIN PRESSURE (psi)	ALTITUDE EQUIVALENT FOR CABIN PRESSURE (ft)
40,000	2.72	140	11.32	7500
35,000	3.40	176	12.00	5500
25,000	5.46	282	14.08	500
15,000	8.30	315	14.70	Sea Level
Sea Level	14.70	760	14.70	Sea Level

Adapted from AMA Commission on EMS.

The partial pressure of ambient oxygen is a constant percentage of ambient pressure. As cabin pressure decreases, the partial pressure of oxygen decreases.

Expected PO_2 Saturation of a Normal Subject at Different Altitudes[3]

ALTITUDE (ft)	ATMOSPHERIC PO_2 (mmHg)	ARTERIAL PO_2 (mmHg)	O_2 SATURATION (%)
0 (sea level)	159	98	97
1,000	153	90	96
2,000*	148	86	95
4,000	137	80	93
6,000	125	64	90
8,000	116	55	86

*Most rotocraft operate at or below this altitude.

Patients with adequate arterial PO_2 before a flight may require supplemental oxygen during flight.

Concentration of Oxygen Required During Flight[4]*

METERS	0	400	1200	1800	2400	3000
FEET	0	2000	4000	6000	8000	10,000
	21	23	25	27	29	32
	30	33	35	38	42	45
	40	44	47	51	55	60
	50	54	59	64	69	75
FIO_2	60	65	70	76	83	90
	70	76	82	90	97	100
	80	87	94	100	PPR	PPR
	90	98	100	PPR†	PPR	PPR
	100	100	PPR	PPR	PPR	PPR

*Concentration of inspired oxygen required during flight to maintain an arterial oxygen pressure of 100 mmHg. Use the altitude equivalent for cabin pressure as the elevation (see Pressure Changes with Altitude).[4]

†PPR—Positive pressure required.

The oxygen-carrying capacity of blood is affected by the atmospheric oxygen pressure as well as by serum hemoglobin level. Both anemia and elevation have effects, and "altitude equivalents" for levels of anemia are described. A healthy adult can tolerate altitudes of 6000 feet without supplemental oxygen. For an anemic adult, the 6000 foot margin is reduced by his altitude equivalent. The difference is the altitude that he can tolerate without supplemental oxygen.

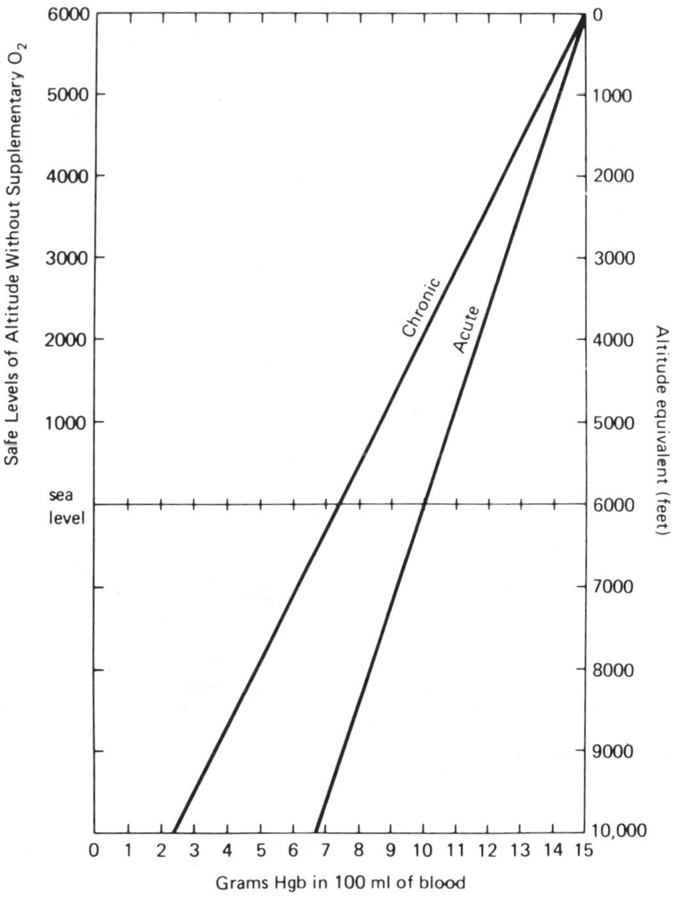

Fig. 1-1. Safe levels of altitude without supplemental O_2 related to grams hemoglobin in 100 ml of blood.[4]

The volume of a gas increases as the pressure around it decreases. As an aircraft gains altitude, gas in closed spaces expands. This change may cause discomfort (middle ear, sinuses), displace vital organs (expanding pneumothorax), or alter equipment (airsplint gets tighter).

Volume Expansion of Gases[4]

ALTITUDE (ft)	ALTITUDE (m)	GAS VOLUME
0	0	1.0
5000	1500	1.2
10,000	3000	1.5
15,000	4500	1.9
18,000	5400	2.0
20,000	6000	2.4

Use the altitude equivalent for cabin pressure as the elevation.

The water vapor content of air decreases with elevation. Outside air that is compressed makes dry cabin air; supplemental humidification is necessary.

During takeoff and landing of fixed-wing craft, the forces of acceleration and deceleration affect intravascular volume. If a patient is head forward during takeoff, acceleration decreases venous return and cardiac output. This effect could be detrimental to a patient with hypovolemia or cardiac failure, but it could be beneficial to a patient with cerebral edema. The patient experiences the reverse effect during landing, or during takeoff if positioned head aft.

Solutions for optimizing position include minimizing the rate of acceleration or deceleration; placing the patient crosswide in the craft; and turning the patient around in midflight. If none of these aids are physically possible, a decision must be made based on the patient's illness, and the conditions for takeoff and landing.

References:

1. AMA Commission on Emergency Medical Services. Medical aspects of transportation aboard commercial aircraft. JAMA 1982;*247*:1007–1011.

2. Fuller D. Flying and intraocular gas bubbles (letter). Am J Ophthalmol 1981:*91*:276–277.

3. Johnson JC. Medical care in the air. Ann Emerg Med 1981;*10*:324–327. (Reproduced with permission.)

4. McNeil EL. Airborne Care of the Ill and Injured. New York: Springer-Verlag, 1983. (Tables and figure reproduced with permission.)

5. Parsons CJ, Bobechko WP. Aeromedical transport: its hidden problems. Can Med Assoc J 1982:*126*:237–243.

6. Roper DL. Air transportation after eye surgery (letter). JAMA 1982;*247*:3315.

Air Transport of the Critically Ill: Problems and Remedial Actions[5]

SYSTEM APPARATUS	CONDITION	PROBLEMS	ACTIONS
Respiratory	Pneumothorax or pneumomediastinum	Air expansion compresses vital organs	Check x-rays and establish chest tube with one-way valve before flight; fly at low altitude
Cardiovascular	Ischemic heart disease; cardiac failure; anemia	Tissue hypoxia	Administer oxygen
	Electronic pacemaker	Electromagnetic signals may be sensed as spontaneous rhythm and inhibit firing	Minimize radio transmission; keep metal objects away from pacemaker; use fixed-rate mode
GI	Pneumoperitoneum Post-operative ileus	Air expansion compresses vital organs Wound dehiscence	NG tube; delay transfer at least 24 hours after surgery; avoid constrictive clothing; fly at low altitude
	Colostomy	Expanded air triggers peristalsis; expanded gas fills bag	Empty bag prior to flight; carry extra bag; release gas by venting bag with a needle—cover needle hole with tape
CNS	Unconscious	Motion sickness and aspiration Convulsions provoked by stimuli	NG tube; antiemetic Give anticonvulsants before flight
		Loss of spontaneous movement	Change patient's position; watch pressure points
	Intracranial air	Air expansion compresses vital organs	Fly at low altitude
Eye	Post-retinal or cataract surgery	Expanding intra-ocular gas forces fluid from eye	Avoid flying for two days after surgery; fly at low altitude; acetazolamide before flight; place head down if pain occurs;
	Penetrating trauma	Global contents may be extruded if cabin pressure drops suddenly	Fly at low altitude

Table continued on following page

Air Transport of the Critically Ill: Problems and Remedial Actions[5] (Continued)

SYSTEM APPARATUS	CONDITION	PROBLEMS	ACTIONS
ENT		Air expansion in middle ear, sinuses, or dental cavities	Use vasoconstricting nasal sprays before flight; give analgesics Have patient swallow, yawn, perform Valsalva maneuver; Fly at low altitude
	Tracheostomy	Os may not fit oxygen equipment	Take a spare tube and adapters
Skeletal	Balanced traction	Weights shift during movement	Change to fixed traction with spring tension
	Cast on edematous limb	Limb ischemia as tissues expand	Split cast; elevate limb
	Stryker frame	Loading is difficult; aspiration if patient vomits	Consider changing to scoop stretcher with traction; check with aircraft about loading; NG tube; antiemetic
	Airsplint; pneumatic antishock trousers	Expansion of air in splint causes limb ischemia	Avoid use if possible; adjust inflation during flight
	Jaws wired	Aspiration if patient vomits	Change wires to elastic bands before flight; carry wire cutters
GU	Loss of bladder control	Cold, wet bedding; macerated skin	Place Foley catheter before flight
Skin	Gas gangrene	Air expansion compresses vital organs	Fly at low altitude
General	Nitrogen saturation (divers)	Air expansion compresses vital organs and causes pain	Avoid flying for a minimum of 8 hrs (preferably 24 hrs.) after a dive Fly at low altitude

Infection	Spread of infection	Isolate patient
Burns	Acquisition of infection	Isolate patient
Immobilization	Thrombophlebitis; inadequate blood volume because of venous stasis	Perform muscle-contracting exercises; Put on elastic stockings; Low dose heparin
Psychiatric		
Uncontrolled violent behavior	Physical threat to aircraft and other passengers	Sedate and restrain before flight
Perinatal		
Neonate	Hypothermia	Transport in incubator; monitor core temperature;
	Physiologic pulmonary shunting	Give oxygen
	Hypoglycemia	IV glucose
Premature labor	Nonsterile, uncontrolled delivery; inadequate care for newborn	Give tocolytic agents before flight; be prepared for delivery
Apparatus		
IV fluids	Air expanding in bottle forces fluids to flow at higher rate; glass bottles break	Change to collapsible bags before flight
Oxygen		Calculate required volume; take extra
Suction devices and monitors		Check for electrical compatibility with aircraft
Lighting		Have battery-powered source available
Endotracheal tube	Expanded cuff causes tracheal ischemia	Adjust cuff pressure during flight
Dry air compressed from outside	Irritated mucous membranes	Humidification

URINE TEMPERATURE: A CLUE TO EARLY DIAGNOSIS OF FACTITIOUS FEVER

The urine temperature is within 1 to 1.5°C of the oral temperature taken simultaneously.

Reference:

1. Murray HW, Tuazon CU, Guerrero IC, et al. Urinary temperature: a clue to early diagnosis of factitious fever. New Engl J Med 1977; *296*:23.

EMERGENCY AIR AMBULANCE

One occasionally cares for a critically ill patient who needs immediate transfer to a specialized care facility some distance away. The United States Air Force, in very selected circumstances, will provide emergency air evacuation service to civilians. There must be (1) an immediate threat to life; (2) a lack of appropriate local medical help; and (3) no adequate commercial air ambulance or other transportation service available.

The Air Force will not fly terminally ill patients or accept requests either on the basis of either lack of funds or family convenience. There is a 24-hour Pentagon phone service that one may call to inquire about this, call 202-697-9560 from 8 A.M. to 5 P.M. Monday through Friday; call 202-695-7220 from 5 P.M. to 8 A.M. Monday through Friday and all day Saturday and Sunday. Ask for the MEDEVAC duty officer. If the Air Force does not believe that the case meets its criteria, it provides the name of the nearest commercial air ambulance firm.

SURVEILLANCE: THE EMERGENCY PHYSICIAN'S ROLE IN ORGAN DONATION

> *"Our own death is indeed unimaginable, and whenever we make the attempt to imagine it, we can perceive that we really survive as spectators. Hence, at bottom no one believes in his own death, or to put the same thing in another way, in the unconscious every one of us is convinced of his own immortality."*
>
> Sigmund Freud

The problems of organ donation are generally focused on kidneys, but corneas, livers, skin, hearts, and lungs are also now routinely being transplanted. In 1979, there were 45,565 patients reimbursed by Medicare for dialysis; 6311 patients were on registries awaiting transplants. In the same year, only 3066 cadaveric kidney transplants were performed.

There are many obstacles to obtaining organs. Forty percent of deaths occur outside of hospitals. Only 15 per cent of potential donors become actual donors. Over 55 per cent of potential donors die by the end of their first hospital day, whereas consent for donation is more likely to be given during the second or third hospital day. If consent for donation is received, 19 per cent of kidneys are lost because of cardiovascular instability. In addition, many cases are under the jurisdiction of a medical examiner or coroner.

The Uniform Anatomical Gift Act, which has been adopted by all states, clarifies the legal aspects of organ donation. It permits donation ante-mortem by the signing of a simple wallet-sized card. A Gallup poll has shown that 70 per cent of Americans are willing to donate organs. Yet, only 1.5 per cent of Maryland drivers signed the donor card on the backs of their driver licenses.

Although the emergency department is not usually an appropriate setting for the diagnosis of brain death, the emergency physician is in an ideal position to identify potential donors. He must be familiar with the selection criteria of the local transplant organization and know how to reach its procurement coordinator. If he does not know what transplant services are available in his area, he should contact the Eye Bank Association of America (6560 Fannin, Level 8, Houston, Texas 77030; phone 713-790-6126), the local kidney society, or the University of Pittsburgh (1-800-24-DONOR).

It is *not* the role of the physician who is caring for the patient to approach the closest relatives to request donation. His concerns are for the welfare of the patient and the patient's family as stipulated in the Uniform Anatomical Gift Act. A health professional uninvolved with the patient's care (preferably someone trained in interpersonal relations with an understanding of retrieval procedures) can approach the family with no question of conflict of interest.

The following criteria for potential donors have been developed from those of six transplant centers and the medical literature. Individual transplant centers may use different standards.

Broad Intercenter Criteria for Organ Donation[2]

1. Sufficient information is available in the donor's medical record to make a decision about suitability as determined by current center-specific practice.

2. Death occurred within a controlled environment where medical personnel were present.

3. Donor's age is from newborn to 65 years.

4. Chronic renal disease and active upper urinary tract infection were absent at the time of death.

5. No history or evidence of disseminated malignancy exists. There is no localized malignancy other than that of the central nervous system, skin, cervix, head, or neck.

6. The terminal course had none of the following:
   a. Prolonged hypotension
   b. Prolonged hyperthermia
   c. Sepsis, systemic infection including hepatitis, peritonitis
   d. Severe electrolyte disturbances
   e. Bowel wound or bowel surgery in the two weeks prior to death
   f. Abnormal urinalysis in the absence of a catheter
   g. Creatinine values >3.5 mg/100 ml or blood urea nitrogen values > 100 mg/100 ml at any time unless attributable to prerenal factors, including the hepatorenal syndrome
   h. Urinary output of < 50 ml/hr (0.5 ml/kg/hr for children) during the six hours before death; or oliguria or anuria defined as < 20 ml/hr (0.25 ml/kg/hr for children) for more than six hours at any time during the terminal course
   i. Ureteral reflux, stones, or hydronephrosis.

Finally, each physician should decide whether he is willing to donate his own organs. If so, he should carry a Uniform Donor Card. One is available through the local Kidney Society, or the one included here may be cut out and used (Fig. 1–2).

Fig. 1-2. Uniform Donor Card. (Reproduced with permission from the Central New York Kidney Disease Society).

UNIFORM DONOR CARD

of _____
Print or type name of donor

In the hope that I may help others, I hereby make this anatomical gift, if medically acceptable, to take effect upon my death. The words and marks below indicate my desires. I give:
    (a) ☐ any needed organs or parts
    (b) ☐ only the following organs or parts

_____
Specify the organ(s) or part(s)

for the purpose of transplantation, therapy, medical research or education.
    (c) ☐ my body for anatomical study if needed
Limitations or
special wishes, if any. _____
KEEP THIS CARD WITH YOUR DRIVER LICENSE

References:
1. Bart KJ, Macon EJ, Humphries AL, et al. Increasing the supply of cadaveric kidneys for transplantation. Transplantation 1981;*31*:383–387.
2. Bart KJ, Macon EJ, Whittier FC, et al. Cadaveric kidneys for transplantation. Transplantation 1981;*31*:379–382. (Appendix reproduced [with modifications] with the permission of the authors and The Williams & Wilkins Co., Baltimore)
3. Kaste M, Palo J. Criteria of brain death and removal of cadaveric organs. Ann Clin Res 1981:*13*:313–317.
4. Sadler AM, Sadler BL, Stason EB. The Uniform Anatomical Gift Act: a model for reform. JAMA 1968;*206*:2501–2506.
5. Stuart FP, Veith FJ, Cranford RE. Brain death laws and patterns of consent to remove organs for transplantation from cadavers in the United States and 28 other countries. Transplantation 1981;*31*:238–244.

```
Signed by the donor and the following two
witnesses in the presence of each other.


_____        _____
Signature of Donor               Date of Birth


_____        _____
City and State                   Date Signed


_____        _____
Witness                          Witness


This is a legal document under the Uniform
Anatomical Gift Act or similar laws.
```

USE ALL YOUR SENSES

The sense of SMELL may help you identify a toxin or condition! Your ability to recognize odors can be enhanced by practice with Dr. Goldfrank's "sniffing bar".[1]

Do not confuse this list with your grocery list!

Odor	Toxin or Condition
Acetone (Russet apples)	Ethanol, isopropyl alcohol, chloroform, lacquer, ketoacidosis
Acrid (pear-like)	Paraldehyde, chloral hydrate
Alcohol	Ethanol, isopropyl alcohol, *Cryptococcus neoformans* meningitis (CSF odor)
Almonds, bitter	Cyanide
Ammonia	Uremia, bladder infection (urine odor), cholera
Apples, rotten	*Clostridium* gas gangrene
Armpits, foul	Paratyphoid fever
Bad breath	Infection, abscess, or malignancy of the pharynx, esophagus, or stomach; acute illness
Brown bread, freshly baked	Typhoid
Beer, stale	Tuberculous lymphadenitis
Butcher shop	Yellow fever
Camembert, overripe	Infection with proteolytic bacteria
Cinnamon	Pulmonary tuberculosis
Cottage cheese	Tophaceous gout

Odor	Toxin or Condition
Disinfectants	Phenol, creosote
Eggs, rotten	Hydrogen sulfide, mercaptans, disulfiram
Feces	Anaerobic infections, intestinal obstruction
Fetor hepaticus	Liver failure
Fish and raw liver	Liver failure, zinc oxide, non-specific vaginitis
Foul	Bromides, steatorrhea
Fruit	Ethanol, isopropyl alcohol, amyl nitrite
Garlic	Dimethyl sulfoxide, organophosphates, phosphorus, arsenic, selenium, tellurium, thallium
Gas (stove gas)	Carbon monoxide (by association)
Grapes	*Pseudomonas* infection
Honey	Pemphigus vulgaris
Mice	*Proteus* infection, diphtheria
Musty	Penicillins, cephalosporins
Maple syrup	Maple syrup urine disease (odor in urine)
Mothballs	Camphor
Peanuts	Vacor (rodenticide)
Putrid	Scurvy, lung abscess, bronchiectasis
Sewer gas	Methane
Shoe polish	Nitrobenzene
Sweet	Marijuana, portacaval shunt, portal vein thrombosis, diphtheria
Vinegar	Glacial acetic acid
Vinyl (pungent)	Ethchlorvynol (Placidyl)
Violets	Turpentine (urine odor)
Wet leaves	Pulmonary tuberculosis
Wintergreen	Methyl salicylate

References:
    1. Goldfrank L, Weisman R, Flomenbaum N. Teaching the recognition of odors. Ann Emerg Med 1982; *11*:684–686.
    2. Gottlieb AJ, Zamkoff KW, Jastremski MS, et al. The Whole Internist Catalog. Philadelphia: WB Saunders, 1980:4.
    3. Smith M, Smith LG, Levinson B. The use of smell in differential diagnosis. Lancet 1982;*2*:1452.

"Doctors are men who pre-scribe medicines of which they know little, to cure diseases of which they know less, in human beings of whom they know nothing."

VOLTAIRE

A BAREFOOT DOCTOR

To provide health care for its huge rural population, the Chinese government trained "lay" people in the principles of Western and traditional Chinese medicine. The instruction book used was *A Barefoot Doctor's Manual,* from which these selections have been taken.

Whereas a large part of the book follows Western style, the descriptions of differential diagnoses and treatments from Chinese tradition remind us that the body and its ailments can be approached from many other perspectives.

The emergency physician should be familiar with such traditional treatments because the marks produced during some treatments may be confused with those of abuse. These practices are not limited to the Chinese; the Vietnamese practice *Cao Gio* (scratch the wind) that uses dermabrasion, which rids the body of "bad winds." Also, some Europeans practice *cupping,* using methods similar to those described here.

Skin Scrape (Kua-sha)

Conditions suited for treatment: Heat stroke, catarrhal headaches, indigestion, painful joints, colic, and so forth.

Technique: First dip an old copper coin in wine or water. Then move the coin over the patient's skin in a back-and-forth movement called "kua-sha." The folk practice often employs the fingers in a pinch-pull movement called "t'i-sha," "chih-sha," "nieh-sha", or "niu-sha."

Usual sites for kua-sha: Sites chosen for kua-sha may include the occipital depression over the neck, both sides of the thoracic vertebrae, both sides of the Adam's apple, the bridge of the nose, the "t'ai-yang" depression (located in the depression of the temples), the "inter-eyebrow" space, the anterior part of the chest, the elbow and knee spaces, and so forth. Scraping action generally goes from top to bottom, first from the back, then to the front along the intercostal spaces. When pinch-pulling is used, the index and middle fingers are used to pluck on the skin until reddish stripes begin to appear.

Precautions: During the kua-sha treatment, be sure to observe the patient's expression. Do not use too much force in case the skin breaks open. If unfavorable changes are noticed, stop the procedure immediately and treat accordingly. The kua-sha instrument must be blunt and smooth, otherwise the skin can easily be cut.

Bloodletting

Bloodletting is a method of treatment employing a triangular needle or small magnetic disk to cut open the site of an injury or an acupuncture point and allow a small amount of blood to flow out.

Conditions suited for treatment: Heat stroke, colic, vomiting and diarrhea, abscesses and swellings, stroke, traumatic injuries, and so forth.

Technique: Select a site for bloodletting. After routine sterilization of the skin area, prick open the skin with the sterilized triangular needle. A small amount of blood is permitted to flow out.

Usual bloodletting sites: For summer stroke and colic select the "shih-hsuan" and "ch'u-tse" points. For vomiting and diarrhea, select the "wei-chung." For traumatic injuries, abscesses, and swellings, bloodletting may be followed by cupping treatment for even better results, i.e., pus drained, swelling reduced, and poisons neutralized.

Cupping (Pa-huo-kuan)

Conditions suited for treatment: Wind-chill moisture–based numbness (arthritis), stomachache, abdominal pain, windchill catarrh, traumatic falls, bruises, abscesses, stroke paralysis, and so forth.

Sites and conditions to be avoided: All skin conditions, bony prominences (in thin patients), sites prone to cramps, areas showing many superficial blood vessels and much hair growth. Also the abdomen, chest, and breasts of pregnant women; and the precordium, tumor, and lymphatic node sites.

Technique: Hold a flaming alcohol sponge with a pair of forceps and quickly flame the inside of a cup, then take it out. At this time, the air inside the cup has become less dense, and the cup is placed instantly over the selected spot, where it will attach firmly to the skin because of the atmospheric pressure outside. This method is quite safe.

Precautions: Generally, use large cups over muscular or fleshy areas and small ones over less fleshy areas. Also, use large cups on healthy young people or new patients still in good physical shape, but use small cups for the old and weak, women, children, and the chronically ill.

Select cupping sites over the localized lesion or swollen spot. Have the patient in a recumbent position during the cupping procedure in case he faints. If the patient feels unwell during treatment, discontinue the cupping procedure immediately. Set duration of the procedure for 10 to 15 minutes, but make sure it is sufficient to induce reddish stripes in the cupping area. Do not use strong pressure on the cup to remove it in case it cuts the skin. To remove, press skin around the edges of the cup. When outside air enters the cup, it will fall off by itself.

References:
1. A Barefoot Doctor's Manual. US Dept. HEW, 1974. DHEW Publications no. (NIH) 75-695:79–81.
2. Du JNH. Pseudobattered child syndrome in Vietnamese immigrant children. Can Med Assoc J 1980;122:394–395.

TATTOOS

"You shall not make any cuttings in your flesh on account of the dead or tattoo any marks upon you."

Leviticus 19:28

Tattoos have suggested deviant tendencies for many years and were proscribed by the Judeo-Christian tradition. During the fifth century in Japan, criminals were branded with tattoos. In the United States, as of 1979, 11 states had laws related to tattooing. It is not surprising that the emergency physician who encounters a heavily tattooed patient might experience feelings of alarm and fear. In the hope that the level of acceptance will increase with the level of understanding, this short description of the significance of tattoos is offered.

Tattooing was practiced as long ago as the Ice Age, 8000 B.C. The soles of the feet are the only areas of the body that are not tattooed in any society.

In a study at a British general hospital, tattooed men were compared with untattooed men. The tattooed men were less likely to be church members, more likely to have relatives with tattoos, and three times as likely to have criminal records. Most (78%) were tattooed before the age of 21 years. Half were completely sober when they were tattooed. The majority (85%) were with friends at the time.

In another study, the US Army tried to find a predictor correlated with motorcycle accidents. The best predictor was the number of tattoos a cyclist wore.

In many societies, tattoos are used as ornamentation and may be placed erotically. For example, women may have tattoos on the shoulder or the "bikini area" to "surprise a lover."

Since obtaining the tattoo is painful, it suggests courage and it is a rite of passage in some societies. Since the design is permanent, it shows dedication. Tattoos are sometimes used as religious or superstitious devices.

In modern western society, tattoos are most often used for identity. In this sense, they are used by people who have lost the sense of self; i.e. institutionalized retarded people, military people, prisoners, gang members, and prostitutes. Symbols for the branches of the armed forces, geographic regions, and gangs point out a relationship to a group. A relationship to another person is revealed with their initials or name. The name may also be that of the wearer.

Some designs represent a characteristic of the wearer. The meaning may be obscure; even the tattooed individual is unable to explain it. Such symbols are more frequently seen among the emotionally disturbed. People who have more than one tattoo are more likely to be schizophrenic. Those whose tattoos are homemade or self-inflicted are more likely to be alienated from society.

The significance of many tattoos is obvious, other designs have no deep meaning, and many are used inappropriately. (Retarded people in one institution use gang signs as a status symbol, although they are not gang members.) Some tattoos have been given different interpretations by different groups, e.g., the bluebird has a different meaning for sailors than for homosexuals. With these cautions, the following "dictionary" may be used to interpret some tattoos.

Design	Meaning
Horseshoe, black cat, four-leaf clover	Luck
Pigs or roosters on feet	Protection against drowning (for sailors)
Bluebird or swallow	First 5000 miles at sea
Bluebird	Homosexual
Fox or snake entering the anus	Homosexual
Question mark (on left ring finger)	Bisexual
Cross, lamb, fish, X, and JN	Christianity; placed on the back by sailors to ensure a decent burial in a foreign land or to induce leniency during a flogging
Rose	Alcoholism; constancy; eroticism
Pachuco mark (cross with rays)	Gang member
Eagle, lion	Gang leader
Dagger	Virility; revenge
Snake	Virility
Eyes on buttocks	Warning; on guard
"13"	Marijuana (M is the 13th letter of the alphabet)
Monkey on shoulder; spider; dots on hand; arrows and syringes	Drug addiction
Single dot	
Cheek, eyelid, thenar web	Homosexual
Cheek	Served time in a state juvenile correction facility
Chin, lower lip	Served time in federal prison
Three dots at the base of thumb	Mort aux vaches (Death to the cows, i.e., police)
Four dots	
The dorsal proximal phalanx of a single finger	Lesbianism
One on each of four fingers	Served a prison sentence
Lily (on shoulder)	Served time in solitary confinement
Picks and chains	Performed forced labor
Butterfly	Thief
Dice; playing cards; girl in wine glass	Gambler
"4" (between breasts; on medial area of the knee; at thenar web)	Prostitute (from four-letter word for intercourse)
Eagle with girl in talons	Pimp

References:

1. Edgerton RB, Dingman HF. Tattooing and identity. Int J Soc Psychiatry 1963;9:143–153.

2. Gittleson NL, Wallfn GDP. The tattooed male patient. Br J Psychiatry 1973;122:295–300.

3. Goldstein N. Laws and regulations relating to tattoos. J Dermatol Surg Oncol 1979;5:913–915.

4. Goldstein N. Psychological implications of tattoos. J Dermatol Surg Oncol 1979;5:883–888.

5. Scutt RWB, Gotch C. Art, sex, and symbol. The mystery of tattooing. New York: AS Barnes, 1974.

CAUSES OF GAS IN SOFT TISSUES

BACTERIAL CAUSES OF CREPITANT CELLULITIS
   Clostridium
   Escherichia coli
   Klebsiella species
   Peptostreptococcus species
   Bacteroides and *Fusobacterium* species
   Streptococcus pyogenes
   Mixed infections with facultative and anaerobic species
OTHER NON-INFECTIOUS CAUSES OF CREPITATION
   Trapped air in traumatic and surgical wounds
   Compressed-air injection
   Gas released from H_2O_2 irrigation of a wound
   Air trapped about the site of an intravenous catheter
   Subcutaneous air secondary to pulmonary barotrauma

Reference:
   Simon HB, Swartz MN. Anaerobic Infections. *In:* Rubenstein E, Federman DD (eds.). Sci Amer Med 1983;7:1.

THE QUAKER AND THE NEWS DEALER — A FABLE

The following fable comes from Edward J. Shahady, M.D. in his excellent discussion of the problems of managing difficult patients, which appeared in the April, 1984 issue of *Consultant.*

A Quaker who lives in a great city is enjoying a visit from a friend who comes from a small country town. One morning they go out to buy a newspaper. On the way, the Quaker tells his friend how much he likes the news dealer and how eager he is to introduce him to his friend. When they arrive at the newsstand, the Quaker greets the news dealer warmly and asks for his newspaper. The dealer, who appears disgruntled, makes no reply, and ungraciously flings the paper onto the counter.

As the Quaker and his friend leave, the friend is shocked. He says, "If I were you, I'd be furious. Here this person is supposed to be your friend, yet he didn't even say hello, and on top of that, he almost threw the paper at you. Why didn't you tell him off? I certainly would have."

The Quaker replies, "Do you want me to allow this person to control the way I act? It was his behavior, not mine, that changed. By reacting angrily, I would be giving him the power to influence my behavior by his own. I choose to act rather than to react."

Moral: Don't let your patient's behavior influence your own by provoking you into an angry reaction. The physician can best manage the problem patient if he does not let the problem patient dictate and control the physician's behavior.

Reference:
   1. Shahady EJ. Uncovering the real problems of crocks and gomers. *Consultant* 1984; April: 33–45. (Reproduced with permission of the author and publisher.)

> *GOMER—Get Out of My Emergency Room.* A derogatory term used by immature physicians who have not reached full understanding of the higher ideals of medicine. Your medical knowledge and skills must be used with caring and compassion if you are truly to be a good physician. Remember all *GOMERS* ultimately die.

COST CONSCIOUSNESS QUIZ

"Good medicine is the cheapest medicine."
A. Gottlieb

Do you know how much money it costs the patient (or his insurance company and you) when you decide to get a simple laboratory examination for "interest"? Below you will find a list of commonly used diagnostic procedures, laboratory tests, and hospital supply items. Fill in your estimate of the cost in the blank provided. The current charges for these items at a university teaching hospital can be found on page 382.

Operating room use, 1 hour	_____	Complete blood count and differential	_____
25% albumin, 50 ml	_____	Blood gases	_____
Lactated ringers, 1000 ml	_____	Electrolytes, BUN, and glucose	_____
Angiocath	_____	Folic acid	_____
Ethilon Suture, 5–0	_____	Magnesium serum	_____
Transthoracic pacing kit	_____	Theophylline level	_____
Cockup splint	_____	Culture sputum and smear	_____
Adult electrodes	_____	HCG pregnancy slide	_____
Kerlix	_____	Urinalysis, regular	_____
Cervical collar	_____	Ankle x-ray	_____
Endotracheal tube	_____	Chest x-ray, PA single	_____
O₂ by mask (daily change)	_____	X-ray, portable machine use	_____
IPPB treatment	_____	CT scan upper abdominal (pancreas, liver)	_____
Long leg cast	_____	Skull series	_____
CVP manometer	_____	Lung scan	_____
Suture tray	_____	ECG	_____

STEROID SENSIBILITY

The use of topical steroids in treating inflammatory skin diseases has increased dramatically. Many varieties are available for prescription with varying degrees of potency. The table compares their relative strengths.

Relative Potency of Topical Glucocorticosteroids

%	
	LOWEST POTENCY
0.25 to 2.5	Hydrocortisone
0.25	Methylprednisolone acetate (Medrol)
0.04	Dexamethasone* (Hexadrol)
0.1	Dexamethasone* (Decaderm)
1.0	Methylprednisolone acetate (Medrol)
0.5	Prednisolone (Meti-derm)
0.2	Betamethasone* (Celestone)
	LOW POTENCY
0.1	Fluocinolone acetonide* (Synalar, Fluonid)
0.01	Betamethasone valerate* (Valisone)
0.025	Fluoromethalone* (Oxylone)
0.025	Triamcinolone acetonide* (Aristocort, Kenalog, Trymex)
0.1	Clocortolone pivalate* (Cloderm)
0.03	Flumethasone pivalate* (Locorten)
	INTERMEDIATE POTENCY
0.2	Hydrocortisone valerate (Westcort)
0.025	Betamethasone benzoate* (Uticort, Benisone)
0.025	Flurandrenolide* (Cordran)
0.1	Betamethasone valerate* (Valisone)
0.05	Desonide (Tridesilon)
0.025	Halcinonide* (Halog)
0.05	Desoximetasone* (Topicort LP)
0.05	Flurandrenolide* (Cordran)
0.1	Triamcinolone acetonide*
0.025	Fluocinolone acetonide*
	HIGH POTENCY
0.05	Betamethasone dipropionate* (Diprosone)
0.1	Amcinonide* (Cyclocort)
0.25	Desoximetasone* (Topicort)
0.5	Triamcinolone acetonide*
0.2	Fluocinolone acetonide* (Synalar HP)
0.05	Diflorasone diacetate* (Florone, Maxiflor)
0.1	Halcinonide* (Halog)
0.05	Fluocinonide* (Lidex, Topsyn)
	HIGHEST POTENCY
0.05	Clobetasol propionate* (Dermovate)

*Fluorinated steroids.

The question of how much topical steroid to apply is addressed next. It is agreed that they should be applied sparingly.

Amount of Steroids Required for a Single Daily
Application

BODY AREA	AMOUNT IN GRAMS
Head (not scalp)	1–2
Trunk (anterior)	3–6
Trunk (posterior)	3–6
Arms (each)	1–2
Legs (each)	3–6
Genito-anal	1–2
Total Body	15–30

Body location influences the degree of absorption as shown in the following table.

Regional Variations in the Percutaneous Penetration
of Hydrocortisone in Man

SKIN AREA	PENETRATION OF HYDROCORTISONE EXPRESSED AS A FACTOR OF THAT FOR THE FOREARM (VENTRAL)
Foot Arch (plantar)	0.14
Ankle (lateral)	0.42
Palm	0.83
Forearm (ventral)	1.0
Forearm (dorsal)	1.1
Back	1.7
Scalp	3.5
Axilla	3.6
Forehead	6.0
Jaw Angle	13.0
Scrotum	42.0

Some other characteristics of topical steroids to consider include:

1. Ointments provide the most effective absorption; patients, however, vastly prefer creams and lotions.

2. Areas that are moist or occluded (face, intertriginous areas, the perineum) afford a less absorptive barrier and therefore a higher systemic absorption.

3. Systemic side effects are more common in children, and this population should be treated initially with the least potent preparations. Stronger agents can be added later if clinically necessary.

References:
    Lester R. Topical formulary for the pediatrician. Pediatr Clin North Am 1983;*30*:74–79.
    (Tables reproduced with permission.)

NOTES ON NARCOTICS

1. All of the narcotics listed in the table can be given either intramuscularly or subcutaneously and produce a similar level of analgesia in equianalgesic doses with the exception of oxycodone (Percodan), which is given orally.

2. With the exception of oxymorphone, nalbuphine (Nubain), and butorphanol (Stadol), all are available as oral medications. When given orally, they are less potent because inconstant absorption and intestinal metabolism result in lower plasma levels. Onset of action is delayed and peak levels are reduced following oral administration. Methadone, levorphanol, oxycodone, and codeine retain about 50 percent of their potency when given orally and stand out as the preferred oral agents. Meperidine given orally retains a third of its activity, whereas morphine and hydromorphone have the lowest oral potency.

3. Rectal administration produces a somewhat lower peak activity with a longer duration of action than does parenteral administration. Hydromorphone and oxymorphone are both available commercially for rectal administration; the other narcotics may be prepared for administration with a suppository. The rectal route should be considered for the therapy of chronic, severe pain.

4. In equianalgesic doses, the side effects of the various narcotics are fairly similar. Hydromorphone, methadone, and meperidine produce less sedation. Oxymorphone produces the greatest degree of respiratory depression, and morphine produces the greatest degree of emesis. The least antitussive activity is seen with meperidine and hydromorphone, which also cause the least constipation.

Reference:

1. Physicians' Desk Reference. 38th edition, Ovadell, NJ: Medical Economic Company, Inc. 1984.

2. Catalano, RB. Semin. Oncology 1975; 2:379.

3. Gottlieb AJ, Zamkoff KW, Jastremski MS, et al. The Whole Internist Catalog. Philadelphia: WB Saunders, 1980:237–238.

4. Marks RM, Sachar EJ. Undertreatment of medical inpatients with narcotic analgesics. Ann Intern Med 1973; 78:173–181.

Narcotics

	EQUIANALGESIC DOSE (mg)*	USUAL ADULT DOSE (mg)*	ORAL-PARENTERAL EFFICACY RATIO	AVERAGE DURATION OF ACTION (hrs)	SUGGESTED ROUTES OF ADMINISTRATION
Morphine	10	5–10	low (1/6)	4–5	IM, SC, IV, PO
Hydromorphone (Dilaudid)	1.5	1.5–2	probably low	3–4	IM, SC, IV, PO
Oxymorphone (Numorphan)	1	1–1.5	1/6	4–6	IM, SC, IV, PR
Methadone (Dolophine)	8–10	5–15	high (1/2)	4–6	IM, SC, PO
Levorphanol (Levo-Dromoran)	2	2–3	high (1/2)	4–6	IM, SC, PO
Meperidine (Demerol)	75–100	50–100	moderate (1/3–1/4)	3	IM, SC, IV, PO
Nalbuphine (Nubain)	10	10	—	3–6	IM, SC, IV
Oxycodone (Percodan)	4.5	4.5 (1 tablet)	high (1/2)	3–6	PO
Codeine	—	40	high (1/2)	4–6	IM, PO
Butorphanol (Stadol)	1	2 mg IM 1 mg IV	—	3–4	IM, IV

*Equianalgesic dose when compared with morphine, 10 mg given subcutaneously.

THE PATIENT WHO WALKS OUT

"Beware of the patient who can't walk out of the
ED on his own at discharge."

Marshall B. Segal, M.D., J.D.

No one likes an unhappy customer, especially when it comes to health care. A familiar event in the emergency department (ED) is the patient who leaves prior to being seen by a physician. These "walk-out patients" place hospitals in potential clinical and legal jeopardy and, more importantly, should lead us to question what we did wrong to provoke their departure.

An interesting study was carried out over a one-year period at The Johns Hopkins Hospital Adult Emergency Room. A total of 426 patients were identified as walk-outs. Of these patients, 179 were matched with a control group; the controls were defined as patients who were similar in sex, race, age, and severity of complaints and who presented within four hours of the walk-out patients. The walk-out patients and their matched controls were interviewed within two weeks after their ED encounter by telephone or in person. The study results are listed as follows:

1. The number of walk-outs represented only one per cent of the total ED population seen over the one-year period.

2. Walk-outs were most common during the evening shift (52%) and least common during the day shift (21%).

3. The majority were single, male, between 18 and 34 years of age (65%) and without health insurance.

4. Walk-outs occurred most frequently on Saturdays.

5. Two thirds left within one hour of signing in.

6. Nearly half presented on the day their symptoms began.

7. At the time of presentation, 57 per cent reported a great deal of pain or discomfort. At the time of follow-up, it was shown that only 15 per cent obtained immediate care at another ED facility that day, and 61 per cent sought no follow-up at all.

8. The follow-up interview revealed that both the controls and the walk-out patients, when questioned subjectively, had recovered equally from their complaints.

9. Of the walk-out patients, 52 per cent stated that their main reason for leaving was that the waiting time was too long.

The investigators concluded that the health of the walk-out patients was not affected and that they recovered as well and as rapidly as the control subjects who were interviewed. Their final recommendations as to how to prevent walk-outs from occurring included:

1. Frequent explanations should be made to the patients as to why they are waiting and how long it is likely to continue.

2. The principles of triage should be explained to unhappy patients.

3. Ancillary diversions should be provided for the patients to improve the waiting time, i.e., televisions, periodicals, and child-care facilities.

4. Periodic telephone follow-up of walk-out patients should be made to provide a useful system for quality control in the Emergency Department.

> *"You should not prevent patients from getting well on their own."*
>
> Osler

Reference:

1. Gibson G, Maiman L, Chase A. Walk-out patients in the hospital emergency department. JACEP 1978;7:47–51.

THE "EYE OF HORUS"

One of the leading figures in the development of early medicine was Imhotep (pronounced I-em-hetep) who lived in ancient Egypt during the III dynasty of Pharaoh Zoser II. The name Imhotep signifies "He who cometh in peace." He initiated a medical cult as early as 2750 B.C. and preceded Aesculapius by many centuries. Health was a major concern for the Egyptians and, as their mythology developed, it became a concern of the deities. Most important of the gods of health and beneficence was Thoth, and it was he who revealed the art of healing to the Egyptians, among them Imhotep (who incidentally became a demigod and eventually a full deity after his death). The basis of mythologic thought, coupled with the scientific advances of this remarkable people, led to the development of a symbol still used in modern medicine—*Rx.*

The Legend:

It is said that Isis, a goddess of beneficent goodness, had two sons —Horus, the good son, and Seth, the demon son. During an attack by Seth, Horus had his eye gouged out, and Isis implored Thoth, the great god of health, to help him. Thoth replaced the eye and its vision, and it was thus that the eye of Horus became an Egyptian symbol for the protection of the gods, health, and recovery.

The Fact

After the Hyksos invasion of Egypt, the old system of weights and measures was replaced by a new decimal system introduced from the East based on the "hnw" (1 hnw = 0.45 liters). Symbols were developed to make the registration of fractions of the hnw easier and are as shown:

▷	1/2 hk.t		◁	1/16 hk.t
○	1/4 hk.t		⌣	1/32 hk.t 1 hk.t = 10 hnw
⌐	1/8 hk.t		│	1/64 hk.t

The physicians, pharmacists, and scribes of the day—well aware of the symbolic nature of the "Eye of Horus"—developed their version of a mnemonic for the various symbols used on their prescriptions.

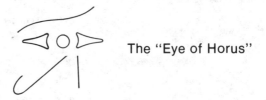 The "Eye of Horus"

Reversed, loosely, this becomes

or,

which is still used by physicians, pharmacists, and scribes today. The final clue to this discovery was provided by Georg Möller in 1911. (Ztschr Aegypt Spr 1911 *48*:99–106).

References:

   1. Green JR. Medical History for Students, Springfield, Illinois: Charles C. Thomas, 1968: 13–19.
   2. Leake, D. The Old Egyptian Medical Papyri, Lawrence, Kansas: University of Kansas Press, 1952:26. (Thanks to Michael Cilip, M.D. for this interesting bit of medical history.)

PRESCRIPTION CHECK LIST

The Right Drug

   1. Have you considered the indications carefully?
   2. Have you reviewed the possible effects?
   3. Is there a potential for drug interaction in the patient?
   4. Are the benefit to risk and benefit to cost ratios favorable for this particular patient?

The Right Information

   5. Does the patient understand why the drug is being given?
   6. Does the patient understand the potential side effects and know which of these, if any, might require expeditious action?
   7. Does the patient understand how, when, and for how long to take the drug? Are you sure?
   8. Are there any specific "do's and dont's" (e.g., use of alcohol) that the patient should be aware of while taking the medication?

The Right Script

9. Is the prescription accurate?

10. Does it conform to what you told the patient?

11. Is it legible?

12. Have you provided enough of the drug to complete the contemplated therapy? Have you limited the quantity dispensed if you are employing the drug in a therapeutic trial?

13. Did you sign the prescription?

14. Is your Bureau of Narcotics and Dangerous Drugs number necessary?

15. Did you use the right form (i.e., triplicate narcotic form, Medicaid)?

And

16. Can the patient get the medication?

17. Can the patient afford the medication?

18. Have you told the patient whether or not to refrigerate the medication?

Prescription Alphabet Soup

D—day (die)
W—week
Q—every (quaque)
H—hours (hora)

BID—twice a day
TID—three times a day
QID—four times a day

caps—capsules
tabs—tablets
oz—ounces
teasp—teaspoon (5 ml)
tbsp—tablespoon (15 ml)

AD—in the right ear
AS—in the left ear
AU in each ear

OD—in the right eye
OS—in the left eye
OU—in each eye

ac—before meals (ante cibum)
Disp—Dispense
gr—grain (granum)
gtt—drop (gutta)
hs—just before sleep (hora somni)
MDD—maximum daily dose
po—by mouth (per os)
pc—after meals (post cibum)
prn—as necessary (pro re nata)
sig—label (signa)
stat—at once (statim)

PRESCRIBING LIQUIDS

Are your patients on long-term liquid medication found to have subtherapeutic or toxic drug levels? Are you threatening them with torture or a lie detector test to reveal their true dosing habits? Stop! Consider the measuring device they're using. One survey found the volume of household teaspoons to range from 1.5 to 8 ml. A casual survey among the authors found the volume of household tablespoons to range from 8.6 to 12 ml. Liquid medications should be prescribed in terms of milliliters and a calibrated cup or syringe should be provided.

Reference:
   1. Sublett JL, Pollard SJ, Kadlec GJ, Karibo JM. Non-compliance in asthmatic children: a study of theophylline levels in a pediatric emergency room population. Ann Allergy 1979;*43*(2):95-97.

FACTS OF HOSPITAL LIFE

"It is a wearisome disease to preserve health by too strict a regimen."

Duc Francois de La Rochefouauld

Dosing schedules for drugs vary among hospitals and even among nursing stations within the same hospital. Drugs ordered to be given "qid" are usually not given at six-hour intervals. More commonly, the schedule will be 10:00 A.M., 2:00 P.M., 6:00 P.M., and 10:00 P.M. or some variation thereof, giving the patient a 12-hour overnight hiatus. Similarly, a "tid" schedule may be 10:00 A.M., 4:00 P.M. and 10:00 P.M.; or a "bid" schedule may be 10:00 A.M. and 4:00 P.M. Patients who take their medications at home often know better than to use such a schedule.

For antiarrhythmics, antianginal therapeutics, many antibiotics, and, in fact, any drug for which it would be undesirable to allow the patient to be unmedicated for any period of time, it may be important to choose a "q6h", "q8h", or "q12h" schedule rather than "qid", "tid", or "bid".

If, on the other hand, exact spacing of doses is not crucial, a "qid" schedule may be more considerate. Patients have enough nocturnal interruptions without also being awakened unnecessarily for medications.

Best of all, discuss dosing schedules with the nurse and the patient before the patient goes home.

TOP TEN UPDATE

Can you guess the top ten selling prescription drugs for the last few years? Compare your list with the following list. It is worthwhile to consider the indications for each drug and to speculate why some of the drugs made it to the top ten.

1981	*1982*	*1983*
1. Tagamet	Inderal	Inderal
2. Inderal	Lanoxin	Dyazide
3. Motrin	Dyazide	Lanoxin
4. Valium	Valium	Valium
5. Diuril	Tylenol with codeine	Lasix
6. Clinoril	Lasix	Tylenol with codeine
7. Keflex	Tagamet	Tagamet
8. Aldomet	Motrin	Ortho-Novum
9. Naprosyn	Ortho-Novum	Motrin
10. Lasix	Keflex	Aldomet

"When a patient on a drug—on any drug—becomes ill the Napoleonic code, rather than the English common law, should apply: The drug should be presumed guilty until proved innocent."

Robert Matz, M.D.

Reference:
   1. The Top 200 Prescription Drugs of 1983. American Druggist Feb. 1984;42–50.

2

RESUSCITATION

RESUSCITATION 35

CPR REVIEW 35

MODIFICATIONS IN CPR FOR INFANTS AND CHILDREN . . . 49

SHOCK 49

ALGORITHMS FOR CARDIAC DYSRHYTHMIAS 54

EARLY CPR—STARTING THE HEART: OUR BIASES 63

THE PEDIATRIC CART: BE PREPARED 68

PEDIATRIC EMERGENCY DRUGS 69

IMMEDIATE MANAGEMENT OF UPPER AIRWAY
OBSTRUCTION 72

RETROGRADE STYLET 74

BLIND NASOTRACHEAL INTUBATION 75

THE ENDOTRACHEAL ROUTE—WHAT TO DO WHEN YOU
CAN'T GET AN IV 76

DRUG CONCENTRATIONS DURING CPR 78

FLOW RATES OF IV CATHETERS 78

IV'S IN PARADISE 80

HAZARDS OF TOPICAL NTG 80

PERICARDIOCENTESIS 80

TEMPORARY PLACEMENT OF BALLOON-TIPPED
PACEMAKERS 82

BASICS OF HEMODYNAMIC MANIPULATION 84

RESPIRATORY VARIATION OF PULMONARY VASCULAR
PRESSURE 86

ACLS: INSTRUCTING THE MEGA-CODE STATION 87

RESUSCITATION

The Advanced Cardiac Life Support (ACLS) course of the American Heart Association (AHA) describes several techniques for artificial ventilation. In one study, unskilled subjects (senior medical students) and semi-skilled subjects (nurse-anesthetist students) ventilated manikins using different equipment. The tidal volumes delivered were averaged and are shown in the graph (Fig. 2-1). Given that the AHA recommends 800-1200cc tidal volume for adults, which method would you choose as the best?

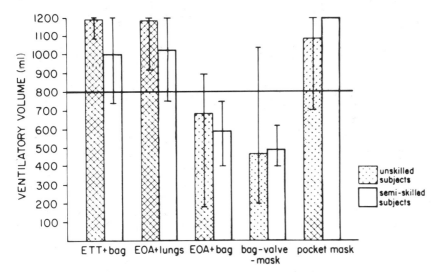

Fig. 2-1. Ventilatory volume delivered by various artificial methods (ETT/Endotracheal tube, EOA—Esophageal obturator airway).[2]

References:
1. American Heart Association. A manual for instructors of basic cardiac life support. Dallas: AHA, 1981:47.
2. Harrison RR, Maull KI, Keenan RL, Boyan CP. Mouth-to-mask ventilation: a superior method of rescue breathing. Ann Emerg Med 1982; *11*:74–76. (Reproduced with permission from the authors and publisher).

CPR REVIEW

Although you are probably certified in Basic Cardiac Life Support, if you do not routinely utilize these skills or practice on a manikin, you probably cannot perform them satisfactorily. Many studies have shown that Cardiopulmonary Resuscitation (CPR) skills deteriorate rapidly after initial training, and that periodic review of the techniques can help to maintain performance skills, ideally with manikin practice, but also by simply reviewing the sequences. The current recommendations of the American Heart Association and the American Red Cross for one rescuer CPR, one and two rescuer CPR, infant resuscitation, and management of complete airway obstruction are provided. Review of these sequences now, and at regular intervals, will help to ensure that you will be able to provide the best possible CPR the next time you are called upon to do so.

One Rescuer CPR (Heartsaver)

STEPS	ACTIVITY AND TIME (Seconds)	CRITICAL PERFORMANCE	RATIONALE
1	Establish unresponsiveness and call out for help. Allow 4–10 sec if face down and turning is required.	Tap, gently shake shoulder. Shout—"Are you OK?" Call out —"Help!" Turn if necessary, supporting head and neck.	Accurate diagnosis is important. This initial call for help is to alert bystanders. Frequently victim will be face down. Effective external chest compression can only be provided with victim flat on back on hard surface.
		Adequate time.	Four to ten seconds gives time for diagnosis and to review mentally the sequence of CPR.
2	Open airway. Establish breathlessness. (Look, listen, and feel.) (3–5 sec)	Kneels properly.	Position for stability and access to the victim.
		Utilize head tilt with chin lift (or head tilt with neck lift).	Airway must be opened to establish breathlessness.
		Ear over mouth, observe chest: look, listen, and feel for breathing.	Many victims may be making respiratory efforts that are ineffective because of obstruction.
3	Four ventilations. (3–5 sec)	Ventilate properly four times and observe chest rise.	Need to expand collapsed lungs but avoid gastric distention.
4	Establish pulselessness. Activate Emergency Medical Service (EMS) System. (5–10 sec)	Fingers palpate for carotid pulse on near side (other hand on forehead maintains head tilt).	The carotid pulse is the easiest to find. It is checked on the near side to avoid pressure on the windpipe.

2

		Know local EMS Number and send a bystander to call EMS. Adequate time.	The sooner ACLS arrives the better chance for survival. It takes 5–10 seconds to find the right place, and the pulse may be very slow or very weak and rapid.
5	Four cycles of 15 compressions and 2 ventilations. (54–66 sec)	Proper rescuer body position.	Stability and access for ventilation and compression.
		Landmark check each time.	To assure proper hand position.
		Position of hands.	Precision in hand placement is essential to avoid serious injury.
		Vertical compression, no bouncing.	To achieve most pressure with least effort.
		Says mnemonic.	Necessary to establish rhythm.
		Proper rate and ratio.	Should attempt to accomplish 60 compressions and 8 ventilations/minute, 50% of compression is downward and 50% is upward.
		Ventilates properly.	Adequate oxygenation must be maintained.
6	Check for return of pulse and spontaneous breathing. (3–5 sec)	Check pulse and breathing.	Victim's status needs to be evaluated after the first minute of CPR and every few minutes thereafter.
7	Resume cycles with 2 ventilations followed by compressions.	Continue CPR in absence of spontaneous pulse and/or respirations.	CPR should be continued until victim responds or rescuer is relieved or exhausted.

One and Two Rescuer CPR

STEPS	ACTIVITY AND TIME (Seconds)	CRITICAL PERFORMANCE	RATIONALE
1	Establish unresponsiveness and call out for help. Allow 4–10 sec if face down and turning is required.	Tap, gently shake shoulder. Shout—"Are you OK?" Call out —"Help!" Turn if necessary, supporting head and neck.	Accurate diagnosis is important. This initial call for help is to alert bystanders. Frequently victim will be face down. Effective external chest compression can only be provided with victim flat on back on hard surface.
		Adequate time.	Four to ten seconds gives time for diagnosis and to review mentally the sequence of CPR.
2	Open airway. Establish breathlessness. (Look, listen, and feel.) (3–5 sec)	Kneels properly.	Position for stability and access to the victim.
		Utilize head tilt with chin lift (or head tilt with neck lift).	Airway must be opened to establish breathlessness.
		Ear over mouth, observe chest: look, listen, and feel for breathing.	Many victims may be making respiratory efforts that are ineffective because of obstruction.
3	Four ventilations. (3–5 sec)	Ventilate properly four times and observe chest rise.	Need to expand collapsed lungs but avoid gastric distention.

2

4	Establish pulselessness. Activate Emergency Medical Service (EMS) System. (5–10 sec)	Fingers palpate for carotid pulse on near side (other hand on forehead maintains head tilt).	The carotid pulse is the easiest to find. It is checked on the near side to avoid pressure on the windpipe.
		Know local EMS Number and send a bystander to call EMS.	The sooner ACLS arrives the better chance for survival.
		Adequate time.	It takes 5–10 seconds to find the right place, and the pulse may be very slow or very weak and rapid.
5	Four cycles of 15 compressions and 2 ventilations. (54–66 sec)	Proper rescuer body position.	Stability and access for ventilation and compression.
		Landmark check each time.	To assure proper hand position.
		Position of hands.	Precision in hand placement is essential to avoid serious injury.
		Vertical compression, no bouncing.	To achieve most pressure with least effort.
		Says mnemonic.	Necessary to establish rhythm.
		Proper rate and ratio.	Should attempt to accompl sh 60 compressions and 8 ventilations/minute, 50% of compression is downward and 50% is upward.
		Ventilates properly.	Adequate oxygenation must be maintained.
6	Check for return of pulse and spontaneous breathing. (3–5 sec)	Check pulse and breathing.	Victim's status needs to be evaluated after the first minute of CPR and every few minutes thereafter.

Table continued on following page

One and Two Rescuer CPR (Continued)

STEPS	ACTIVITY AND TIME (Seconds)	CRITICAL PERFORMANCE	RATIONALE
7	First rescuer resumes CPR with two ventilations followed by compressions.	Resume as single rescuer.	CPR must not be interrupted.
8	Second rescuer identifies himself, checks pulse for effective compressions. (5 sec)	Second rescuer says, "I know CPR". Palpates carotid pulse.	Second rescuer identifies knowledge and willingness to assist. First rescuer accepts assistance. Second rescuer evaluates effectiveness of compressions.
9	Second rescuer calls out "Stop compressions" and checks for spontaneous pulse and breathing. (5 sec)	Second rescuer—5 sec spontaneous pulse and breathing check.	Provides a second assessment of pulse and breathing and verifies the need for continued CPR.
10	Second rescuer ventilates once. States "No pulse. Continue CPR".	Ventilates properly and observes chest rise.	Oxygen should be delivered to the lungs prior to chest compression.
11	First rescuer resumes compressions.	Two-rescuer rate and ratio.	Second rescuer ventilation triggers change of rate and ratio.

2

12	Minimum of two cycles of five compressions and one ventilation. (8–10 sec) Switch and repeat until examiner is satisfied.	Correct rate of compression.	When performed without interruptions, 60 compressions per minute can maintain adequate blood flow and pressure. The rate avoids fatigue and allows optimal ventilation with quick interposition on upstroke of fifth compression.
		Says mnemonic.	
		Interposes breath.	
		No pause for ventilations.	
13	Compressor calls for switch when needed.	Calls for switch.	Signal for change must be clear to avoid confusion.
14	Simultaneous switch.	Gives breath on fifth compression.	Switch must be performed quickly and smoothly to maintain effective CPR.
	Rescuer at head moves to chest.	Moves to the chest. Finds correct hand position ready for chest compression.	Check for return of spontaneous pulse and/or breathing to verify need for continued CPR.
	Compressor moves to the head.	Gives fifth compression.	Oxygen should be delivered to the lungs prior to resuming chest compression.
		Moves to the head. 3–5 sec pulse check.	
		Ventilates once.	
		States, "No pulse, continue CPR".	
		Monitors compression effectiveness.	Verifies effective chest compression.

Infant Resuscitation

STEPS	ACTIVITY AND TIME (Seconds)	CRITICAL PERFORMANCE	RATIONALE
1	Establish unresponsiveness and call out for help (including turning). (4–10 sec)	Tap, gently shake shoulder and see if infant responds. Call out—"Help!" Turn if necessary.	Diagnosis must be equally accurate in children and infants. With this emotionally charged situation, time must be taken to establish the diagnosis of unresponsiveness or breathing difficulty.
		Infant horizontal.	Horizontal position aids effective circulation.
		Adequate time.	Four to ten seconds gives time for diagnosis and to review mentally the sequence of CPR.
2	Open airway. Establish breathlessness. (Look, listen, and feel.) (3–5 sec)	Tip head back. Do not hyperextend.	Hyperextension can collapse trachea or cause cervical spine injury.
		Put ear over mouth and look toward chest to look, listen and feel for breathing.	Many victims may be making respiratory efforts that are ineffective because of obstruction.

3	Four ventilations. (3–5 sec)	Cover mouth and nose, give four breaths in rapid succession, enough to observe chest rise.	Lung capacity of infant smaller than adult, more pressure is required. Avoid over-inflating to prevent gastric distention.
4	Establish pulselessness and activate EMS System. (5–10 sec)	Fingers palpate for brachial pulse in infant. Know local EMS number and send a bystander to call.	Brachial pulse easier to feel in infant than carotid. The faster ACLS arrives the better the chance for survival.
5	Ten cycles of five compressions and one ventilation. Continue uninterrupted. (30 sec)	Two fingers on midsternum for compressions at rate of 100 compressions per minute.	Infants (rate of 100/min) need a more rapid chest compression rate with breaths interposed every five compressions.
6	Check for return of spontaneous pulse and breathing. (3–5 sec)	Check pulse and breathing properly.	Frequent reassessment of the victim's condition is necessary.

Complete Airway Obstruction:
Part 1 — Conscious Victim (Sitting or Standing)

STEPS	ACTIVITY AND TIME (Seconds)	CRITICAL PERFORMANCE	RATIONALE
1	Rescuer asks: "Can you speak?" (2–3 sec)	Rescuer must identify complete airway obstruction by asking victim if he is able to speak.	It is essential to recognize the signs and take immediate action. If the victim is able to speak or cough effectively, do not interfere with his attempts to expel the foreign body.
2	Four back blows (3–5 sec) *Do not apply actual back blows to other students.*	Deliver four sharp blows rapidly and forcefully to the back between the shoulder blades; support the victim's chest with other hand.	Back blows may have the effect of dislodging the foreign body. Chest support is necessary to prevent the victim from falling forward. Whenever possible, the victim's head should be lower than his chest to make use of the effect of gravity.

2

3	Four abdominal thrusts (4-5 sec)	Stand behind victim and wrap your arms around his waist. Grasp one fist with your other hand and place thumb side of your fist in the midline between the waist and ribcage. Press fist into abdomen with quick inward and upward thrusts.	Manual thrust maneuver should move the foreign body upward in the airway. Each back blow or manual thrust should be delivered with the intent of relieving the obstruction.
	OR		
	Four chest thrusts (4-5 sec) *Do not apply actual manual thrusts to other students.*	Stand behind victim and place your arms under victim's armpits to encircle the chest. Grasp one fist with other hand and place thumb side of fist on breastbone. Press with quick backward thrusts.	Chest thrusts are more easily delivered than are abdominal thrusts when the abdominal girth is large, as in gross obesity or in advanced pregnancy.
4	Repeat above sequence until successful. (Steps 2-3)	Alternate the above maneuvers in rapid sequence until successful or the victim becomes unconscious.	Time is of the essence; the two techniques are rapidly repeated alternatively until obstruction is relieved or unconsciousness occurs.

Complete Airway Obstruction:
Part II—Victim Who Becomes Unconscious

STEPS	ACTIVITY AND TIME (Seconds)	CRITICAL PERFORMANCE	RATIONALE
1	Position the victim and call for help. Allow 4–10 sec if face down and turning is required.	Turn victim supine if necessary. Call out for help. Support head and neck. Adequate time.	Initial call is to alert bystander. Victim must be properly positioned in case CPR is required. Support head and neck to prevent injury.
2	Open airway and attempt to ventilate. (3–5 sec) (Repositioning of the head and a second attempt to ventilate is optional and acceptable.)	Kneel properly—utilize head tilt with chin lift (or head tilt with neck lift). Attempt ventilation. (Airway still obstructed.)	Lack of oxygen or falling and jarring motion may loosen foreign body enough to permit ventilation.
3	Activate EMS System. (2 sec)	If second person is present he should activate EMS System. Know local EMS number.	Advanced life support capability may be required.
4	Four back blows (4–6 sec)** *Do not apply actual back blows to other students.*	Roll victim toward you, using your thigh for support. Give four forceful and rapidly delivered blows to back between shoulder blades.	Continually check for success. Each back blow or manual thrust should be delivered with the intent of relieving the obstruction.
5	Four abdominal thrusts (5–6 sec)	Position yourself with your knees close to victim's hip. Place heel of one hand in the midline between the waist and	Kneeling at victim's side gives the rescuer greater mobility and access to the airway. The sequence of back blows and

OR	4 chest thrusts (5-6 sec) *Do not apply actual manual thrusts to other students.*	ribcage and second hand on top. Press into abdomen with quick inward and upward thrusts. This maneuver may be done astride the victim. / abdominal thrusts is more effective than either method when used alone.
		Same hand position as that for applying external chest compression. Exert quick downward thrusts. / Chest thrusts are preferred in the presence of large abdominal girth (advanced pregnancy and obesity). Quick downward thrusts generate effective airway pressures.
6	Check for foreign body using finger sweep. (6-8 sec)	Turn head up, open mouth with jaw-lift technique and sweep deeply into mouth along cheek with hooked finger. May need to remove dentures. / A dislodged foreign body may now be manually accessible if it has not been expelled. Dentures may need to be removed to improve fingersweep.
7	Attempt to ventilate. (3-5 sec)	Utilize head tilt with chin lift (or head tilt with neck lift). Attempt ventilation. (Airway still obstructed.) / By this time another attempt must be made to get some air into the lungs.
8	Repeat above sequence until successful. (Steps 4-7)	Alternate the above maneuvers in rapid sequence until successful. / Persistent attempts are rapidly made in sequence in order to relieve the obstruction.

**NOTE: Although the sequence of back blows followed by manual thrusts is preferred, the reverse sequence of manual thrusts followed by back blows is acceptable.

References:

1. Grogono AW, Jastremski MS, Johnson M, Russell RF. Educational graffiti: better use of the lavatory wall. Lancet 1982; *1*:1175-1176.
2. Montgomery WM, Herrin TJ, Lewis AJ (eds.). Basic life support for physicians. Dallas: American Heart Association, 1982. (Performance sheets reproduced with permission of the American Heart Association.)

Modifications in CPR for Infants and Children

TECHNIQUE	ADULT	CHILD	INFANT
Opening the airway	Maximum backward tilt of the head with neck-lift or chin-lift.	Moderate backward tilt of the head with neck-lift or chin-lift.	Minimum backward tilt of the head with neck-lift or chin-lift.
Rescue breathing	Mouth-to-mouth or mouth-to-nose; 12–15/min.	According to size of child; 15–20/min.	Mouth-to-mouth and nose; 20/min.
Circulation			
Compression point	Lower ⅓ of sternum	Lower ½ of sternum	Mid-sternum
Compression with	Two hands, one on top of the other	Heel of one hand	Two fingers
Compression depth	4–5 cm	2.5–3.5 cm	1.5–2.5 cm
Compression rate	60/min	80–100/min	100/min
Ratio of compressions to ventilations	5:1	5:1	5:1

MODIFICATIONS IN CPR FOR INFANTS AND CHILDREN

The basic principles of cardiopulmonary resuscitation for adults are well known to most emergency department personnel. These principles are, for the most part, the same for children. Adjustments must be made, however, to compensate for the anatomical differences encountered in infants and children. The pertinent modifications are described in the table on the opposite page.

SHOCK

"Shock, a momentary pause in the act of death."
John Collis Warren

Shock is the clinical syndrome of tissue hypoperfusion that is often fatal if not immediately recognized and expeditiously managed. A diverse spectrum of primary processes can produce the clinical state of shock. A useful classification system of shock is that of Weil and Shubin: hypovolemic; cardiogenic; obstructive; and distributive.[4]

Hypovolemic and cardiogenic shock account for most cases of shock. Obstructive shock refers to cases with an adequate volume and pump, but physical obstruction to perfusion, such as a pulmonary embolus or cardiac tamponade. Distributive shock includes conditions such as malignant hypertension, sepsis, and anaphylaxis, in which the primary pathophysiology is at the microvascular level, resulting in maldistribution of perfusion.

The emergency physician will often be responsible for the initial resuscitation of patients in shock. An organized management plan, applied consistently, should provide the most favorable outcome. The emergency resuscitation algorithm for hypotension presented next from the Harbor-UCLA Medical Center has been prospectively tested in a large clinical trial. Patients managed by personnel using the algorithm were found to have shorter resuscitation times, lower arterial pressure time deficits (defined as time MAP < 80), and fewer shock-related complications than the randomly treated control patients.

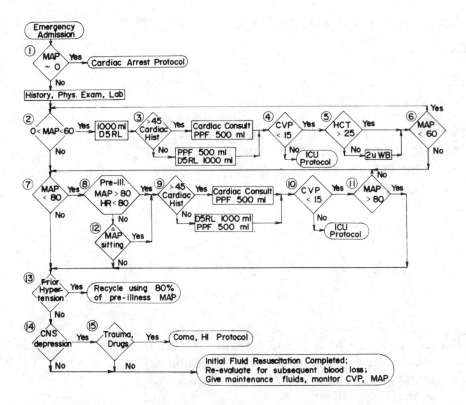

Fig. 2-2. Clinical algorithm for the initial resuscitation.[1]

Step 1. If the MAP (mean arterial pressure) is 0 or nearly 0, determine presence of cardiac arrest and begin CPR. If the patient has an MAP less than 20 mmHg, alert personnel for a possible cardiac arrest.

Step 2. If the MAP is less than 60 mmHg, immediately start D5RL (5% glucose in lactated Ringer's solution), 1000 ml, and run it as rapidly as possible, especially if the MAP is less than 50 mmHg.

Step 3. If the patient is less than 45 years of age and does not have history of cardiac disease, place a CVP line and start another D5RL, 1000 ml, plus 500 ml of plasma-protein fraction (PPF) or artificial colloid through a third IV line.

Step 4. Monitor the CVP at frequent intervals during the rapid infusion of these three solutions so as not to exceed values greater than 15 cm H₂O. If the CVP is greater than 15 cm H₂O, directly to the ICU protocol.

Step 5. If the hematocrit value is less than 25 per cent, give two units of type-specific blood. Later, when crossmatched blood is available, transfusions of whole blood or packed red blood cells should be given to maintain hematocrit value greater than 33 per cent.

Step 6.   Rapid restoration of the MAP to 60 mmHg is the titration end-point for fluids in this section of the Algorithm; if the MAP is less than 60 mmHg, recycle from *Steps 2 to 6.* If an MAP greater than 60 mmHg has been achieved, proceed to *Step 7.*

Step 7.   If the MAP is less than 80 mmHg, go to *Step 8;* if not, proceed to *Step 13.*

Step 8.   If the MAP is less than 80 mmHg, ask the patient, the patient's family, or examine a previous hospital record to evaluate the patient's "normal" pre-illness control MAP. If the normal MAP is less than 80 mmHg, and the heart rate is greater than 80 beats/min, measure orthostatic blood pressure (*Step 12*).

Step 9.   As in *Step 3,* the cardiac patient requires less salt and water but more colloid. If the age of the patient is greater than 45 years or there is a history of cardiac disease, give 500 ml of colloid; if the patient's age is less than 45 years, and there is no history of cardiac disease, give D5RL, 1000 ml, plus 500 ml of colloid.

Step 10.   Fluids may be given safely if the CVP is less than 15 cm H_2O; if the latter is exceeded, go to the ICU protocol and continue to give fluids as needed to restore circulatory integrity provided wedge pressure of 18 mmHg is not exceeded.

Step 11.   If the MAP is greater than 80 mmHg without exceeding a CVP greater than 15 cm H_2O, the objective of this cycle has been achieved; if the MAP is less than 80 mmHg, recycle *Steps 7 to 11.*

Step 12.   Orthostatic blood pressure is measured; if there is a change in the MAP of greater 10 mmHg (sitting or standing) it is presumptive evidence of a blood volume deficit of at least 1000 ml.

Step 13.   After the MAP has been restored to the normal value (> 80 mmHg), it is still necessary to be sure the pre-illness blood pressure was normal. If prior hypertension was observed, the physician should repeat *Steps 7 to 13* using 80 per cent of the pre-illness value as the criterion for the adequacy of resuscitation.

Step 14.   Examine the patient for evidence of CNS depression, drug poisoning, and drug abuse.

Step 15.   Examine the patient for evidence of head injury or other trauma. If there are positive signs, the patient should be treated in accordance with a coma–head injury protocol.

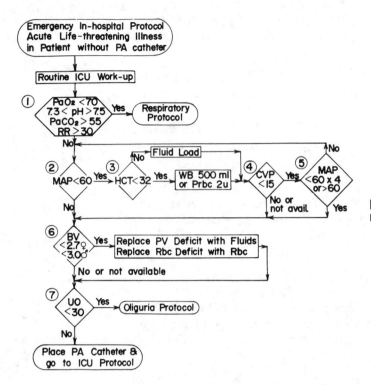

Fig. 2-3. ICU algorithm for patients who do not have a pulmonary arterial catheter.[3]

Step 1.   Routine ICU work up, including arterial blood gas levels, chest x-ray, ECG, CBC and differential, urinalysis, and routine blood chemistry and electrolyte levels, should be repeated stat, unless recently done. If blood gas levels are abnormal, they should be corrected in accordance with a respiratory protocol.

Step 2.   If the MAP is less than 60 mmHg, go to hematocrit *Step 3;* if the MAP is greater than 60, order blood volume measurement.

Step 3.   If the hematocrit is less than 32 per cent, give one unit whole blood or two units packed RBCs; if hematocrit is greater than 32 per cent give a fluid load of 1000 ml D5RL if the patient is primarily dehydrated; 500 ml of PPF or other colloid when hypovolemia is considered the important clinical problem, or 25 gm of 25 per cent albumin if the patient appears to be hypovolemic but water overloaded with expanded extracellular water and peripheral or pulmonary edema.

Step 4.   Fluid load is monitored using CVP measurements; if CVP is less than 15 cm H_2O, proceed to *Step 5.*

Step 5.   If the fluid loading increases MAP greater than 60 mmHg, proceed to *Step 6*; if not, recycle up to four times, or until MAP reaches 60 mmHg.

Step 6.   Measure blood volume and optimize to 3.0 L/M² in males and 2.7 L/m² in females by replacement of plasma volume and red cell mass. If blood volume measurements are not available, or if these optimal values have been obtained, proceed to *Step 7.*

Step 7.   Measure hourly urinary output; if output is less than 30 ml/hr, go to oliguria protocol. If output is greater than 30 ml/hr, place a pulmonary arterial catheter and monitor cardiorespiratory variables.

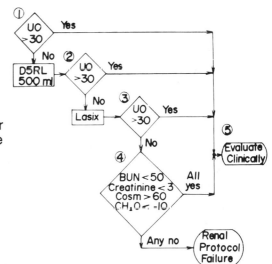

OLIGURIA PROTOCOL

Fig. 2-4. Oliguria algorithm subroutine for management of patients with sudden acute oliguria.[3]

Step 1.   If urine output is greater than 30 ml/hr, proceed to *Step 5* and re-evaluate; if output is less than 30 ml/hr, and the patient is not clinically water overloaded, as evidenced by peripheral or pulmonary edema, positive fluid balance, and basilar rales, give D5RL, 500 ml intravenously, over a 1 to 2 hour period.

Step 2.   If fluid load has increased urinary output to greater than 30 ml/hr, proceed to *Step 5* and re-evaluate; if no response to fluid load, give furosemide (Lasix), 20 mg, and proceed to *Step 3.*

Step 3.   If furosemide has improved urinary output to greater than 30 ml/hr, proceed to *Step 5* and re-evaluate; if there is no response, measure BUN, creatinine, urinary and plasma osmolality, osmolar clearance, and free water clearance (CH_2O) values.

Step 4.   If BUN is greater than 50 mg/100 ml, creatinine level is greater than 3 mg/100 ml and increasing, osmolar clearance is less than 60 ml/min, or CH_2O is greater than -10 ml/hr, place on renal failure protocol.

Step 5.   Evaluate clinically for other evidence of renal impairment and fluid-electrolyte imbalance.

References:

1. Hopkins JA, Shoemaker NC, Chang PC, et al. Clinical trial of an emergency resuscitation algorithm. Crit Care Med 1983; *11*:621–629. (Reproduced with permission of the authors and The Williams & Wilkins Co. Baltimore.)

2. Jastremski MS. Managing shock. Geriatrics 1983; *38*:49–57.

3. Shoemaker WC. Pathophysiology and therapy of shock syndromes. *In*: Shoemaker WC, Thompson WL, Holbrook PR, eds. Textbook of Critical Care. Philadelphia: WB Saunders, 1983. (Reproduced with permission.)

4. Weil MH, Shubin H. Proposed Reclassification of Shock States with Special Reference to Distribution Defects. *In:* Hinsyae LN, Cox BG, eds. The Fundamental Mechanisms of Shock. New York: Plenum Press, 1972.

"Sometimes, though life is
   cold in every vein,
And Death o'er all the
   powers may seem to reign,
Th' electric fluid, Nature's
   purest fire,
The soul reviving vigour can
   inspire;
Breathe through the frame a
   vivifying strife,
And wake the torpid powers
   to sudden life:
Yet more—this shock of life
   is oft the test,
Though all who look may be
   of doubt possest;
Let fly the sudden shock,
   if life remain;
Spasms and contractions
   instantly are plain.
No longer doubt, no more
   the case debate,
You see the body in a
   liveing state."

GEORGE DYER

George Dyer. Annual Report of the
Royal Humane Society of London. London:
Nichols & Sons, 1802.

ALGORITHMS FOR CARDIAC DYSRHYTHMIAS

The following algorithms contain the current recommendations of the American Heart Association for the management of cardiac rhythm disturbances responsible for cardiac arrest. Although one might disagree with some specific points of therapy made in these algorithms, as a whole, they represent a consensus of the nation's experts on the optimal approach to these problems based on currently available data. The other, and perhaps more important, reason to use these algorithms in your resuscitations is that they will ensure a standardized, consistent, and expeditious approach to the management of cardiac arrest. These algorithms have been taken from the American Heart Association Advanced Cardiac Life Support Providers course. If you have not already done so, we would strongly urge you to take part in one of these courses to further improve your resuscitation skills.

Monitored Ventricular Fibrillation

Monitored Arrest

Ventricular fibrillation? ━ No ► to appropriate algorithm

▌
Yes
▼

Establish unresponsiveness and pulselessness
▼

Call for help; precordial thump
▼

Check pulse
▼

Change in rhythm? ━ Yes ► to appropriate algorithm

▌
No
▼

Defibrillate 200–300 joules delivered energy
▼

Check pulse
▼

Change in rhythm? ━ Yes ► to appropriate algorithm

▌
No
▼

Recharge defibrillator immediately 200-300 joules
delivered energy and defibrillate
▼

Check pulse
▼

Change in rhythm? ━ Yes ► to appropriate algorithm

▌
No
▼

CPR, place IV line, and intubate trachea if necessary
+
Epinephrine 0.5–1.0 mg IV or intratracheal + may need bicarbonate IV 1 mEq/kg
▼

To* in Unmonitored Ventricular Fibrillation Algorithm

Unmonitored Ventricular Fibrillation

Recognition: unresponsive, apneic, pulseless

▼

Call for help; initiate CPR

▼

ECG monitor available

▼

Ventricular fibrillation
(or ventricular tachycardia without pulse) ▬ No ► To Asystole or
Electromechanical
Yes   Dissociation Algorithm

▼

Defibrillate 200–300 joules delivered energy

▼

Check pulse

▼

Change in rhythm? ▬ Yes ► to appropriate algorithm

No

▼

Recharge defibrillator immediately 200–300 joules and defibrillate

▼

Check pulse

▼

Change in rhythm? ▬ Yes ► to appropriate algorithm

No

▼

Continue CPR; place IV line; intubate trachea

▼

Epinephrine, 0.5–1.0 mg IV or intratracheal
+
Sodium bicarbonate, 1 mEq/kg (75 mEq initial dose—average-size adult)
or, preferably, according to ABGs

▼

*Defibrillate 360 joules delivered energy (maximal output)

▼

Check pulse

▼

---

*Reference point for **Monitored** Ventricular Fibrillation Algorithm

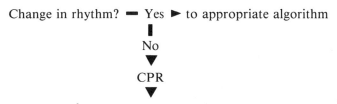

Change in rhythm? ▬ Yes ► to appropriate algorithm
∎
No
▼
CPR
▼
(Frequently evaluate adequacy of ventilation,
oxygenation, and chest compression)
†Bretylium, 350 – 500 mg or 5 mg/kg IV bolus
▼
Defibrillate 360 joules of delivered energy
▼
Check pulse
▼
Change in rhythm? ▬ Yes ► to appropriate algorithm
∎
No
▼
CPR
▼
Bretylium 700 – 1,000 mg or 10 mg/kg IV bolus
▼
CPR; sodium bicarbonate IV according to ABGs or one-half original
dose if no ABGs available (if 10 minutes have elapsed)
▼
Defibrillate 360 joules delivered energy
▼
Check pulse
Change in rhythm? ▬ Yes ► to appropriate algorithm
∎
No
▼
CPR
▼
Repeat epinephrine, 0.5–1.0 mg IV every five minutes and bicarbonate at
one-half dose or according to ABGs
and/or
Repeat bretylium, 10 mg/kg IV bolus as needed

---

†Some may prefer at this point to use lidocaine, 100 mg (or 1 mg/kg) IV bolus followed by
additional boluses, 50 mg (or 0.5 mg/kg) at 5- to 10-minute intervals (total dose of boluses not to
exceed 225 mg) and an infusion of 2–4 mg/min; or procainamide, 20 mg/min (100 mg/5 min) up to
1 g followed by an infusion of 1–4 mg/min before proceeding to bretylium.

Asystole*

CPR
▼
Intubate, ventilate, establish IV if necessary
▼
Epinephrine, 0.5–1.0 mg IV or intratracheal
Repeat at five-minute intervals as needed
▼
Sodium bicarbonate, 1 mEq/kg (or 75 mEq IV as initial dose average-size
adult); repeat at ten-minute intervals at one-half original dose or,
preferably, according to ABGs
▮
CPR
▼
Atropine, 1.0 mg IV
▮
CPR
▼
Check pulse
▼
Change in rhythm? ▬ Yes ► to appropriate algorithm
▮
No
▼
CPR
▼
Calcium chloride, 10% solution 5 mL IV; repeat every ten minutes as needed
▮
CPR
▼
Check pulse
▼
Change in rhythm? ▬ Yes ► to appropriate algorithm
▮
No
▼
CPR
▼
Repeat epinephrine IV, bicarbonate IV, calcium chloride IV as previously
▼
Consider isoproterenol infusion 2 to 20 *ug*/min
(see "Early CPR—Starting the Heart" page 65 before using it.)
▮
CPR
▼

---

*If patient is hypothermic, core temperature should be normalized. Be aware that what
appears to be asystole may be fine ventricular fibrillation and could respond to countershock.

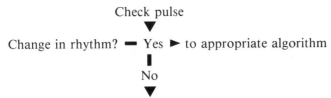

Check pulse
▼
Change in rhythm? ━ Yes ► to appropriate algorithm
▌
No
▼
Repeat epinephrine IV, bicarbonate IV, calcium chloride IV as above
▼
Consider pacemaker

Electromechanical Dissociation

Consider hypovolemia, cardiac tamponade, cardiac rupture, or tension pneumothorax as cause. Reassess ventilation, oxygenation.

CPR
▼
Epinephrine, 0.5–1.0 mg IV or intratracheal
Repeat at five-minute intervals as necessary
▼
Sodium bicarbonate, 1 mEq/kg (or 75 mEq IV as initial dose average-size
adult); repeat at ten-minute intervals at one-half original dose or,
preferably, according to ABGs
▼
Change in rhythm
and/or return of pulse? ━ Yes ► to appropriate algorithm
▌
No
▼
CPR
▼
Calcium chloride, 10% solution 5 ml
Repeat at ten-minute intervals as needed
▼
Change in rhythm
and/or return of pulse? ━ Yes ► to appropriate algorithm
▌
No
▼
CPR
▼
Repeat epinephrine IV, bicarbonate IV, calcium chloride IV as previously
▼
Isoproterenol infusion 2–20 μg/min
(Despite presence of rhythm, continue CPR if no palpable pulse present)
Consider trial of volume infusion

Bradycardia

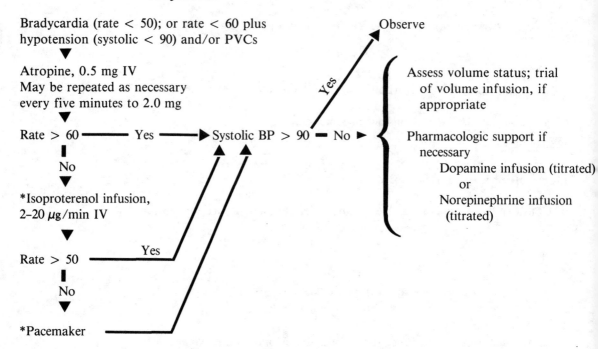

Bradycardia (rate < 50); or rate < 60 plus
hypotension (systolic < 90) and/or PVCs
▼
Atropine, 0.5 mg IV
May be repeated as necessary
every five minutes to 2.0 mg
▼
Rate > 60 ——— Yes ———▶ Systolic BP > 90 ━ No ▶
▮
No
▼
*Isoproterenol infusion,
2–20 μg/min IV
▼
Rate > 50 ——— Yes
▮
No
▼
*Pacemaker ———

Observe

Assess volume status; trial
 of volume infusion, if
 appropriate

Pharmacologic support if
 necessary
   Dopamine infusion (titrated)
   or
   Norepinephrine infusion
    (titrated)

*If bradycardia requires maintenance of isoproterenol drip, pacemaker should be considered.

Ventricular Tachycardia

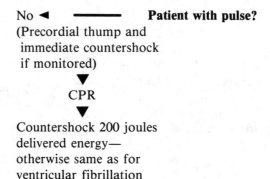

No ◄ ——— **Patient with pulse?**
(Precordial thump and
 immediate countershock
 if monitored)
▼
CPR
▼
Countershock 200 joules
delivered energy—
otherwise same as for
ventricular fibrillation

Patient with pulse?

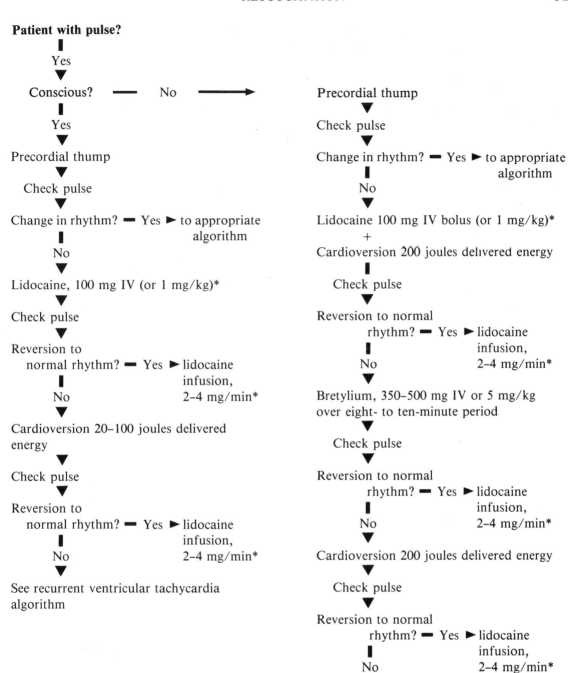

Yes

Conscious? — No ——→

Yes

Precordial thump

Check pulse

Change in rhythm? ➡ Yes ▶ to appropriate
                                algorithm

No

Lidocaine, 100 mg IV (or 1 mg/kg)*

Check pulse

Reversion to
    normal rhythm? ➡ Yes ▶ lidocaine
                                infusion,
    No   2–4 mg/min*

Cardioversion 20–100 joules delivered
energy

Check pulse

Reversion to
    normal rhythm? ➡ Yes ▶ lidocaine
                                infusion,
    No   2–4 mg/min*

See recurrent ventricular tachycardia
algorithm

Precordial thump

Check pulse

Change in rhythm? ➡ Yes ▶ to appropriate
                                algorithm
No

Lidocaine 100 mg IV bolus (or 1 mg/kg)*
              +
Cardioversion 200 joules delivered energy

Check pulse

Reversion to normal
        rhythm? ➡ Yes ▶ lidocaine
                            infusion,
    No   2–4 mg/min*

Bretylium, 350–500 mg IV or 5 mg/kg
over eight- to ten-minute period

Check pulse

Reversion to normal
        rhythm? ➡ Yes ▶ lidocaine
                            infusion,
    No   2–4 mg/min*

Cardioversion 200 joules delivered energy

Check pulse

Reversion to normal
        rhythm? ➡ Yes ▶ lidocaine
                            infusion,
    No   2–4 mg/min*

See recurrent ventricular tachycardia
algorithm

*A second loading dose of 0.5 mg/kg should be given in 5 to 10 minutes.

Recurrent Ventricular Tachycardia
(after maximum lidocaine infusion)

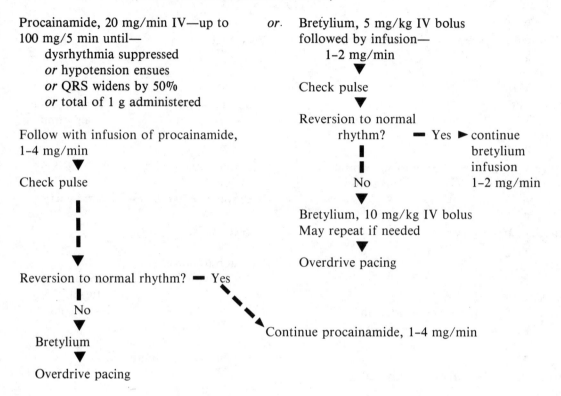

Procainamide, 20 mg/min IV—up to
100 mg/5 min until—
    dysrhythmia suppressed
    or hypotension ensues
    or QRS widens by 50%
    or total of 1 g administered

Follow with infusion of procainamide,
1–4 mg/min
▼
Check pulse

▼

Reversion to normal rhythm? — Yes

No
▼
Bretylium
▼
Overdrive pacing

or. Bretylium, 5 mg/kg IV bolus
followed by infusion—
    1–2 mg/min
▼
Check pulse
▼
Reversion to normal
    rhythm? — Yes ► continue
                  bretylium
                  infusion
No   1–2 mg/min
▼
Bretylium, 10 mg/kg IV bolus
May repeat if needed
▼
Overdrive pacing

Continue procainamide, 1–4 mg/min

Supraventricular Rhythm With Pulse

Following termination of ventricular
fibrillation or ventricular tachycardia
▼
IV (if not in place)
▼
Lidocaine, 100 mg IV bolus (1 mg/kg) after termination of ventricular
tachycardia or ventricular fibrillation followed by lidocaine
infusion of 2–4 mg/min*
▼
Ventilate as necessary
Intubate if not done and patient unresponsive
▼
Oxygenate 100% O_2
▼
Support circulation as necessary

---

*A second loading dose of lidocaine (0.5 mg/kg) should be given in five to ten minutes. If recurrent ventricular tachycardia or ventricular fibrillation is not suppressed by lidocaine, consider procainamide, bretylium, or overdrive pacing. Do not use propranolol to slow sinus tachycardia that occurs in the immediate postresuscitative period. Consider causes of sinus tachycardia (hypovolemia, pump failure, catecholamine excess).
Reference:
1. McIntyre KM, Lewis AJ, eds. Textbook of Advanced Cardiac Life Support. Dallas: American Heart Association, 1983:295–301. (Reproduced with permission. American Heart Association.)

EARLY CPR — STARTING THE HEART: OUR BIASES

"Some people think that doctors and nurses can put scrambled eggs back into the shell."
Dorothy Canfield Fisher

DO'S — In Order of Priority

1. *Diagnose clinically and stat!* If patient looks dead, i.e., no breathing, no pulse, that's enough—start CPR stat.

2. *Ventilate and oxygenate!* Mouth-to-mouth, mouth-to-mask, or bag-to-mask. Don't wait. Reposition the mandible and head to open the airway. Use an oropharyngeal airway and 100 per cent oxygen when possible. Suction prn (endotracheal intubation comes later). Ventilatory rate should be about 12 to 15 per minute. Make the chest expand with each breath. If it doesn't, check the airway—check that oxygen is actually flowing.

3. *External Chest Compression (ECC)!* Rate of about one per second. Place a firm board under the chest. Keep pressing without pausing for ventilation. You should get a pulse palpable in femoral or carotid artery.

4. *Defibrillate* if in ventricular fibrillation (VF) (or ventricular tachycardia)! Give 200 to 400 joules externally in an adult, 2 joules/kg in a child. Defibrillate stat before starting ECC/CPR if a monitored arrest exists and the delay is less than one minute. If the arrest is monitored and observed promptly, a "sternal thump" may convert VF effectively if delivered early, but try it only once or twice. Spend less than five seconds on a "thump."

5. *Attach EKG leads and insert IV line!* Done rapidly by third or fourth person on the team. Consider arterial catheter later (see no. 9).

6. *Give a vasoconstricting drug!* The prime drug in CPR. You must get the coronary perfusion pressure, i.e., the diastolic pressure produced by the ECC above 30 mmHg (as Crile emphasized in 1906). It rarely happens without drugs, because peripheral vasoconstriction must be effectively induced. An inotropic effect may not be important at this moment. That's why CPR is so very different from the treatment of low cardiac output states and dysrhythmias. Epinephrine also greatly enhances the cerebral perfusion produced by ECC.

Use epinephrine and give intravenously if feasible, or endotracheally, 10 ml, at least, of 1:10,000 epinephrine (1 mg). For children give at least 0.01 mg/kg (i.e., 0.1 ml of 1:10,000/kg). Repeat at least every five minutes by the clock.

7. *Give sodium bicarbonate!* Up to 1.0 mEq/kg body weight if the cardiac arrest is longer than five minutes in duration. Acidosis makes epinephrine less effective. Repeat half in ten minutes, then wait

for arterial blood gas levels and pH. Bicarbonate replacement = base deficit of arterial blood X ¼ body weight (kg). Give half of this amount and recheck pH and $PaCO_2$. Excess bicarbonate produces dangerous degrees of CSF acidosis, blood hyperosmolarity, and metabolic alkalosis.

8. *Intubate the trachea!* Now is a suitable time to intubate because the really urgent needs have been attended to. Some patients will be recovering so quickly that they will not need intubation. It should be done by someone with experience, who will check the equipment, intubate in less than 15 seconds, and make sure the tube is in the trachea and not in the esophagus.

9. *Insert the arterial monitoring line!* Take a sample for blood gas values and other laboratory work, then connect the line to a pressure monitor. Diastolic pressure of External Chest Compression must be kept above 30 mmHg. This step may be the most important single factor for successful cardiac resuscitation.

10. *Monitor any interruption to CPR!* Whenever ventilation or External Cardiac Compression is halted, have one person designated to call, clearly, each five-second interval until CPR is started again. Write the times and durations of pauses on the ECG strip or CPR chart.

11. *Keep doing External Cardiac Compression* until a good blood pressure is measured. A weak pulse must be supported by cardiac compression and continued drugs. Electromechanical dissociation is a common reason for death after the heart is restarted. Don't desert the circulation now. It may only need a little more help to succeed.

12. *Keep checking the blood pressure* after you have stopped External Cardiac Compression, even if the pulse feels good. A systolic BP of 50 to 60 mmHg may give a palpable pulse, but that's not a "surviving pressure." Get the BP to greater than 100 mmHg, at least.

13. *Give IV fluid at maximum rate if hypovolemia caused arrest* (e.g., blood loss from aneurysm rupture or major trauma). Time is terribly short now—seconds make a difference. Push lactated Ringer's (as Crile advised in 1906) (or 0.9 % saline) by every available means. Use at least three IV catheters. One should be the biggest catheter that can be put into the biggest available vein. Cut-down should rarely be necessary except in children. Gravity drip is much too slow. One person on each line should push fluid as fast as possible by pump, syringe, or pressurized bag. Once the first 3 to 4 liters are infused, the volume should be enough to give a modest cerebral circulation with CPR. Also consider compression of the venous reservoir by MAST suit (as Crile used in 1903), or knee-hip flexion to compress the abdominal venous reservoir. Control bleeding by local pressure if possible. Immobilize fractures "as they lie" to avoid further tissue damage and pain.

14. *Deflate the stomach* if it has become distended (to avoid vomiting); pass stomach tube by nose or mouth.

15. *Open the chest.* "Slash" the fourth or fifth left intercostal space below the nipple if a palpable pulse cannot be achieved by External Chest Compression. If tamponade is likely, as with a stab or bullet wound of the chest, open the chest and pericardium promptly—don't wait. The heart becomes an obstructing valve when an atrium is compressed from the outside by blood or clot. You must clear the pericardium very quickly, and only then can CPR be effective. (Endotracheal intubation is needed for ventilation when the chest is open). Open chest compression gives a higher cardiac output than closed chest compression.

16. *Cooperate.* You are a part of a team. Coordinate with your physician leader. The nurse-in-charge must be clearly identified and should assign all nursing tasks. Keep your voice at normal volume. Loud voices mean poor communication.

17. *Practice.* Dry runs are essential to achieve good teamwork. You must ask questions if you are not sure of your part or of any detail.

18. *Check equipment regularly* before CPR is needed. See the attached check list (pages 67–68).

19. *Get certified by the American Heart Association* (AHA) in both basic CPR and advanced CPR. The AHA runs excellent courses and supplies well chosen diagrams and illustrations. We should support these important coordinating efforts, and use the AHA protocol for CPR.

DONT'S

1. *Don't try to intubate the trachea as the first move.* Oxygen is needed so urgently—use mouth-to-mouth, mouth-to-mask, or bag-to-mask administration. Leave tracheal intubation to an expert, who will take less than 15 seconds to intubate. Nonexperts waste crucial time, frequently intubate the esophagus, often try to intubate too early in the CPR, and persist beyond reason in their unsuccessful attempts. They can be a menace to the patient.

2. *Don't give peripheral vasodilator drugs* before the heart has restarted—*NEVER, EVER*—because they may lower the coronary perfusion pressure to much less than 30 mmHg and prevent the heart from starting. Isoproterenol has a disastrous record in experimental CPR; coronary pressure averaged 12 mmHg (see Pearson and Redding, 1965). Dopamine also may have a diastolic hypotensive effect, so avoid it before the heart has restarted. Vasodilating drugs also compromise cerebral perfusion. Once the heart is beating at a reasonable rate, an entirely different set of problems arises, and positive inotropic

drugs with a peripheral vasodilator effect may prove invaluable—but not in cardiac arrest before the heart has started.

3. *Don't stop cardiac compression to check the pulse.* If you cannot palpate two pulses, one from the heart and one from the cardiac compression, which is all you need to know, keep on compressing regardless of what the ECG shows. The ECG does *not* indicate cardiac output.

4. *Don't stop cardiac compression for more than five seconds for any observation.* It's "iatrogenic arrest"; it's unwarranted. You may rarely need a five-second pause to identify the ECG signals, but it takes five to ten compressions to re-establish an effective perfusion after each pause. Study the ECG *strip* after cardiac compression is restarted if you must, but not the oscilloscope when chest compression is stopped. Ventilation, cardiac compression, and vasoconstriction are desperately needed—don't stop them to indulge your intellectual curiosity.

5. *Don't stop CPR for more than 15 seconds to intubate the trachea,* no matter who does it. It becomes "induced apnea." Don't be too immature to return to bag and mask if you take more than 15 seconds. It's the patient's brain, not your pride that matters.

6. *Don't use a sternal thump more than once or twice.* If it is used in the first seconds of ventricular fibrillation or ventricular tachycardia, it can be very effective, but don't let it delay defibrillation more than a few seconds.

7. *Don't overventilate with mouth-to-mouth or bag-to-mask administration.* Ventilate enough to make the chest obviously expand with each breath—that's good—but overventilation blows up the stomach and makes vomiting likely. Inhaled vomitus can be disastrous.

8. *Don't stop cardiac compression just because the heart has started to beat.* The beat may be inadequate for survival but still give a palpable pulse. Don't stop compression until the cardiac output is sufficient to give a good measured blood pressure, which may still accompany a poor cardiac output.

9. *Don't give catecholamines through a very peripheral vein.* It causes severe vasospasm in that area.

10. *Don't depend on a gravity drip in the IV line* if the patient has an inadequate blood volume. A gravity drip delivers fluid much too slowly. Push the fluids by pump, syringe, or pressure bag and use three IV lines.

11. *Don't think you can measure the BP by feeling the pulse.* This method is very inaccurate (as Cushing showed in 1903). Once the heart is restarted, BP should be measured and recorded—even an accurate BP is a poor index of cardiac output and blood volume.

12. *Don't mix catecholamines with sodium bicarbonate or calcium chloride* in the IV—the catecholamines are inactivated.

13. *Don't shout.* Loud voices make communicating difficult and increase tension. If you don't have something important to say, keep quiet and listen. Don't be unprofessional; don't chatter about other things while you are in the CPR area.

14. *Don't leave the patient in the emergency room or a ward bed once the heart has been restarted.* As soon as he is stable, head for an ICU taking a portable monitor and defibrillator with you.

Checklist

Is each item working? Does every important item have a spare?

1. *Oxygen*—Are the tanks full? Check connections with ventilating equipment.

2. *Facemasks, ventilator bags*—Do they connect properly and are they at hand in all sizes? Oropharyngeal airways of all sizes at hand?

3. *Suction*—Is the wall-mounted suction apparatus working? Is the portable suction apparatus working? Are rigid tonsil (Yankauer) and long flexible tubes both available with spares?

4. *Laryngoscope*—Are fresh batteries available? Does the blade attach to the handle? Are infant and pediatric blades available? Is the light bulb firmly screwed in? Are extra batteries, bulbs, and tongue blades available?

5. *Endotracheal tubes*—Are infant, child, and adult sizes (3–8.5 mm ID) at hand? Are malleable introducer guide-wires for endotracheal tubes available? Are Magill forceps available?

6. *Defibrillator.* Practice how you charge and fire it. Different models have different controls—practice with each one. On-the-job learning really is inexcusable here. Be sure you know the *OFF* setting for the synchronizer button. Alternatively, does the machine have an automatic release of charge after 30 seconds of full charge?

7. *IV tubing sets and packs of D5W and lactated Ringer's.* Are they available (avoid micro-drip sets, except for catecholamine drips)? Are CVP sets and blood filters available? Are all important medications ready in prefilled syringes (e.g., epinephrine, sodium bicarbonate, calcium chloride, and for later use, atropine, lidocaine, dopamine, isoproterenol, and bretylium)?

8. *Instruments for thoracotomy.* Scalpel with large blade, long thoracic scissors, long hemostats, needle holders and forceps, sutures, rib spreader, sterile towels, and so forth should always be available in a room with good operating room–type light, a table, and ventilating equipment. If you have to send for these items during CPR, it's too late.

9. *Pressure monitor and transducers for arterial pressure line.* Practice how to connect them. Has the monitor calibration been checked recently?

10. *Electrical IV-infusion pump.* Do you know how to connect it and how to run it?

Organized by Eoin Aberdeen, MD. (With special thanks to George Crile, Sr. Isn't it time we caught up to him?)
References:
1. Crile G. A research into means of controlling the blood pressure. Boston Med Surg J. 1903;*148*:247–250.
2. Crile G, Douey DT. Experimental research into resuscitation of dogs killed by anesthetics and asphyxia. J Exp Med 1906;*8*:713–725.
3. Redding JS, Pearson JW. Resuscitation from ventricular fibrillation. Drug therapy. JAMA 1968;*203*:255–260.
4. American Heart Association. Textbook of Advanced Cardiac Life Support. Dallas: 1983.

THE PEDIATRIC CART: BE PREPARED

As any craftsman knows, having the proper tools makes any job much easier to perform. In our pediatric emergency room, one of our most valued and most often utilized pieces of equipment is the resuscitation cart. The contents of the cart are known to all emergency department personnel and are checked each day for completeness. Here's a convenient check list for the preparation of an appropriate life-support system for children.

Medications

(Concentrations and volume unit doses vary from manufacturer to manufacturer).

(3)	Epinephrine	1:10,000 prefilled syringe
(3)	Sodium bicarbonate	10 ml prefilled syringe (1 mEq/ml)
(1)	Sodium bicarbonate	50 ml ampule (1 mEq/ml)
(2)	Calcium chloride	5 ml ampule (10 % solution)
(1)	Atropine	Prefilled syringe (1 mg/10 ml)
(1)	50% Dextrose	50 ml prefilled syringe
(1)	Lidocaine	Mini jet (10 mg/ml)
(1)	Bretylium	Ampule (500 mg/10 ml)
(2)	Fursemide	2 ml ampule (10 mg/ml)
(1)	Diphenhydramine	1 ml ampule (50 mg/ml)
(2)	Mannitol	50 ml ampule (12.5 g/50 ml)
(2)	Ampicillin	1 ampule (1 g/ampule)
(2)	Chloramphenicol	1 ampule (1 g/ampule)
(2)	Pancuronium	1 ampule (10 mg/5 ml)

Ventilatory Equipment

1. Laryngoscope handles, one small, one large
2. Spare bulbs and batteries for laryngoscope
3. Laryngoscope blades
    A. Miller 0, 1, 2, 3
    B. Macintosh 1, 2, 3
4. Oropharyngeal airways: Sizes 00, 0, 1, 2, 3
5. Nasopharyngeal airways: French sizes 12, 16, 20, 24
6. Suction catheters: French sizes 5, 8, 10, 12, 14
7. Endotracheal tubes (ID sizes)
    A. Uncuffed: 2.5, 3.0, 3.5, 4.0, 4.5,
        5.0, 5.5, 6.0, 6.5, 7.0
    B. Cuffcd: 6.5, 7.0, 7.5, 8, 8.5
8. Stylets: One adult, one child
9. Magill forceps
10. Self-inflating resuscitation bag with intact pop-off valve
11. Infant and child face masks
12. (6) tongue blades
13. Lubricant, tincture of benzoin, 1-inch tape

Intravenous Equipment

1. Pediatric armboards and tourniquets
2. 1-inch tape, Betadine and alcohol wipes
3. 500 ml bags of D_5W, normal saline, and lactated Ringer's
4. (2) pediatric T-connectors
5. (2) 3-way stopcocks
6. Plastic intravenous catheters: (4) 24G, (4) 22G, (2) 20G, (2) 18G, (2) 16G
7. Butterfly needles: (4) 25G, (4) 23G, (4) 21G

PEDIATRIC EMERGENCY DRUGS

All emergency department personnel will at some time be called upon to managc thc rcsuscitation of a child. The following two tables provide a quick reference for immediate use. The first lists the most commonly employed life-support medications; the second lists a problem-oriented formulary.

Cardiovascular Resuscitation Drugs For Children

MEDICATION	INITIAL DOSE
NaHCO$_3$ (1 mEq/ml)	1–2 mEq (1–2 ml)/kg
Epinephrine 1:10,000	0.01 mg (0.1 ml)/kg[a]
Atropine (1.0 mg/ml)	0.02 mg (0.02 ml)/kg[a]
Calcium chloride 10%	20 mg (0.2 ml)/kg
Lidocaine 2%	1 mg (0.05 ml)/kg[a]
Dopamine (40 mg/ml) 60 mg (1.5 ml) in 100 ml D5W = 600 μg/ml	1 ml/kg/h = 10 μg/kg/min[b]
Epinephrine 1:1000 6 mg (6 ml) in 100 ml D5W = 60 μg/ml	1 ml/kg/h = 1 μg/kg/min[c]
Isoproterenol 1:5000 0.6 mg (3.0 ml) in 100 ml D5W = 6 μg/ml	1 ml/kg/h = 0.1 μg/kg/min[d]
Lidocaine 4% 120 mg (3 ml) in 100 ml D5W = 1200 μg/ml	1 ml/kg/h = 20 μg/kg/min[e]
Defibrillation	2 watt-sec/kg

[a]May be given via endotracheal tube.

[b]Moderate dose: predominantly beta effects.

[c]High dose: alpha and beta effect.

[d]Low dose.

[e]Moderate dose.

Reference:

1. Holbrook PR, Mickell J, Pollack MM, Fields AI. Cardiovascular resuscitation drugs for children. Crit Care Med 1980;*8*:588-589. (Reproduced with permission of the authors and publisher.)

Problem-Oriented Formulary for Childhood Emergencies

CLINICAL PROBLEM	DRUG	DOSE
Hypotension or Septic Shock	Lactated Ringer's	10–20 ml/kg IV
	Normal Saline	10–20 ml/kg IV
	Plasma-Protein Fraction (PPF)	10–20 ml/kg IV
	Albumin (25%)	1 gm/kg or 4 ml/kg IV
	Dopamine	2–20 μg/kg/min
	Methylprednisolone	30 mg/kg IV

Problem-Oriented Formulary for Childhood Emergencies (Continued)

CLINICAL PROBLEM	DRUG	DOSE
Hypertensive Crisis	Diazoxide	2–5 mg/kg IV push over 30 sec (may repeat)
	Hydralazine	0.15–0.25 mg/kg IM or IV push
	Nitroprusside	0.5–8 µg/kg/min IV infusion
Hypoglycemia	Dextrose (50%)	1–2 ml/kg IV push
	Glucagon	0.3 mg/kg SC, IM, IV (maximum 1 mg) (1 unit = 1 mg = 1 ml)
Anaphylaxis	Diphenhydramine	2 mg/kg IM, IV slow push
	Epinephrine	1:1000, 0.01 ml/kg SC (maximum 0.3 ml) 1:10,000, 0.1 ml/kg IV (maximum 5 ml) slow push
Status Epilepticus	Diazepam	0.1–0.3 mg/kg IV push
	Phenobarbital	10–20 mg/kg at maximum rate of 30 mg/min IV
	Phenytoin	10–20 mg/kg at maximum rate of 50 mg/min IV
Congestive Heart Failure	Digoxin	2 years of age or less, 0.025 mg/kg IM or IV; > 2 years of age, 0.02 mg/kg IM or IV; give in divided doses over 24 hours
	Furosemide	1 mg/kg IV, IM, or PO
Tetralogy of Fallot Hypoxic Spells	Morphine Sulfate	0.1–0.2 mg/kg SC, IV, or IM
	Propranolol	0.05–0.1 mg/kg IV push (maximum, 5 mg)
Status Asthmaticus	Epinephrine	1:1000, 0.01 ml/kg SC (maximum 0.3 ml)
	Terbutaline	0.01–0.04 mg/kg SC
	Aminophylline	Loading Dose, 4–6 mg/kg IV over 20 min

IMMEDIATE MANAGEMENT OF UPPER AIRWAY OBSTRUCTION

"Everything is always worse than you thought it was going to be."

Murphy

Acute upper airway obstruction is a life-threatening emergency that requires prompt intervention. Transtracheal catheter ventilation is a relatively simple technique that can be initiated rapidly. It usually provides adequate oxygenation and ventilation until a more definitive procedure, such as tracheal intubation or tracheostomy is accomplished. A simple system for transtracheal catheter ventilation can be constructed from materials that should be readily available in an emergency department or intensive care unit. All one needs is a 14 gauge intravenous catheter-over-needle assembly, a bag-valve–mask device, and the adapter from a 3.0 mm internal diameter pediatric endotracheal tube assembled as shown in Figure 2-5.

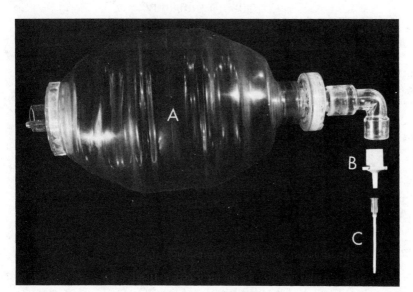

Fig. 2-5. *A:* bag-valve device; *B:* 3.0 mm endotracheal tube adapter; and *C:* 14 gauge catheter.[2]

The catheter is inserted into the trachea at the cricothyroid membrane. The catheter-over-needle assembly is attached to an empty 10 cc syringe and inserted in the midline of the cricothyroid membrane, pointed down toward the lungs at an angle of approximately 45° (Fig. 2-6.) A negative pressure is applied to the syringe while the needle is being inserted, so that air will be aspirated into the syringe when the trachea is entered. When it is entered, the catheter is advanced over the needle, and the needle is withdrawn from the catheter. The syringe

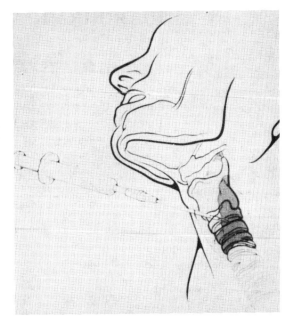

Figure 2-6. Insertion of transtracheal catheter.[1]

is then attached directly to the catheter and aspirated to ensure that there is still a free flow of air to indicate that the catheter remains in the trachea. The bag-valve device and the 3.0 mm endotracheal tube adapter are then attached to the hub of the catheter, allowing the patient to be ventilated and oxygenated.

An additional advantage of this technique is that the positive pressure produced in the trachea by ventilation with the bag-valve device may sometimes actually expel an obstructing foreign body and solve the problem. Complications of the procedure include hemorrhage, esophageal perforation if the needle is advanced too far, and subcutaneous or mediastinal emphysema if ventilation is attempted when the catheter tip is not properly positioned in the trachea.

This technique will not be effective in total upper airway obstruction because exhalation must occur through the upper airway. However, almost all upper airway obstructions are partial, i.e., they are complete in inspiration but not in expiration, so that this technique usually is effective. Expiration may be assisted by using manual chest compression to increase intrathoracic pressure.

References:
1. White RD, Goldberg AM, Montgomery WM. Adjuncts for airway control and ventilation. *In*: McIntyre KM, Lewis AJ, eds. Textbook of Advanced Cardiac Life Support. Dallas: American Heart Association, 1981:IV-8. (Reproduced with permission from the American Heart Association.)
2. Stinson TW. A simple connection for transtracheal ventilation. Anesthesiology 1977; *47*:232.

RETROGRADE STYLET

If the larynx cannot be visualized and intubation is necessary, a retrograde stylet may be used to guide the endotracheal tube. Choose a 24-inch, through-the-needle catheter. Insert the needle introducer through the cricothyroid membrane (Fig. 2–7A). Advance the catheter through the needle and out through the nose or mouth (Fig. 2–7B). Slide the endotracheal tube over the free end of the catheter through the larynx (Fig. 2–7C). Hold the endotracheal tube in place while withdrawing the needle and catheter. Advance the endotracheal tube to the depth required.

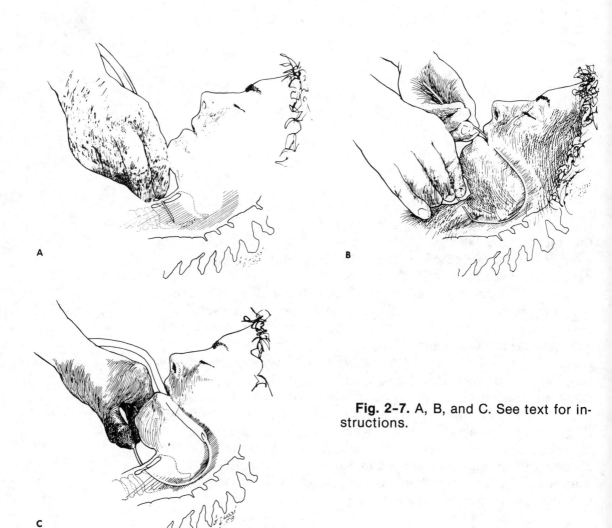

Fig. 2–7. A, B, and C. See text for instructions.

Reference:
1. Linscott MS, Horton WC. Management of upper airway obstruction. Otolaryngol Clin North Am 1979;*12*:351–373. (Figures reproduced with permission.)

BLIND NASOTRACHEAL INTUBATION

There are many descriptions of the technique for orotracheal intubation, but descriptions of the technique for nasotracheal intubation are hard to find.

Indications

Nasotracheal intubation is indicated for a patient with spontaneous respirations who requires airway protection or ventilation. It is particularly suited for the following:

1. A patient with trismus or biting.
2. A patient who may have a fracture of the cervical spine.
3. A patient who is awake.*
4. A patient who is sitting.
5. A patient who is nonfasting.

---

*Excellent anesthesia is required for the awake patient. One author's personal experience with two nasal intubations showed them to be very painful procedures.

Contraindications

Contraindications for nasotracheal intubation include any patient with apnea, coagulopathy, possible basilar skull fracture, or obstructions of the upper airway (foreign body, large polyps, malignancy, epiglottitis).

Complications

All problems associated with orotracheal intubation are possible with nasotracheal intubation, plus retropharyngeal perforation, nasal bleeding or necrosis, sinusitis, damage to adenoids or turbinates, introduction of nasal flora into the airway, and inadequate ventilation. (The work of breathing progressively increases as the tube size falls below 7.5 mm internal diameter. This last effect may prevent some patients from being weaned from the respirator.)

Procedure

1. Select a tube. Use a cuffed tube 1 mm smaller than the one you would choose for oral intubation. It is important that the tube be well curved. Tubes may be stored in cylindrical containers to accentuate the curve. The curve on the tip of the Endotrol® tube can be varied by the lever on the operator's end. If repeated attempts are necessary, use a new tube, because the plastic softens with heat and the tube loses its shape. As an alternative, cooling the tube in ice may allow you to reshape it to the desired form.

2. Select the wider nostril by observing the patient sniff.

3. Induce nasal vasoconstriction and anesthesia with phenylephrine and lidocaine or cocaine. Lubricate the distal catheter with an anesthetic ointment (lidocaine jelly). (Translaryngeal anesthesia is optional: Results of series in which it was not used are good. It involves injecting 2 ml of lidocaine, 2 to 4 per cent, with epinephrine through the cricothyroid membrane.)

4. If it is not contraindicated, flex the neck and extend the head.

5. Insert the tube into the wider nostril. With the beveled edge toward the nasal septum, hold the tube parallel to the nasal floor (perpendicular to the plane of the face). Insert with gentle pressure. When the tip reaches the posterior nasopharynx, rotate the tube so that its curve corresponds to the curve of the airway. (The tip of an Endotrol® tube can be directed anteriorly.) Advance the tube through the vocal cords as the patient inspires. Correct placement is indicated by movement of air through the tube and by the loss of vocalization. Placement is further verified by auscultation of the lungs during positive pressure ventilation.

6. If the tube is not in place, withdraw the tip to the posterior oropharynx and re-advance. (Magill forceps and a laryngoscope may be used to draw the tip of the tube anteriorly into the larynx.)

References:
    1. Danzl DF, Thomas DM. Nasotracheal intubations in the emergency department. Crit Care Med 1980;*8*:677–682.
    2. Elder CK. Naso-endotracheal intubation: advantages and technic of "blind intubation." Anesthesiology 1944;*5*:392–399.
    3. Gold MI, Buechel DR. A method of blind nasal intubation for the conscious patient. Anesth Analg. 1960;*39*:257–263.
    4. Iserson KV. Blind nasotracheal intubation. Ann Emerg Med 1981;*10*:468–471.

THE ENDOTRACHEAL ROUTE: WHAT TO DO WHEN YOU CAN'T GET AN IV

Several important drugs can be given through an endotracheal tube, permitting absorption through the large surface area of the lungs (65 m²) into the alveolar circulation (98% of cardiac output). Compared with intravenous administration, the endotracheal route generally gives blood levels that are initially lower but more prolonged.

Though the intravenous route is preferred, the endotracheal route is an alternative for administration of epinephrine, lidocaine, atropine, and naloxone (Narcan). In addition, studies in dogs suggest that this route is suitable for diazepam (Valium).

2

Techniques

Dose	Use at least as much as you would for the IV route (i.e., the high side of the range of recommended doses).
Volume	Dilute to 5–10 ml. Studies in dogs suggest that normal saline is preferable to sterile distilled water as the diluent.
Position	The patient should not be in Trendelenburg.
Equipment	Verify that the endotracheal tube has been placed correctly. Draw the diluted drug into a syringe. Choose a catheter (as used for central venous pressure lines) long enough to reach through the endotracheal tube to its distal end. Attach the catheter to the syringe or insert the needle of a prefilled syringe into the catheter.
Instillation	Place the catheter deep into the endotracheal tube. Squirt the drug into the bronchi. Then, flush the catheter with air.
Removal	As the catheter is removed, cover the endotracheal tube to prevent the drug from being forced out by chest compression or cough.
Ventilate	Bag 5 to 10 times to distribute the drug.
Instillation (Alternative Technique)	In a letter to the *Annals of Emergency Medicine* (1983; *12:*196), Feferman and Leblanc suggest that a more efficient way to administer drugs endotracheally is to insert an 18 gauge needle into the side of the endotracheal tube. Medications can then be injected into the tube through the syringe without disrupting ventilation or losing them back out through the tube. The injection should be made during the inspiratory phase to help ensure that the drug will travel into the lungs.

References:
   1. Barsan WG, Ward JT, Otten EJ. Blood levels of diazepam after endotracheal administration in dogs. Ann Emerg Med 1982;*11*:242–247.
   2. Feferman I, Leblanc L. A simple method for administering endotracheal medication [letter]. Ann Emerg Med 1983;*12*:196.
   3. Ganong F. Review of medical physiology. Los Altos, California; Lange, 1975:483.
   4. Greenberg MI, Baskin SI, Kaplan AM, Urrichio FJ. Effects of endotracheally administered distilled water and normal saline on the arterial blood gases of dogs. Ann Emerg Med 1982;*11*:600–604.
   5. Greenberg MI, Roberts JR. Drugs for the heart by way of the lungs. Emerg Med 1980; 209–212.

DRUG CONCENTRATIONS DURING CPR

The American Heart Association Advanced Cardiac Life Support course advocates the use of a peripheral vein as the first choice for access to the circulation for drug administration during CPR. However, a recent study has raised serious questions about the effectiveness of peripherally administered drugs during cardiac arrest, because of the low flow and venous stasis associated with chest compression. Figure 2–8 shows the concentrations of cardio-green dye in the femoral artery following injection into either an antecubital or subclavian vein during cardiopulmonary resuscitation. The central administration of the dye provided both earlier and much higher peak concentrations of the dye. These findings suggest that drugs administered by the central route would be much more likely to be effective than drugs administered peripherally during CPR.

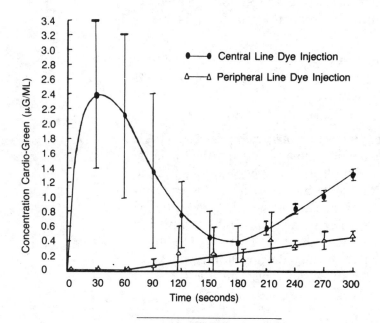

Fig. 2–8. Concentration of cardio-green dye in the femoral artery during CPR.

Reference:

1. Kuhn GJ, White BC, Swetnam RE, et al. Peripheral vs. central circulation times during CPR: a pilot study. Ann Emerg Med 1981;*10*:417–419. (Figure reproduced with permission from the authors and publisher.)

FLOW RATES OF IV CATHETERS

The ability to rapidly infuse intravenous fluids and blood products for hemorrhagic shock in the trauma victim or in the GI bleeder, for example, depends on a variety of factors. The usual dictum to "establish two IVs" is incomplete unless the following factors are considered.

1. *IV catheter diameter.* The larger the inside diameter of the catheter, the faster the flow rate.

2. *IV catheter length.* The longer the catheter, the slower the flow rate. A subclavian catheter will have a slower flow rate than a shorter peripheral IV of the same gauge.

3. *IV tube length.* The longer the tube from the IV solution to the catheter, the slower the flow.

4. *Fluid viscosity.* The greater the viscosity, the slower the flow rate. Crystalloid solutions run faster than does whole blood. Packed red blood cells will infuse faster when they are first diluted with normal saline.

5. *Fluid pressure.* Flow rates can be increased by using an infusion pump or pressure cuff.

Several studies have been published that compare the flow rates for different infusion setups. The findings are summarized in the following table. As expected, the fastest flow rate was obtained with the catheter with the largest bore, i.e., the 9 French Introducer with infusion cuff. In addition, for catheters of the same size, the flow rates may differ significantly depending on the manufacturer. ·

IV Catheter Infusion Rates

	CRYSTALLOID (ml/min)		PACKED RBCS WITH INFUSION CUFF (ml/min)	
	Gravity	Infusion cuff	Diluted	Normal
Central Venous Catheters				
USCI 9 French Introducer	247	566	343	124
USCI 8 French Introducer	243	540	324	–
Deseret Angiocath 14 gauge, 5¼-inch	157	341	210	63
Deseret Intracath 16 gauge, 8-inch	70	–	–	–
Peripheral IVs				
Argyle Medicut 14 gauge, 2-inch	194	484	287	96
Deseret Angiocath 14 gauge, 2-inch	173	405	257	–
Argyle Medicut 16 gauge, 2-inch	151	353	220	–
Deseret Angiocath 16 gauge, 2-inch	108	231	158	–
B-D Longdwell 16 gauge, 2½-inch	102	–	–	–
Argyle Medicut 18 gauge, 2-inch	86	–	–	–
Deseret Angiocath 18 gauge, 2-inch	62	–	–	–

References:
1. Dailey RH. Flow rate variance of commonly used IV units. JACEP 1973;*2*:341–342.
2. Dula DJ, Muller HA, Donovan JW. Flow rate variance of commonly used IV infusion units. J Trauma 1981:*21*: 480–482.
3. Graber D, Dailey RH. Catheter flow rates updated. JACEP 1977;*6*:11.
4. Mateer JR, Thompson BM, Aprahamian C, Darin JC. Rapid fluid resuscitation with central venous catheters. Ann Emerg Med 1983;*12*:149–152.

IV'S IN PARADISE

Take a young green coconut, five to six months old. (See your favorite botany text for guidelines on determining the age of the nut.) Raise strips of the husk and tie them into a knot. The loop that's formed is used to hang the coconut. Sterilize the surface of the nut. Remove the husk with a sterile knife until the inner shell is reached. Puncture the shell with a sterile needle, attach it to an infusion line, and commence infusion.

The coconut provides approximately 600 ml of fluid of pH 4.8 and specific gravity of 1.019, containing 8 mEq calcium, 3 mEq magnesium, 2 mEq sodium, 21 mEq potassium, 25 mEq chloride, 24 mg phosphate, 2 gm protein, and 17 gm sugar.

Reference:
1. Iqbal QM. Direct infusion of coconut water. Med J Malaysia 1976;*30*:221–223.

HAZARDS OF TOPICAL NTG

Nitroglycerin can be given transcutaneously, either as an ointment in a lanolin-petroleum base or as a package for sustained release. Patients often wear these preparations over the precordium for the subjective benefit of having medicine close to the heart. If a patient wearing nitroglycerin over the left side of the chest is defibrillated, an electrical arc can form. Nitroglycerin ointment has high resistance (low conduction), and the discharge is transmitted across the ointment; sustained-release patches have an aluminum covering that attracts the charge from the defibrillation paddles. In addition to startling everyone present, the electrical arc decreases the amount of current delivered to the patient and thus may prevent successful defibrillation.

Such problems can be avoided by advising patients to wear nitroglycerin away from the chest or by removing the nitroglycerin patch before defibrillating.

References:
1. Babka JC. Does nitroglycerin explode? NEJM 1983;*309*:379.
2. Parke JD, Higgins SE. Hazards associated with chest application of nitroglycerin ointments. JAMA 1982;*248*:427.

PERICARDIOCENTESIS

"Diseases, desperate grown
By desperate appliances are reliev'd
Or not at all."

Shakespeare

When evaluating patients with penetrating or blunt chest injuries and those in shock or with electromechanical dissociation after CPR, the physician must consider pericardial tamponade. The presence of a high central venous pressure (CVP) with persistent hypotension following fluid resuscitation is indicative of this disorder. At this point, pericardiocentesis with removal of as little as 20 to 30 ml of blood from the pericardium may be lifesaving.

2

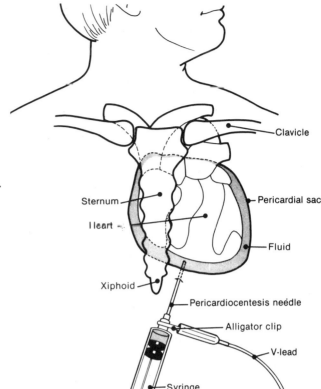

Fig. 2-9. Technique of pericardio-centesis.

Clavicle

Pericardial sac

Sternum

Heart

Fluid

Xiphoid

Pericardiocentesis needle

Alligator clip

V-lead

Syringe

Prepare and drape the patient in the usual manner. Infiltrate the skin with 1 per cent xylocaine about 1 cm to the left of the xyphoid. Infiltrate deeply to the costal arch. Next, connect the limb leads of an electroradiograph to the patient and attach one end of a sterile double alligator clip to the V lead of the ECG machine and the other end to an 18-gauge spinal needle that is attached to a 10 ml syringe. Insert the needle into the anesthetized tract at an angle of 30 degrees to the skin, aiming for the patient's left shoulder (Fig. 2–9). Apply a

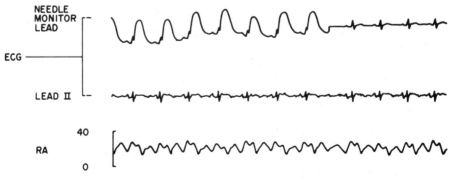

NEEDLE
MONITOR
LEAD

ECG

LEAD II

RA

40

0

Fig. 2-10. The monitor lead shows the ECG tracing obtained from the pericardial needle. The first eight beats illustrate the marked ST segment elevation injury pattern seen when the needle is in contact with the epicardium. The last four beats show the ECG when the needle is in the free pericardial space. The bottom tracing is of the right atrial pressure.

slight negative pressure to the syringe and watch the ECG tracing as you advance the needle. When the needle enters the pericardium, you will feel a "pop." If the ECG develops an injury pattern of ST-segment elevation (Fig. 2–10), this indicates epicardial contact and you must withdraw the needle slightly with continued application of negative pressure. If fluid is recovered, aspirate until the patient's unstable hemodynamic state has improved or until no further fluid can be aspirated. A catheter may also be passed through the needle into the pericardial space for continued drainage of fluid, if needed.

References:
1. Kravis TC. Atlas of emergency procedures. *In*: Kravis TC, Warner CG, eds. Emergency Medicine, A Comprehensive Review. Rockville: Aspen Systems Corporation, 1983:1083–1085. (Figure 2–9 reproduced with permission from Aspen Systems Corporation, 1983.)
2. McIntyre KM, Lewis AJ, eds. Textbook of Advanced Cardiac Life Support. Chicago: American Heart Association, 1981:XIV 11–16.
3. Shabetai R. Pericardiocentesis. *In:*Shebetai R. ed. The Pericardium. New York: Grune & Stratton, Inc., 1981:325–347. (Figure 2–10 reproduced with permission from the author and publisher.)

TEMPORARY PLACEMENT OF BALLOON-TIPPED PACEMAKERS

Whenever possible, it is preferable to insert cardiac pacemakers under direct fluoroscopic guidance. However, there are several situations, mainly sudden cardiac arrest or symptomatic bradycardia, that may neccessitate insertion of a balloon-tipped catheter at the bedside.

After vascular access is achieved by placing an introducer in the internal jugular, subclavian, or femoral vein, a number 3 French, balloon-tipped pacing catheter is inserted via the introducer into the respective vessel (Fig. 2–11). The distal electrode of the pacing catheter

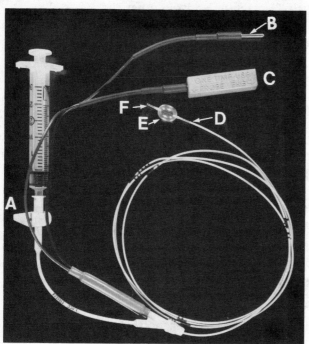

Fig. 2-11. Balloon-tipped pacing catheter. *A:* proximal balloon port; *B:* proximal electrode lead; *C:* distal electrode lead; *D:* proximal electrode; *E:* balloon; *F:* distal electrode.

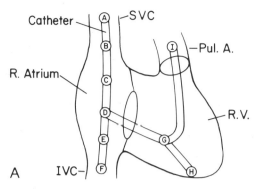

Fig. 2-12 A. Intracavity locations (A-I) corresponding to intracavity ECG tracings below.

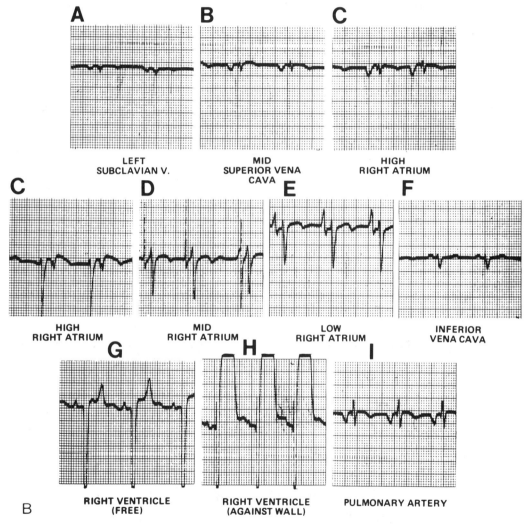

B

Fig. 2-12 B. As the pacing catheter approaches the right atrium, the amplitude of the P waves increases progressively. Since atrial depolarization is inferiorly directed in this patient, P waves recorded above the atria have a negative deflection, whereas those low in the atria and in the inferior vena cava are positive. As the catheter enters the ventricle, the QRS amplitude increases markedly, and a QS complex is inscribed. When the catheter tip touches the endocardial surface, marked ST-segment elevation is seen. As the electrode passes into the pulmonary artery, the QRS amplitude diminishes, and a negative P wave is inscribed since the catheter tip is again above the level of the atria.

is then attached to the V lead of a well-grounded ECG machine using double alligator clips. The limb leads must also be attached to the patient in the usual manner (be sure all connectors are well insulated). The remaining connector for the proximal pacing electrode is left unconnected. The distal tip is now a unipolar exploring electrode.

Figure 2–12 demonstrates the intracavity tracings (see 2–12B) obtained from various locations (see 2–12A) during insertion of an exploring transvenous electrode. Recognition of these patterns will allow determination of the positions of the catheter during insertion.

Once good endocardial contact is made, the catheter is attached to the pacer box by connecting the distal electrode lead to the negative terminal and the proximal electrode lead to the positive terminal. Then, the pacing threshold should be checked and the pacer repositioned, if necessary, to obtain a satisfactory threshold (< 2 ma).

References:
1. Bing OHL, McDowell JW, Hartman J, Messer JV. Pacemaker placement by electrocardiographic monitoring. N Eng J Med 1972;*287*(13):651. (Figure 2-12 B reproduced with permission of the authors and publisher.)
2. Hawthorne JW, McDermott J, Poulin FK. Cardiac pacing. *In*: Johnson RA, Haber E, Austen WG, eds. The Practice of Cardiology. Boston: Little Brown & Company, 1980:219–257.

BASICS OF HEMODYNAMIC MANIPULATION

The Starling ventricular function curve is a classic way of looking at cardiac function. Conceptualization of a hemodynamic manipulation, in terms of its effect on the Starling curve, is a useful trick to help the neophyte begin to understand the complexities of hemodynamic manipulation in the critically ill. A Starling curve is constructed by plotting some measure of preload against some measure of cardiac pumping performance. The pulmonary artery wedge pressure is the usual clinical measure of left ventricular preload. Stroke volume, which can be obtained by division of the thermodilution cardiac output by the heart rate, is a common measure of left ventricular pumping function. Left ventricular function will be at a single point on a single curve at any given time but has the potential for moving both along a given curve or to a different curve, depending on the status of the various determinants of cardiac function. In Figure 2–15, *A* represents a normal function curve and *B* represents the depressed function curve of a failing ventricle.

There are three basic hemodynamic manipulations used to improve cardiac function and thus perfusion. Preload optimization places the ventricle at its most favorable point on a single function curve. The optimal preload is the cardiac filling pressure that gives the

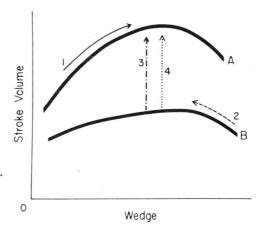

Fig. 2-13. Starling ventricular function curve.

highest cardiac output. Hypovolemic patients should be given volume (manipulation 1) until the optimal wedge pressure is achieved. This optimum will usually be a wedge pressure of 10 to 12 mmHg in patients with normal left ventricular function, and 14 to 18 mmHg in patients with depressed left ventricular function. The failing ventricle will usually have a preload above the desired range, which is lowered to the optimal level using either diuretics or a drug that dilates the venous capacitance bed, such as nitroglycerin (manipulation 2). Contractility augmentation (manipulation 3) increases the strength of myocardial contraction, and the ventricle functions more normally as shown in the curve. Drugs such as dopamine and dobutamine are usually used in the acute situation to achieve contractility augmentation. Contractility augmentation improves cardiac performance at the cost of an increased myocardial oxygen demand, which may be an important drawback in the patient with coronary artery disease. The final hemodynamic manipulation is afterload reduction (manipulation 4). Afterload reduction, achieved with arterial dilators such as nitroprusside or hydralazine, decreases the impedance to the injection of blood from the ventricle, and allows the ventricle to function on a more normal performance curve with the added benefit of decreasing myocardial oxygen demands.

Critically ill patients often may require multiple interventions simultaneously. However, if you keep these basic principles in mind, and remember that the most important end point is restoration of tissue perfusion, you will be well on your way to a comfortable understanding of the hemodynamic management of critically ill patients.

Reference:

1. Jastremski MS. Hemodynamic monitoring: concepts every clinician should know. Consultant 1982;*22*:96–111. (Figure reproduced with permission of the publisher.)

RESPIRATORY VARIATION OF PULMONARY VASCULAR PRESSURES

"The indication for the use of a flotation catheter is any situation in which a physician would consider placing a central venous pressure line for the purpose of cardiovascular monitoring."

Swan

Hemodynamic data obtained with the Swan-Ganz catheter are routinely used to make major therapeutic decisions in the critically ill. When using this tool to manage critically ill patients, one must be aware that changes in intrathoracic pressure produced by changes in the respiratory cycle can cause considerable variation in the measured pulmonary vascular pressures. Figure 2–14 shows the pulmonary artery wedge pressure reading from a patient being ventilated in the intermittent mandatory ventilation (IMV) mode. Patients being ventilated with IMV have a mixture of spontaneous breaths that lower intrathoracic pressure and positive pressure ventilator breaths that raise intrathoracic pressure. A reading taken at point *A* would be erroneously low. A reading at point *C* would be erroneously high. The correct wedge pressure is obtained by reading the pressure at point *B*, end expiration, when intrathoracic pressure is in a steady state unaffected by respiration.

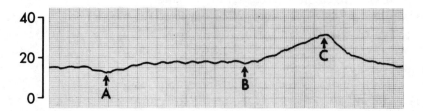

Fig. 2–14. Pulmonary artery wedge pressure tracing from a patient on IMV. *A* represents the patient's spontaneous inspiration (wedge pressure equals 13 mmHg). *B* is the end expiratory point at which intrathoracic pressure is stable (wedge pressure equals 18 mmHg). *B* is the "real" wedge, i.e., the point at which pressures always should be measured. *C* represents the positive pressure inspiration from the ventilator (wedge pressure equals 32 mmHg).

Reference:

    1. Jastremski, MS. Hemodynamic monitoring: concepts every clinician should know. Consultant 1982;*22*:96–111. (Figure reproduced with permission of the publisher.)

> ## A SKILLFUL TEACHER
> When a superior man knows the causes which make instruction successful, and those which make it of no effect, he can become a teacher of others. Thus in his teaching, he leads and does not drag; he strengthens and does not discourage; he opens the way but does not conduct to the end without the learners' own efforts. Leading and not dragging produces harmony. Strengthening and not discouraging makes attainment easy. Opening the way and not conducting to the end makes the learner thoughtful. He who produces such harmony, easy attainment, and thoughtfulness may be pronounced a skillful teacher.
>
> CONFUCIUS
> 550–478 B.C.

2

ACLS: INSTRUCTING THE MEGA-CODE STATION

A. Prepare
   1. Tell students specifically what they are expected to know well ahead of time. For example, should they know dosages? How to mix drips? This instruction can be done by mail before the course begins.

   2. Instructors must know the information contained in the algorithms and descriptive material. All instructors should be coordinated in their teaching material.

3. Prepare scenarios. The instructor's manual has them. Some are elaborate, involving several arrhythmias. Others are incorrect (e.g., stimulating a hypothermic heart). Instructors can devise their own scenarios. Give details including whether the patient is on a cardiac monitor or has an IV, and what personnel are available. Remember that airway obstruction is part of ACLS. It's best to avoid traumatic arrest: ACLS training is not directed there.

4. Know the equipment. Be familiar with the manikin, the monitor and defibrillator, and the arrhythmia generator you will be using.

B. Decide What You Want To Teach
1. The mega-code station synthesizes the knowledge and skills from the rest of the course into a coordinated, team approach to the management of cardiac arrest. Time limitations may help you decide whether individual students should have to handle several clinical problems or whether groups of students should have to handle individual clinical problems. With the latter method, the group as a whole experiences several problems. The skill of leadership is not covered elsewhere and it should be emphasized at the mega-code station.

2. Complications can be introduced (e.g., intubating the esophagus, putting drugs in the wrong boxes so that the wrong drug is given, touching the manikin during defibrillation), and pressure can be added (background noises, interruptions). These complications can be educational, but make sure they are not distracting from the learning experience.

C. Know Your Group
1. Know names and backgrounds. The emphasis will vary with the group's background. Emergency medical technicians (EMTs) may want more technical skills; physicians may want more theory.

2. If you recognize one person as being well prepared, choose him to go first or to handle more difficult situations. If a group member seems poorly prepared, give him situations that are easy to handle. Don't embarrass anyone; the negative attitude that this behavior generates can impede learning.

3. Define each person's role clearly.

4. Keep the station fun, but don't get sloppy.

3

TRAUMA

INITIAL ASSESSMENT OF THE TRAUMA PATIENT 90

ASSESSING SEVERITY OF INJURY: THE TRAUMA SCORE . 93

THE GLASGOW COMA SCALE 95

THE TRUMA RECORD 95

TREATMENT OF SHOCK IN THE TRAUMA PATIENT 101

WHEN SECONDS COUNT—UNCROSSMATCHED BLOOD . 102

PEDIATRIC TRAUMA 105

OVERLOOKED INJURIES IN MULTIPLE TRAUMA 106

PNEUMATIC ANTISHOCK TROUSERS 107

PERITONEAL LAVAGE IN THE DIAGNOSIS OF THE
ACUTE ABDOMEN IN TRAUMA 103

STAB WOUND TO THE ABDOMEN 111

THORACIC AORTIC TRANSECTION 112

CHEST TUBE STABILIZATION 113

BLAST INJURY 114

MANAGEMENT OF PELVIC FRACTURE 116

BLADDER AND URETHRAL INJURIES IN
PELVIC FRACTURE 116

REPLANTATION 118

REMOVAL OF PROTECTIVE HEADGEAR 119

ZIPPER INJURIES 120

"The bottom line is that the emergency physician's responsibility is to transfer the care of the viable trauma patient expeditiously to a surgeon competent in further managing the patient's injuries. The general surgeon's responsibilities are to either assume that care or assist in expediting the transfer of the viable trauma patient to a more competent surgical colleague."

GERRIS R. HEDGES, M.D.

INITIAL ASSESSMENT OF THE TRAUMA PATIENT

The patient with serious injuries is a challenging problem for the emergency physician. Often, the steps taken in the first minutes with the patient will have a profound influence on the final outcome. In order to offer the best chance for a favorable outcome, the physician must proceed systematically through the initial assessment, evaluating the patient's injuries and establishing priorities for treatment. The initial assessment is divided into four phases:

1. *Primary Survey:* Injuries that threaten life or limb are identified.

2. *Resuscitation Phase:* These life-threatening injuries are treated.

3. *Secondary Survey:* A systematic, in-depth evaluation of the patient from head to toe is performed with continuous reassessment of the patient's condition.

4. *Definitive Care Phase:* Less serious injuries are managed.

The ABC's of the Primary Survey

*A*irway management with cervical spine (C-spine) control.
*B*reathing.
*C*irculation with hemorrhage control.
*D*isability—neurologic status.
*E*xpose—completely undress the patient.

A—**Airway Management with C-Spine Control.** The first priority is to establish a patent airway. Because manipulation of the neck can convert a fracture without neurologic deficit to a fracture-dislocation with neurologic deficit, airway management must be accomplished without hyperextension of the neck. Orotracheal intubation is therefore discouraged. Spine injury must be considered in any patient with injury above the clavicles and is adequately assessed only by obtaining a cross-table lateral cervical spine x-ray with visualization of all seven cervical vertebrae. Absence of neurologic deficits does not rule out C-spine injury.

Maneuvers that can be used to obtain a patent airway, listed in order of increasing intervention, include: (1) chin lift, (2) oral airway insertion, (3) blind nasotracheal intubation, and (4) needle or open cricothyroidotomy.

B—**Breathing.** Once a patent airway is assured, the adequacy of ventilation must be assessed. During the primary survey, three injuries must be looked for that most often compromise air exchange, i.e., tension pneumothorax, open pneumothorax, and flail chest.

C—**Circulation with Hemorrhage Control.** The circulation should be assessed by evaluation of the patient's pulse, noting the rate, quality, and site obtained. A general rule for estimating systolic pressure is: Radial pulse present (80 mmHg); femoral pulse present (70 mmHg); and carotid pulse present (60 mmHg).

At this point, exsanguinating hemorrhage should be identified and controlled. Control is accomplished immediately with direct pressure on the wound. Subsequent transfer of the patient to the operating room for definitive control may be necessary.

D—**Disability (Neurologic Status).** Early neurologic evaluation establishes a baseline against which any change in the patient's condition is measured. During the primary survey the patient's level of consciousness and pupillary size and reaction should be evaluated. Further neurologic examination should be done during the secondary survey.

E—**Expose—Completely Undress the Patient.** It is mandatory to remove *all* clothing. Remember to check the back for significant injuries.

> "Cutting clothing is destructive, but leaving injuries unidentified may have far graver consequences."
>
> NORMAN MCSWAIN, M.D.

Resuscitation Phase

During this phase of the initial assessment, correction of the life-threatening injuries identified in the primary survey should be initiated. Correction includes treatment of tension and open pneumothorax, flail chest, and shock. While phases are separated for the purposes of this presentation, lifesaving therapy should be instituted at the time the problem is identified rather than waiting until the end of the primary survey.

Secondary Survey

Once resuscitation measures have been instituted, the secondary survey, i.e., a systematic, complete physical examination, is performed. At this point, necessary x-rays are obtained. Remember to examine the patient's back. A Foley catheter and nasogastric (NG) tube should be placed at this time. Contraindications to Foley catheter placement are blood at the urethral meatus, scrotal hematoma, or free-floating prostate. In these cases, a retrograde urethrogram should be done first in order to identify disruption of the urethra. In the case of a maxillo-facial fracture, the NG tube should be passed through the mouth, to avoid cannulization of the central nervous system (CNS).

Definitive Care Phase

Treatment is now initiated for injuries identified in the secondary survey.

Other Things to Do

1. *Obtain a history.* The most important responsibility is to ascertain the events surrounding the injury. Other data to consider are the patient's past history, medications, and allergies. A useful mnemonic is to take an AMPLE history.

    A—*A*llergies
    M—*M*edications
    P—*P*ast illnesses
    L—*L*ast meal
    E—*E*vents of the injury

2. *Re-evaluate the patient.* As you proceed to examine and treat the patient, continually monitor the patient's response and watch for deterioration, which may indicate inadequate treatment or unrecognized injury.

3. *Keep a record.* Baseline information, as well as the change in response to specific interventions, should be meticulously recorded.

Reference:
    1. American College of Surgeons Committee on Trauma. Advanced Trauma Life Support Course, 1981.

ASSESSING SEVERITY OF INJURY: THE TRAUMA SCORE

Several indexes have been developed to help quickly assess the severity of injury of trauma patients. The Trauma Score (TS), developed by Champion and coworkers,[1] is an example. It may be used to predict outcome from an injury, to perform triage in the field, to evaluate changes in a patient's status over time, or to evaluate trauma care in different facilities. The TS is presented next along with a sample calculation for a patient. In addition, a graphic representation of the probability of survival for a given trauma score is presented.

Trauma Score

PHYSICAL SIGN	VALUE	POINTS	SCORE
Respiratory Rate			
Number of respirations in 15 sec ×4	10-24	4	
	25-35	3	
	> 35	2	
	< 10	1	
	0	0	_____
Respiratory Effort			
Shallow—markedly decreased chest movement or air exchange	Normal	1	
Retractive—use of accessory muscles or intercostal retraction	Shallow or retractive	0	_____
Systolic Blood Pressure			
Systolic cuff pressure—either arm, auscultate or palpate	> 90	4	
	70-90	3	
	50-69	2	
	<50	1	
	No carotid pulse	0	_____
Capillary Refill			
Normal—refill within 2 sec	Normal	2	
Delayed—more than 2 sec	Delayed	1	
None—no capillary refill	None	0	_____
Glasgow Coma Scale			
(See page 95)	14-15	5	
	11-13	4	
	8-10	3	
	5-7	2	
	3-4	1	_____

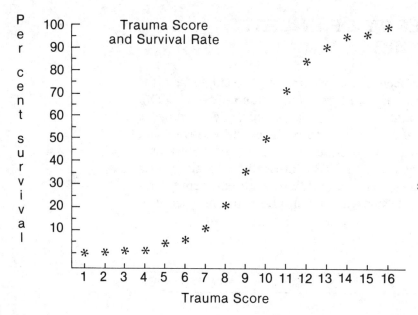

Fig. 3-1. Trauma score and survival rate.

Example: | Points
Respiratory Rate = 28 — 3
Respiratory effort = shallow — 0
Systolic Blood Pressure = 80 — 3
Capillary Refill = <2 sec — 2
Glasgow Coma Scale = 10 — 3
Total — 11
Probability of Survival = 71 per cent

Reference:
1. Champion HR, Sacco WJ, Carnazzo AJ, et al. Trauma score. Crit Care Med 1981;*9:* 672–676. (Reproduced with permission from the authors and The Williams & Wilkins Co., Baltimore.)

THE GLASGOW COMA SCALE

In evaluating the comatose patient, serial determinations of the level of coma are more important than any single determination in providing information about the course of the patient's disease or response to therapy. A useful tool for evaluation is the Glasgow Coma Scale (GCS). As the initial physician to assess the condition of the patient in coma, the emergency physician's evaluation is of utmost importance to establish the patient's initial status. The GCS provides some indication of the trauma patient's prognosis. Those patients having a score of less than seven generally do poorly.

Glasgow Coma Scale

EYE OPENING	SCORE
Spontaneous	4
To sound	3
To pain	2
No response	1
BEST VERBAL RESPONSE	
Oriented	5
Disoriented	4
Inappropriate words	3
Incomprehensible sounds	2
None	1
BEST MOTOR RESPONSE	
Obeys commands	6
Response to pain	
Localizes	5
Withdraws	4
Decorticate	3
Decerebrate	2
No response	1

Reference:
1. Teasdale G, Jennet B. Assessment of coma and impaired consciousness: a practical scale. Lancet 1974; 2:81.

THE TRAUMA RECORD

The trauma service personnel at the University of Virginia School of Medicine, Charlottesville, have been kind enough to allow us to share their *Trauma Record Form* with you. Use of such a preprinted medical record for the trauma victim has helped reduce omissions in the evaluation of the trauma patient, has greatly improved the quality of information retained in the patient's permanent record, and has taken less time than a classic free-form, unstructured admission note.

Examination of the Multiple Trauma Victim

PHYSICAL FINDINGS

	Normal	Abnormal

PRIMARY SURVEY
1. Assess Ventilation
   a. Assess responsiveness
   b. Inspect and palpate for unilateral and bilateral
      chest movement
   c. Listen for and feel breath sounds

BP _____ P _____ R _____

2. Examine Circulation
   a. Palpate pulse (quality, rate, rhythm)
   b. Color of skin

R   L

3. Search for External Bleeding
   a. Inspect disrobed anterior area of trunk
      and extremities

R

4. Calculate Trauma Score

Trauma Score

		Points Scored
Respiratory Rate	Rate/minute	
	36	2
	25–35	3
	10–24	4
	1–9	1
	None	0
Respiratory Expansion	Normal	1
	Shallow	0
	Retractive	0
Systolic Blood Pressure (mmHg)	90 or more	4
	70–89	3
	50–69	2
	0–49 or less	1
	No Pulse	0
Capillary Return	Normal	2
	Delayed	1
	None	0

Table continued on following page

3

Glasgow Coma Score (GCS)	*Points*
Eye Opening	
Spontaneous	4
To voice	3
To pain	2
None	1
Verbal Response	
Oriented	5
Confused	4
Inappropriate words	3
Incomprehensible words	2
None	1
Motor Response	
Obeys commands	6
Localizes (pain)	5
Withdraw (pain)	4
Flexion (pain)	3
Extension (pain)	2
None	1

Total

Total	*Score*
14–15	5
11–13	4
8–10	3
5–7	2
3–4	1

History

Previous illness
Allergy
Immunization status
Medications

Examination of the Multiple Trauma Victim (Continued)

	PHYSICAL FINDINGS	
	Normal	*Abnormal*

SECONDARY COMPREHENSIVE SURVEY

1. Head

a. Inspect scalp and face for wounds, swelling, ecchymosis, and fractures

b. Perform otoscopic examination of nose and ears (CSF leak, hemotympanum)

c. Examine eyes and record:
  Eye movement
  Size of pupils
  Reaction of pupils to light
  Visual acuity

d. Inspect mouth for malocclusion, carious and missing teeth, lacerations

e. Check for facial fractures
  Palpate nose
  Inspect septum for hematoma
  Palpate zygomatic arches and infra-orbital ridges
  Check stability of midface and mandible

2. Neck

a. Inspect for wounds, hematoma, swelling, and venous distention

b. Palpate for subcutaneous emphysema and tracheal deviation

3. Chest

a. Inspect for wounds, swelling, hematoma, and ecchymosis

b. Observe chest and its movements (prominent hemithorax, paradoxical, etc.)

c. Palpate for fractures and subcutaneous emphysema. Check thoracic cage stability using anterior-posterior and lateral compressions

d. Percuss chest (hyperresonant, dull)
e. Auscultate for breath and heart sounds

4. *Abdomen*
   a. Inspect for wounds, swelling, hematoma, and ecchymosis
   b. Auscultate for bowel sounds
   c. Palpate for tenderness, guarding (voluntary vs. involuntary), rebound, and masses (bladder, etc.)
   d. Check stability of pelvis by compressing iliac wings and symphysis pubis

5. *Musculoskeletal*
   a. Observe posture (decerebrate, decorticate, etc.) and identify wounds, swelling, ecchymosis, and hematoma
   b. Palpate each extremity for tenderness and fractures
      Record pulses
   c. Record muscle strength and sensation bilaterally

| | Arm | | Leg | |
	R	L	R	L
Pulses				
Motor				
Sensation				

6. *Genitalia and Perineum*
   a. Inspect penis (blood at meatus) and perineum (ecchymosis)
   b. Perform rectal examination
      Record position of prostate
      Anal sphincter activity
      Rectal sensation

7. *Back ("logroll patient" after spinal injury ruled out)*
   a. Inspect for wounds, ecchymosis, hematoma, swelling, fractures
   b. Palpate spinal vertebrae, ribs and pelvis for tenderness and fractures

Table continued on following page

3

Examination of the Multiple Trauma Victim (Continued)

DIAGNOSTIC WORK-UP

Venous Blood Studies		*Arterial Blood Studies*	*Urinalysis*	*Peritoneal Lavage*
WBC	CO_2	pH	Color	WBC
RBC	CPK	P_{CO_2}	pH	RBC
Hgb	AMY	P_{O_2}	SG	
Hct	ALC	P_{O_2}/F_{IO_2}	Protein	
BUN	PTT	Base deficit	WBC	
Glu	PT		RBC	
Na	Blood Type		Glucose	
Cl	Cr		Other	
K				

X-ray

ECG

Clinical Impression

Physician _____ Nurse _____

TREATMENT OF SHOCK IN THE TRAUMA PATIENT

Shock in the critically injured patient is primarily hypovolemic, secondary to blood loss. Exceptions are patients with tension pneumothorax, cardiac tamponade, or myocardial contusion. With tension pneumothorax, the rise in intrathoracic pressure impedes venous return. When cardiac tamponade is present, the fluid in the pericardial sac impedes cardiac filling. The end result in all cases is decreased cardiac output and shock.

Treatment of hypovolemic shock involves volume replacement in amounts adequate to reverse the patient's hemodynamic instability. One of the best ways to judge the adequacy of this therapy is urinary output. It should be maintained at about 1 ml/kg/hr. Failure of the patient to improve with fluid therapy indicates either insufficient volume replacement or ongoing blood loss. In the absence of external hemorrhage, lack of improvement implies bleeding into the chest or abdomen and may require immediate surgical intervention to control the hemorrhage.

There are four classes of acute hemorrhage, depending on the amount of blood loss that has occurred. These are summarized in the table.

*Classes of Acute Hemorrhage**

	CLASS I	CLASS II	CLASS III	CLASS IV
Blood Loss in ml	up to 750	1000–1250	1500–1800	2000–2500
Blood Loss in %†	up to 15	20–25	30–35	40–50
Pulse Rate‡	72–84	>100	>120	140 or greater
Blood Pressure§	118/82	110/80	70–90/50–60	<50–60 systolic
Pulse Pressure (mmHg)	36	30	20–30	10–20
Capillary Blanch Test	Normal	Positive	Positive	Positive
Respiratory Rate	14–20	20–30	30–40	>35
Urine Output (ml/hr)‖	30–35	25–30	5–15	Negligible
CNS-Mental Status	Slightly Anxious	Mildly Anxious	Anxious and Confused	Confused and Lethargic
Fluid Replacement (Use 3:1 rule for fluid resuscitation)	Crystalloid	Crystalloid	Crystalloid + Blood	Crystalloid + Blood

* Committee on Trauma, American College of Surgeons, Advanced Trauma Life Support Course, 45, 1981. (Reprinted with permission of the American College of Surgeons.)
† % of blood volume in a standard 70 kg male
‡ Assume normal of 72/min
§ Assume normal of 120/80
‖ Assume normal of 40–50 ml/hr

Initial Therapy

1. *Crystalloid.* Lactated Ringer's is the fluid of choice for initial volume replacement. As a general guide, you will need to give three times the volume of estimated blood loss as crystalloid.

2. *Blood.* As noted in the classification of hemorrhage, Class III or IV hemorrhage will require blood replacement in addition to crystalloid. It should begin as soon as possible. If time permits, type-specific crossmatched blood should be used. If life-threatening hemorrhage exists, however, type-specific uncrossmatched blood should be given. If this is not available, Type O should be given. For males, Type O-positive blood is given. For females of childbearing age, Type O-negative blood is used to prevent Rh sensitization. (See When Seconds Count—Uncrossmatched Blood, next).

3. *MAST.* (See page 107).

WHEN SECONDS COUNT – UNCROSSMATCHED BLOOD

Definitions. Know what your order means.

Type. The recipient's ABO type is determined by mixing recipient cells with known anti-A, anti-B, and anti-AB sera. In the reverse procedure, recipient serum is mixed with cells known to be A, B, or O. Any discrepancy in the results of these two procedures must be investigated.

The Rho(D) type is determined by mixing recipient cells with known anti-D serum.

It takes five to ten minutes to determine type-specific blood for transfusion.

Screen. Red blood cells that contain the antigens most often involved in iso-immunization are tested against recipient serum. These antigens look for "unexpected" antibodies, and the process takes at least 45 minutes.

Hold. Blood is reserved for one patient and is unavailable for transfusion to another.

Crossmatch. This procedure helps identify minor antibodies. In the major crossmatch, the serum of the recipient is mixed with cells of the donor. In the minor crossmatch, which is optional, cells of the recipient are mixed with serum of the donor. The mixtures are suspended in various matrices or pre-treated with proteolytic enzymes. Some samples are examined directly; others are incubated at room temperature or at 37°C. Samples are finally centrifuged, then examined for hemolysis or agglutination. Agglutination may be enhanced by the addition of antiglobulin serum. A full crossmatch requires a minimum of 45 minutes.

Abbreviated Crossmatch. Blood is released before incubation or enhancement of agglutination. The abbreviated crossmatch takes five to ten minutes to complete after the initial type and screen.

Use of Uncrossmatched Blood

I.   General. The American Association of Blood Banks recommends that only packed red blood cells (PRBCs) be used for uncrossmatched blood. Though this reduces many problems, 20 per cent of whole blood plasma still remains in preparations of PRBCs. The physician must sign a release stating that he accepts responsibility for giving a patient blood that has not been fully crossmatched.

II.   Type O. "Universal donor" blood can be transfused to any recipient, because the red blood cells have no A or B antigens. Although plasma has anti-A and anti-B antibodies, they are usually diluted and neutralized.

Problems
1. "Dangerous universal donors" have high titer antibodies. Their plasma may cause acute reactions in A, B, and AB recipients. During the Korean War, 35 per cent of Type O blood had high antibody titers and could not be used as universal donor blood.
2. If large quantities (15–20 units) of Type O blood are transfused, recipient RBCs are selectively destroyed.
3. If large quantities of Type O blood are transfused and type-specific blood is given later (within two weeks), type-specific RBCs may be hemolyzed.

III. The Rh factor. Whereas Rho(D)-negative blood is preferable for use as a universal donor, Rho(D)-positive blood can be used if the patient has not been previously immunized by transfusions or pregnancy. During the Viet Nam conflict, O-Rho(D)-positive blood was used as the universal donor, saving the rare O-Rho(D)-negative blood for type-specific use. "Immunization may occur if the patient is Rh-negative, but it is better to have a living immunized patient than a dead one with no antibodies."[3] In addition, RhoGAM can be administered to prevent Rh sensitization.

IV. Type specific. Blood is matched according to ABO and Rh types. Even this limited typing takes time, and pressure to hurry the procedure may increase errors. No ABO or Rho(D) antibodies to the recipient's RBCs are transfused with the plasma.

V. "Universal Recipient." Patients with Type AB blood may receive blood of other types. Type O blood is least desirable, since its serum has both anti-A and anti-B antibodies.

Who Needs a Full Crossmatch?

Patients who have been pregnant, those who have received transfusions previously, and neonates need full crossmatches.

In the first two cases, the patients may have been sensitized to red blood cell antigens other than Rho(D). Neonates have ABO-antibodies transferred passively from their mothers.

References:
1. Blood Bank, The University of Chicago Medical Center. Emergency Transfusion Request Form. Chicago, 1980.
2. Barnes A. Transfusion of universal donor and uncrossmatched blood. Bibl Haematologica 1980; *46*:132–142.
3. Huestis DW, Bove JR, Busch S. Practical Blood Transfusion. 3rd ed. Boston: Little, Brown & Company, 1981: 165–166, 178, 205–208, 210–212.
4. Oberman HA, Barnes BA, Friedman BA. The risk of abbreviating the major cross-match in urgent or massive transfusion. Transfusion 1978; *18*:137–141.

PEDIATRIC TRAUMA

Accidents are the main cause of death among children. Mortality of young victims of trauma may be reduced by an organized, knowledgeable approach to their care. Although the principles of adult trauma apply, specifics of management vary according to the patient's body size. Orotracheal tube specifications, for instance, can be estimated from the child's age using the table below.

Vital signs are valuable indicators of a patient's status. However, they must be interpreted in light of the patient's age (see pages 282, 283).

Early airway management may require an endotracheal tube.

Pediatric Orotracheal Tube Specifications[3]

AGE	FRENCH SIZE	INTERNAL DIAMETER (ID) (mm)	LENGTH (cm)	ID OF 15 mm MALE CONNECTOR (mm)
Newborn ($<$ 1.0 kg)	11–12	2.5	10	3
Newborn ($>$1.0 kg)	13–14	3.0	11	3
1–6 mo	15–16	3.5	11	4
6–12 mo	17–18	4.0	12	4
12–18 mo	19–20	4.5	13	5
18–36 mo	21–22	5.0	14	5
3–4 yrs	23–24	5.5	16	6
5–6 yrs	25	6.0	18	6
6–7 yrs	26	6.5	18	7
8–9 yrs	27–28	7.0	20	7
10–11 yrs	29–30	7.5	22	8
12–14 yrs	32–34	8.0	24	8

Breathing. A child's thorax is easily compressed by a dilated stomach. The early use of a nasogastric tube is in order. If a chest tube is required, use the largest one that can be accommodated by the intercostal space.

Circulation. A cutdown may be required for venous access. Fluid volumes for maintenance and resuscitation are shown in the tables.

Maintenance Fluid Volume Requirements
*— $D_5\frac{1}{4}NS$[*1]*

WEIGHT (kg)	AMOUNT OF FLUID
0–10	100 ml/kg/24 hr
11–20	1000 ml + 50 ml/kg/24 hr (times no. of kg $>$ 10)
21–40	1500 ml + 20 ml/kg/24 hr (times no. of kg $>$ 20)
$>$40	2500 ml/24 hrs (adult requirement)

*10 per cent dextrose solution for the neonate.

Blood Products—Volume for Intravenous Administration (ml/kg bolus)[1]

Lactated Ringer's	20
Whole blood	20
Plasma	20
5% albumin	20
Packed RBCs	10
25% albumin	4

For peritoneal lavage, use 10–15 ml/kg lavage fluid. Criteria for positive results are based on concentrations and therefore are the same as for adults.

During resuscitation, the child is exposed and loses heat; therefore beware of hypothermia.

References:

1. Eichelberger MR, Randolph JG. Pediatric trauma: an algorithm for diagnosis and therapy. J Trauma 1983;*123*:91–97. (Tables reproduced with permission of the authors and The Williams & Wilkins Co., Baltimore.)

2. Jorden RC. Pediatric trauma resuscitation. *In*: Rosen P, Baker FJ, Braen GR, et al. (eds.). Emergency Medicine. St. Louis: C.V. Mosby Co., 1983:124–126.

3. Downes JJ, Raphaely RC. Pre- and postanesthetic care and cardiopulmonary resuscitation. *In*: Behrman RE, Vaughn VC III, McKay RJ, Nelson WE (eds.). Nelson Textbook of Pediatrics 12th ed. Philadelphia: WB Saunders, 1983:258. (Table reproduced with permission of the authors.)

OVERLOOKED INJURIES IN MULTIPLE TRAUMA

"Don't carry a coffin by yourself; call a consultant."
Marshall B. Segal, M.D., J.D.

In the management of multiply injured patients, fractures and other orthopedic injuries are often overlooked while attention is directed to more serious injuries. The following is a list of commonly overlooked problems. A careful physical examination, as part of the secondary survey (see Initial Assessment of the Trauma Patient, page 90), will help to successfully identify most of these injuries.

Overlooked Injuries in Multiple Trauma

Basilar skull fracture
Zygomatic arch and orbital fractures
Odontoid process fracture
C7 vertebral injury
Posterior dislocation of the shoulder
Scaphoid, lunate, and paralunate dislocations
Radial head fracture
Digital fractures
"Seat-belt" fracture (T12, L1)
Pelvic fracture
Femoral neck fracture
Posterior dislocations of the femoral head
Tibial plateau fracture
Fracture of the talus

Reference:

1. Iverson LD, Clawson DK. Manual of Acute Orthopedic Therapeutics. Boston: Little, Brown & Co., 1982:6–7. (Reproduced with permission.)

PNEUMATIC ANTISHOCK TROUSERS

Pneumatic antishock trousers control bleeding by putting direct pressure on external wounds and by reducing vascular wall tension and flow. They increase cardiac filling pressure and peripheral vascular resistance.

Their use is indicated for hypotension (systolic, BP < 80), whether its cause is subdiaphragmatic bleeding, drugs, spinal anesthesia or cord trauma, coagulopathy, anaphylaxis, or pericardial tamponade. The trousers can also be used to immobilize the pelvis or lower extremities and to increase arterial pressure during CPR. They may be helpful for cases of clinical shock with systolic BP between 80 and 100; for supradiaphragmatic bleeding (while increasing flow to the bleeding site, they also increase flow to the cardiopulmonary and cerebral systems); or for cardiogenic shock (Killip's Class III).

Antishock trousers are contraindicated for patients with pulmonary edema or congestive heart failure, burns that would be covered, and tension pneumothorax. Use of the abdominal compartment is contraindicated in patients during the third trimester of pregnancy and in patients with bleeding esophageal varices. The trousers may be contraindicated in patients with underlying renal or pulmonary disease, or in patients with a suspected fracture of the lumbar spine. The use of the abdominal compartment is relatively contraindicated in evisceration or during the first and second trimesters of pregnancy.

The cardiovascular effects of pneumatic antishock trousers are shown in the table "External Counterpressure-Induced Physiologic Changes."

Pneumatic trousers are formed of three compartments and differ according to manufacturer. They are fastened by Velcro straps or by zippers on the legs with a belt on the abdomen. They have gauges to measure the compartmental pressure or valves that release at 104 mmHg.

Clothing should be removed from the patient's abdomen and legs before the trousers are applied, to allow access to the perineum. The trousers may be slid under the patient if immobilization is necessary, or the patient may be placed on the trousers. The leg compartments are inflated first. If the patient's BP becomes adequate, there is no need to proceed with inflation of the abdominal compartment.

The pressure on pneumatic trousers should not be released in the field. (If intra-abdominal bleeding is suspected, deflation should be done in an operating room prepared for laparotomy.) Total deflation time should be 20 to 30 minutes. Only one compartment is released at a time. If release causes the BP to drop more than 5 mmHg, deflation is stopped until fluids are administered to restore the blood pressure.

Both metabolic and respiratory acidosis may result from the use of antishock trousers—the first, because of impaired perfusion under the garment; the second, because of diaphragmatic restriction. Limb ischemia may lead to a compartment syndrome or necrosis. There may be decreased renal perfusion or decreased vital capacity; both must be monitored closely. The trousers have the technical disadvantage of covering areas that may need to be examined. There have been several recent reports of spinal cord injury caused by movement of patients with lumbar fractures during placement of antishock trousers.

External Counterpressure-Induced Physiologic Changes[4]

PARAMETER	RELATIVE CHANGE
Central Venous Pressure	Increases
Pulmonary Capillary Wedge Pressure	Increases
Stroke Volume	Increases
Heart Rate	Decreases
Cardiac Output	Increases (in hypovolemic patients)
Systemic Blood Pressure	Increases
Peripheral Resistance	
Total	Variable
Local	Increases
Arterial Blood Flow	
Supradiaphragmatic	Increases
Infradiaphragmatic	Decreases
Metabolic Function	Lactic acidosis possible
Renal Function	No significant change
Respiratory Function	
Vital Capacity	Decreases
Lung Blood Volume	Increases

References:
　　1. Krome R. Initial approach to the trauma patient. *In:* Tintinalli J (ed.). Study Guide in Emergency Medicine. ACEP, 1976:16–1.
　　2. McSwain NE. Pneumatic trousers and the management of shock. J Trauma 1977. *17*(9): 719–724.
　　3. Pelligra R, Sandberg EC. Control of intractible abdominal bleeding by external counter-pressure. JAMA 1979; *241*(7):708–713.
　　4. Wasserberger J, Balasubramanium S, Ordog G. Pneumatic antishock trousers: a widening spectrum of new uses. ER Reports 1981; *2*(23):105–110. (Table reproduced with permission of the authors and the publisher.)

PERITONEAL LAVAGE IN THE DIAGNOSIS OF THE ACUTE ABDOMEN IN TRAUMA

Diagnosis of the acute abdomen in the injured patient remains a difficult problem. When restricted to clinical criteria alone, accuracy has been reported at between 42 and 87 per cent. Powell and coworkers[2] reported a clinical accuracy rate of 65.5 per cent in 955 patients in a combined series study. Clinical assessment is hampered by the presence of altered sensorium as a result of head injury, alcohol or other drug use, and severe pain. Children and mentally impaired patients are also a challenge in diagnosing intra-abdominal injury. In addition, the patient with acute spinal cord injuries may have associated intra-abdominal injuries, but no abdominal pain, rigidity, or guarding. According to Powell's review, a missed or delayed diagnosis of intra-abdominal injury results in a 15 to 58 per cent mortality. The presence of head trauma is particularly important. When it is associated with abdominal trauma, it carries a 56 per cent mortality and 26 per cent of these deaths are attributable to undiagnosed abdominal injuries.

Many procedures have been used to increase the accuracy of diagnosis of abdominal injuries. Technetium-99m scanning of the liver and spleen is one such technique. It has a 99 per cent accuracy rate in diagnosing liver injuries and a 97 per cent accuracy rate in diagnosing spleen injuries. Arteriography is also particularly helpful, especially in evaluating retroperitoneal injuries, but is usually not available on a timely basis. Other techniques have included laparoscopy and, more recently, CT scanning of the abdomen.

None of these procedures have been as effective in diagnosing intra-abdominal trauma as peritoneal lavage. It is simple, convenient to perform and accomplished with minimal equipment. A midline incision is made in the infra-umbilical region after the skin and subcutaneous tissue are injected with local anesthesia with epinephrine. The midline fascia is incised and the peritoneum exposed. The peritoneal dialysis catheter is then passed into the abdomen, either using the trocar to penetrate the peritoneum or incising the peritoneum and passing the catheter without the trocar. Blind infra-umbilical puncture of the fascia and peritoneum has also been described. If the initial aspiration through the catheter is negative for blood, 1000 ml (10–15 ml/kg for children) of normal saline is instilled into the abdomen, allowed to mix, and then removed by gravity drainage. Criteria for a positive peritoneal lavage are summarized as follows.

Criteria for Positive Peritoneal Lavage

GROSSLY BLOODY INITIAL RETURN
CELL COUNT
    > 100,000 RBCs/mm^3
    > 500 WBCs/mm^3
PRESENCE OF OTHER MATERIAL IN THE FLUID
    Bile
    Food particles
    Bacteria
    Feces
DRAINAGE OF LAVAGE FLUID THROUGH A CHEST TUBE OR
    FOLEY CATHETER

Several comments regarding this technique should be made. The presence of abdominal distention or previous abdominal incisions dictates the passage of the catheter with direct visualization to avoid injury to the intestine. In the presence of a pelvic fracture, false-positive results, which may occur because of passage of the catheter through an anterior retroperitoneal hematoma, may be minimized by making the incision in the supra-umbilical region. In infants and small children, a 14 gauge plastic needle may be used instead of a dialysis catheter. The stomach and bladder should be emptied before lavage is performed.

The gravid uterus is a relative contraindication; if necessary, the procedure may be done above the umbilicus with direct visualization and incision of the peritoneum, passing the catheter without using the trocar.

The accuracy rate for diagnostic peritoneal lavage is high with low false-positive, false-negative, and complication rates. Powell combined 31 series, involving 10,358 patients with blunt trauma, and reported an overall accuracy rate of 97.3 per cent. The false-positive rate was 1.4 per cent, and the false-negative rate was 1.3 per cent. The complication rate is less than 1 per cent. When the criteria for positive results include a lowered RBC count (positive if $> 50,000/mm^3$), similar results are obtained for penetrating trauma.[1] Complications of the procedure include local wound problems, inadequate fluid return, injury to the intestine, bladder puncture, laceration of iliac vessels, and disruption of retroperitoneal hematomas.

Peritoneal lavage does have its limitations. Serious injuries, such as ruptured diaphragm, intestinal perforation, or retroperitoneal injuries, may be missed. Blind reliance on the procedure may delay treatment in the 1.3 per cent of patients with false-negative results. Finally, peritoneal lavage is not indicated when the diagnosis is certain or laparotomy is planned.

In summary, diagnostic peritoneal lavage is a safe, reliable technique for the evaluation of the abdomen in the trauma patient, with an accuracy of 97 per cent. False-positive and false-negative rates are 1.4 and 1.3 per cent, respectively. With the use of proper technique, complications can be minimized to less than 1 per cent.

References:
1. Alyono D, Morrow CE, Perry JF Jr. Reappraisal of diagnostic peritoneal lavage criteria for operation in penetrating and blunt trauma. Surgery 1982; *92*:751–757.
2. Powell DC, Bivins BA, Bell RM. Diagnostic peritoneal lavage. Surg Gynecol Obstet 1982; *155*:257–264.

3

STAB WOUND TO THE ABDOMEN

The traditional approach to a patient with penetrating injury to the abdomen is mandatory exploratory laparotomy. Over the past three decades, however, a selective approach has been shown to be a safe way to manage such patients, especially stab wound victims. Some methods of evaluation of these patients are presented here.

The most immediate threat to the victim of a stabbing is hemorrhage, which mandates an aggressive initial approach. Standard resuscitation that includes airway management and intravenous fluids is initiated. Failure to respond to such measures demands immediate operation. In the hemodynamically stable patient, further evaluation may be undertaken. Two problems are evaluated: Has the peritoneum been penetrated, and if so, is there visceral injury that must be treated?

A variety of methods are used to aid this evaluation. The starting points are the history and physical examination. Whereas the presence of peritoneal signs is helpful, one fourth to one third of patients with significant injury may have a normal examination on admission. Frequent, serial examinations provide more information. X-rays are generally not helpful, except to localize a bullet or bone injuries from a gunshot wound. In the presence of hematuria, an IVP is mandatory. Sinography does not consistently demonstrate peritoneal penetration and should not be done.

When there is a clear indication for exploration, such as hemorrhage, evisceration, or signs of peritoneal irritation, no further evaluation is necessary. Otherwise, wound exploration and diagnostic peritoneal lavage provide useful information to aid in management.

After sterile preparation and infiltration with local anesthetic, the stab wound is extended to allow visualization of the underlying fascia. When the fascia is not violated, the wound can be closed and the patient discharged. If this finding is equivocal, or if peritoneal penetration is identified, the patient should be admitted for further evaluations, including frequent, serial examinations, and watching for development of peritoneal signs or hemorrhage. In addition, many surgeons recommend diagnostic peritoneal lavage at this point. If the results are negative, the patient is discharged after 24 hours of careful observation.

Peritoneal lavage is also helpful in evaluating patients with stab wounds to the lower part of the chest. The presence of greater than 5000 RBCs/ml in the lavage fluid indicates that the diaphragm has been penetrated and laparotomy is indicated.

References:
1. Jackson GL, Thal ER. Management of stab wounds of the back and flank. J Trauma 1979; 19:660–664.
2. McAlvanah MJ, Shaftan GW. Selective conservatism in penetrating abdominal wounds: a continuing reappraisal. J Trauma 1978; 18:206–212.
3. Nance FC, Wennar MH, Johnson LW, et al. Surgical judgement in the management of penetrating wounds of the abdomen: experience with 2212 patients. Ann Surg 1974; 179:639–646.
4. Thompson JS, Moore EE, Van Duzer-Moore S, et al. The evolution of abdominal stab wound management. J Trauma 1980; 20:478–484.

THORACIC AORTIC TRANSECTION

Thoracic aortic transection occurs as a result of shearing forces acting on the aorta during severe deceleration, such as might occur after a fall or in a motor vehicle accident. A tear at the root of the aorta is fairly common and usually immediately fatal. The most common site of disruption, in patients who survive long enough to reach the emergency department (ED), is just distal to the left subclavian artery at the site of the ligamentum arteriosum. Survival in these patients depends on an intact adventitia, for when this goes, the patient exsanguinates.

When treating patients who reach the ED, a high index of suspicion is necessary to make the diagnosis. Whereas certain signs, including differential radial pulses, no femoral pulses, and paraplegia (secondary to disruption of the blood supply to the spinal cord), may be present, the physical examination is usually not helpful. The diagnosis is suggested by the chest x-ray and confirmed by the aortogram. Certain x-ray findings, which follow, are helpful in suggesting the possibility of an aortic tear and should be followed by an aortogram for a definitive diagnosis. The most important of these findings is the widened mediastinum. When the chest x-ray is taken in the supine position with an AP film, the mediastinum may appear widened because of the technique alone. Therefore, if the patient's condition permits, the chest x-ray should be repeated with a standard upright PA film. Aortography remains the definitive study for diagnosis of this problem; the roles of CT scanning and digitally enhanced arteriography have yet to be established for this injury.

X-ray signs of thoracic disruption:
1. widened mediastinum
2. loss of aortic knob
3. apical pleural cap
4. trachea deviated to right
5. esophagus deviated to right (nasogastric tube)
6. downward displacement of left mainstem bronchus
7. clavicle or first rib fracture.

References:
1. Cole DC, Knopp R, Wales LR, Morishima MS. Nasogastric tube displacement to the right as a sign of acute traumatic rupture of the thoracic aorta. Ann Emerg Med 1981; *10*: 623–26.
2. Mattox KL, Pickard L, Allen MK, Garcia-Rinaldi R. Suspecting thoracic transection. JACEP 1978; 7:12–15.

CHEST TUBE STABILIZATION

Insertion of a chest tube is a procedure often performed in the emergency department. After its placement, it is important to secure the tube properly. Figure 3-2 shows a simple method that requires no special equipment, provides an airtight seal, and ensures precise approximation of wound edges.

3

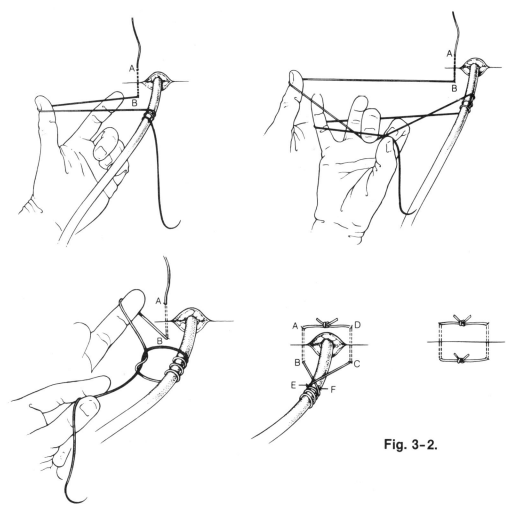

Fig. 3-2.

Fig. 3-2. After inserting a suture at point A and bringing it out through point B, wrap it several times around the tube about 2 to 3 cm from the entry site (left). Holding the suture steady with your left hand, use your right hand and the needle end of the suture to form a square knot (center, left) and guide the knot into place (center). Then pass the suture through the skin at points C and D on either side of the incision and tie the two suture ends to make a horizontal mattress stitch (center, right). When you're ready to remove the tube, cut the suture at the knot (E-F), withdraw the tube, and tie the cut suture ends together to close the incision, making sure the wound edges are in good approximation (right).

Reference:
1. Simon R, Bailey T, Abraham E, Brenner B. A new technique for securing a chest tube. Ann Emerg Med 1982; 2:620–621. (Figure reproduced with permission of the authors and publisher.)

BLAST INJURY

Blast injury refers to the trauma resulting from an explosion. With the unfortunate rise of terrorism, the incidence of these injuries is no longer limited to wartime. Injuries from an explosion may be classified according to the mechanism of injury. *Primary blast injuries* are those that result directly from the sudden rise in atmospheric pressure—the blast wave—caused by the explosion. *Secondary blast injuries* are those that result from the flying debris caused by the blast. When the blast wave throws an individual against surrounding objects, *tertiary blast injuries* result. Finally, *burns,* either from the explosion itself or from the fires ignited by the blast, may occur.

The extent of primary blast injury depends on a variety of factors, including the duration, intensity, and rate of rise of the peak pressure wave; the distance from the blast; and the density of the propagating medium (water transmits the blast wave better than air, resulting in more severe injury for a given blast). Pulmonary complications of primary blast injury include hemorrhage and air embolism. Initially, the pressure in the fluid-filled vascular tree is greater than in the alveoli, causing disruption of the tissue and bleeding into the alveoli. This pressure gradient is then reversed, forcing air into the ruptured vessels.

Data from a review of 305 fatalities caused by explosions in Northern Ireland are summarized in the accompanying table. In addition, the injuries of 1532 patients who presented to the Accident and Emergency Department of Royal Victoria Hospital in Belfast are provided. Several observations can be made from these series:

1. Obviously, those with more serious injuries were more likely to be among the fatalities. Of those surviving to reach the hospital, only 9 (0.6%) died; 5 of them had sustained internal injuries.

2. Amputations were common in those who died, with lower extremities more often involved than upper. Of those surviving to reach the hospital, 4 of 20 patients with amputations died.

3. Clothing seems to be of protective value. Head lacerations occurred in 63 per cent of those with lacerations, while only 10 per cent suffered trunk lacerations.

4. In survivors, primary blast injury to the lungs was rare, occurring in only 2 patients.

Injuries in Blast Fatalities

INJURY	PER CENT
Brain damage	66
Skull fracture	51
Lung contusions	47
Eardrum rupture	45
Liver laceration	34
Spleen laceration	29
Eye injury	
non-penetrating	20
penetrating	19
Kidney lacerations	9

Injuries in Blast Survivors

INJURY	PER CENT
Lacerations	40
Abrasions	18
Bruises	13
Fractures	4
Burns	3
Concussions	2
Amputations	1

References:
1. Haddon WA, Rutherford WH, Merrett JD. The injuries of terrorist bombing: a study of 1532 consecutive patients. Br J Surg 1978; *65*:525–531.
2. Hill JF. Blast injury with particular reference to recent terrorist bombing incidents. Ann R Coll Surg Engl 1979; *61*:4–11.

MANAGEMENT OF PELVIC FRACTURE

Pelvic fracture as a result of trauma is a serious injury, with mortality ranging from 10 to 30 per cent. Much of this mortality is related to the presence of associated injuries, but a significant proportion of patients die of exsanguination from lacerated pelvic vessels. Gilliland and coworkers[1] identified several factors that are associated with increased mortality. The initial blood pressure and hemoglobin concentration were significantly lower in the nonsurvivors compared with survivors. In addition, nonsurvivors required more blood transfusions and clotting factor replacement than did survivors.

Initially, standard resuscitation and evaluation procedures are instituted. Remember that genito-urinary trauma is common with pelvic fracture, and incidence is related to the severity of injury. Urinary catheterization in males is contraindicated if urethral injury is suspected; signs of this injury include scrotal hematoma, bleeding from the urethra, and prostate displacement noted on rectal examination. When intra-abdominal injury must be ruled out, diagnostic peritoneal lavage may be performed through a supra-umbilical, open approach. Negative peritoneal lavage is extremely reliable in this setting. The false-positive rate, due to an increased RBC count in the presence of pelvic fractures, is quite high in the range of 15 to 25 per cent. This high rate may be due to passage of the catheter through an anterior retroperitoneal hematoma or tears in the peritoneum overlying a posterior hematoma. Therefore, positive peritoneal lavage results must be evaluated with caution. Transfemoral arteriography can be helpful at this point both for diagnosing intra-abdominal or pelvic vessel bleeding, and for treating pelvic bleeding with embolization.[2] In addition to embolization of bleeding pelvic vessels, prolonged application of military antishock trousers (MAST) has been successful in controlling exsanguinating hemorrhage from pelvic fracture.

Reference:
1. Gilliland MD, Ward RE, Barton RM, et al. Factors affecting mortality in pelvic fractures. J Trauma 1982; *22*:691–693.
2. Gilliland MD, Ward RE, Flynn TC, et al. Peritoneal lavage and angiography in the management of patients with pelvic fractures. Am J Surg 1982; *144*:744–747.

BLADDER AND URETHRAL INJURIES IN PELVIC FRACTURE

Pelvic fracture is a serious injury with frequent, concurrent injuries of both pelvic and extra-pelvic organs. Genito-urinary trauma is the second most frequent intra-pelvic complication of pelvic fracture after hemorrhage from vascular injury, and should be suspected in any patient with pelvic fracture. Injuries include urethral injuries, bladder rupture, and, rarely, upper genito-urinary tract injuries. The incidence of urinary tract trauma increases with the severity of injury to the pelvis, with an incidence as high as 50 per cent in crush injuries, for example.

Urethral injury is a serious problem that carries a significant risk of long-term morbidity, including stricture, impotence, incontinence, and fistula. Urethral injury is extremely rare in females. Clinical findings associated with urethral injury are: (1) Blood at the urethral meatus; (2) scrotal, perineal, or perianal hematoma; (3) high-riding or floating prostate; (4) inability to void; and (5) resistance when passing a Foley catheter (attempted in the absence of other signs of urethral injury).

Presence of any one of these signs is an indication for urethrography. *Foley catheterization is contraindicated until urethral injury has been ruled out.* Once suspected, diagnosis must be confirmed by retrograde urethrography. Ideally, this is done under fluoroscopy with the patient in the oblique position. A single, portable AP x-ray will suffice if the patient's condition precludes fluoroscopy. A 14 French Foley catheter is passed a short distance into the urethra and the balloon is inflated with 1–2 cc of air. Eight to 10 ml of a dilute, water-soluble contrast medium (e.g., 30% Hypaque) is injected into the urethra and may be repeated up to a total of 30 to 40 ml. If no urethral injury is identified, cystography is then performed by filling the bladder with 300 to 400 ml of contrast dye. Strict aseptic technique is mandatory.

Foley catheterization prior to urethrography is contraindicated for several reasons. Passage of the Foley catheter may convert a partial tear to complete disruption. The urethra may have been stretched, and inflating the balloon of the catheter in the proximal urethra is possible even with the Foley catheter inserted to its full extent, thus further damaging the injured urethra. Finally, the Foley catheter may be successfully passed into the bladder, leading to the false impression that no urethral injury exists. Treatment of urethral injury is initial suprapubic cystostomy and delayed repair; primary repair results in a higher incidence of late complications.

Bladder rupture is another common urinary tract injury associated with pelvic fracture. Most ruptures (80 per cent) occur extraperitoneally whereas 20 per cent occur intraperitoneally. Extraperitoneal rupture is usually a result of direct puncture of the bladder by the bone fragments associated with anterior pelvic fractures. Intraperitoneal rupture, on the other hand, is usually a result of the bladder's bursting from a sudden increase in pressure in an already distended bladder. Signs of bladder rupture often develop late, and diagnosis depends on contrast studies such as cystography and intravenous pyelogram. Early surgical repair is the treatment of choice, although selected cases of minor rupture have been treated successfully with simple catheterization.

References:
1. Billowitz E. Pelvic Fractures. *In*: Chipman C (ed.). Emergency Department Orthopedics. Rockville, Maryland: Aspen Systems Corporation, 1982:75–96.
2. Weems WL. Management of genitourinary injuries in patients with pelvic fractures. Ann Surg 1979; *189*:717–723.

REPLANTATION

With the advent of microscopic surgery, replantation of limbs became a reality in the early 1960's. Since such treatment is available only in specialized centers, the local emergency department must stabilize a patient who has an amputation and protect the amputated part as well as the stump until he can receive definitive care.

General care of the patient includes fluid resuscitation, treatment of other injuries, tetanus prophylaxis, and broad-spectrum antibiotic coverage.

Irrigate the stump with lactated Ringer's, apply a sterile gauze pressure dressing, and elevate the stump. Do not apply antiseptics.

A limb that is totally or partially amputated is threatened by hypoxia. Cooling it decreases the metabolic rate and oxygen requirement.

Irrigate the amputated part with lactated Ringer's, wrap it in dry, sterile gauze and place it in a dry, sterile container. Put that container in a second container holding wrapped ice.

Irrigate a partially amputated extremity with lactated Ringer's, dress it with dry sterile gauze and splint the junction. Secure ice in plastic bags and place them around the distal extremity.

The amputated or devascularized extremity should not come in direct contact with ice, as frostbite-type injuries may occur.

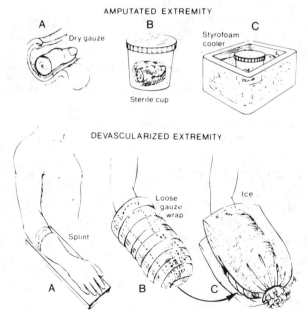

Fig. 3-3. Method for cooling an amputated extremity or a partially amputated, devascularized extremity.

Reference:

1. Morgan RF, Reisman NR, Curtis RM. Preservation of upper extremity devascularization and amputations for replantation. Amer Surg 1982; *48*:481–483. (Figure reproduced with permission of the authors and Lippincott, Harper and Row.)

REMOVAL OF PROTECTIVE HEADGEAR

A safety helmet may guard the head and face during trauma but provides little protection to the cervical spine. Improper removal of protective headgear from an injured person can aggravate cervical cord damage if the neck has been fractured. If the patient is unconscious, if his neck hurts, or if the helmet shows signs of trauma, you should treat the patient as if he has a cervical spine fracture. The illustrations show how an injured patient's safety helmet can be removed while continuous neck traction is maintained throughout the procedure.

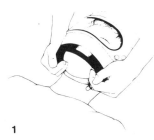

1

To prevent aggravation of cervical spine injuries, supply in-line traction by placing your hands on each side of the helmet with your fingers on the mandible. This will keep head and neck stable, even if the helmet strap is loose.

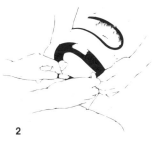

2

Maintain in-line traction and have an assistant remove or cut the helmet's chin strap.

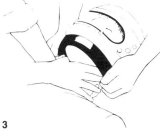

3

Keeping your hands in place, have your assistant cup the mandible with one hand and apply pressure on the back of the neck with the other. With in-line traction now supplied from below, you're free to remove the helmet.

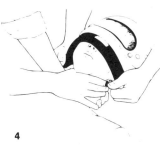

4

Exert lateral traction on both sides of the helmet to clear the ears and gently pull it off. If the helmet provides full facial coverage, you'll have to tilt it back to pull it over the nose. If the patient wears glasses, be sure to take them off before removing the helmet.

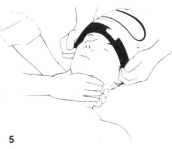

5

In-line traction is maintained throughout the process to keep the head and neck immobile.

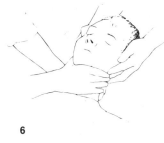

6

After removal, resume in-line traction from above by placing your hands on either side of the patient's head with your palms over his ears.

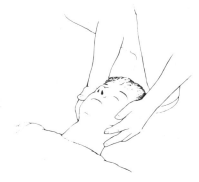

7

Keep your hands in this position to maintain in-line traction until you have the patient secured to a backboard to prevent any motion of the cervical spine during transport.

Fig. 3-4.

Reference:

1. McSwain NE. To doff a helmet. Emerg Med 1982; August: 104–105. (Figure reproduced with permission of the American College of Surgeons and the publisher.)

ZIPPER INJURIES

The penile foreskin may be caught in a zipper, causing the patient pain and embarrassment. Local swelling, the patient's anxiety, and his resultant lack of cooperation may inhibit efforts at freeing the entrapped skin. Local or general anesthesia may be required so the skin may be freed by manipulation or removed by circumcision. A third method is to open the zipper by squeezing the median bar with a bone cutter (Fig. 3–5). This technique can also be used to free entrapped labia (in females, obviously).

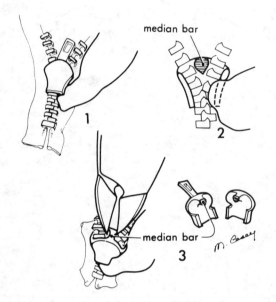

Fig. 3– 5. Technique for zipper removal.

Reference:

1. Flowerdew R, Fishman IJ, Churchill BM. Management of penile zipper injury. J Urol 1977; *117*:671. (Figure reproduced with permission of the authors and The Williams & Wilkins Co., Baltimore.)

4

ENVIRONMENTAL HAZARDS AND POISONS

POISONING BY MARINE LIFE 122

MUSHROOM POISONING 125

LICE—PEDICULOSIS 127

MANAGEMENT OF ANIMAL BITES 128

RABIES PROPHYLAXIS 131

THE GENERAL APPROACH TO THE POISONED PATIENT . . 134

THE ANTIDOTE, PLEASE 135

ACETAMINOPHEN OVERDOSE 140

OVER-THE-COUNTER ACETAMINOPHEN PRODUCTS 142

ASPIRIN OVERDOSE 142

IRON POISONING 144

THE DUST OF ANGELS 145

ORGANOPHOSPHATE POISONING 146

MANAGEMENT OF CAUSTIC INGESTIONS 148

OVER-THE-COUNTER DRUG ABUSE 152

YOU'D BETTER WATCH OUT 153

WORK MAY BE HAZARDOUS TO YOUR HEALTH 154

RADIATION DOSE EFFECTS 163

INITIAL MANAGEMENT OF RADIATION INJURY 164

DISASTER MANAGEMENT: EVACUATION 170

HOW HOT IT FEELS 170

HEAT INJURY IN LONG DISTANCE RUNNING 171

HYPERTHERMIA 172

FROSTBITE 175

POISONING BY MARINE LIFE

Most venomous marine organisms are docile and sting or bite only when provoked. The consequences of hostile encounters with them may be envenomation, puncture wounds, lacerations, and, rarely, serious systemic reactions. Venoms of marine organisms are short-acting and thermolabile. Most of the clinical signs and symptoms are cholinergic in nature. Tetanus prophylaxis is an important measure in the management of all wounds.

Injuries sustained from jellyfish, coral, sea urchins, catfish, and stingrays are discussed here.

Jellyfish

This large group of organisms are members of the phylum Coelenterata, which means "inside cavity." In essence, they are little more than a digestive cavity with tentacles. The common jellyfish is a gelatinous, translucent mass of material 6 to 8 inches in diameter, with floating or streaming tentacles. It may be bluish-red or colorless.

The Portuguese man-of-war is a distinctive coelenterate; it is a colony of polyps that forms a blue, balloon-like mass raised above the water's surface. The man-of-war is found commonly, but not exclusively, in warmer climates.

These organisms depend on currents, winds, and tides for transport. They are able to control tentacles by contracting them. Each tentacle contains numerous venomous, stinging nematocysts. The toxin resides in the fluid in the nematocyst. When the tentacle touches its prey, the nematocyst releases a coiled thread as well as its toxin.

Even a dead Portuguese man-of-war contains potent venom for several days after being washed up onto the beach.

Clinical Manifestations and Therapy

The sting of jellyfish is extremely painful. Erythema, small papular eruptions, pustular and desquamative lesions, and lymphadenopathy may all occur. In addition, systemic symptoms, such as headache, weakness, muscle spasms, anaphylaxis, and respiratory depression may be encountered. The Portuguese man-of-war is the only jellyfish that commonly causes systemic reactions.

General treatment is outlined next. Systemic illness may require further therapy, i.e., treatment of anaphylaxis or respiratory depression.

1. Remove tentacles, spines, or any foreign bodies as quickly as possible. As long as tentacles remain on the skin, they will discharge nematocysts. Care must be used, such that the treating individual is not stung.

2. Wash the wound with alcohol to fix the remaining nematocysts, thus preventing their discharge.

3. Jellyfish often cause allergic reactions, and generalized urticaria and intense pruritus are common. Initially, parenteral diphenhydramine, 25 to 50 mg intramuscularly, or a steroid may be needed. At discharge, patients should be given a prescription for an antihistamine or a steroid, or both, for outpatient use.

4. It is not uncommon for patients to have recurrence of urticarial lesions in the area of their initial stings for up to two weeks after the initial injuries. Therefore, follow-up is recommended for all patients with jellyfish stings.

4

Coral

The organism responsible for formation of coral is the coral polyp. These are soft-bodied organisms varying from microscopic to several millimeters in size that secrete substances composed of calcium carbonate. The microscopic nematocysts of these organisms can produce painful wounds.

The major wounds resulting from encounters with coral include severe abrasions and lacerations caused by its stony skeleton. These wounds are typically slow to heal. The initial reaction to a coral cut is the emergence of red welts and itching around the wound site. Left untreated, a coral cut may develop within several days into an ulcer with a septic, sloughing base. The wounds are often avulsion-type injuries contaminated with pathogenic bacteria found in shore waters. The wounds also may contain tiny particles of sediment or coral.

Therapy

For wounds caused by stinging coral, the procedure is similar to that for jellyfish. If accompanied by lacerations, use a local anesthetic and thoroughly inspect and probe the wound for foreign bodies. All dead tissue requires debridement and the wound requires copious irrigation. Prophylactic antibiotics may be indicated.

Facial wounds should be considered for primary closure; however, extremity wounds are best treated by simple dressings.

Sea Urchins

These marine animals resemble a pincushion because of their numerous straight, pointed spines protruding from a spherical center. They are found among coral reefs, on ocean bottoms, and washed up on shore. The extremely brittle spines may break off when you attempt to remove them from the patient's skin. Discomfort ranges from mild to moderate in severity. These spines may fragment within the skin and migrate into a joint or lodge against a nerve, causing excruciating pain.

Therapy

Treatment hinges first on the removal of the spines. The venomous substances in sea-urchin spines are thought to be heat labile, and warm soaks for approximately one hour may relieve discomfort. Cleansing the wound and assuring adequate tetanus prophylaxis are the next steps.

Catfish

Contact with marine catfish can produce instant stinging and throbbing in an affected area or an entire limb. The slimy coating on the surface of the catfish's body contains a protein that has anticoagulant and neurotoxic properties. The material will enter via the puncture or sting site produced by the whisker-like projections on the creature's head.

Therapy

Treatment involves immersion of the affected part into water as hot as the patient can stand for 30 to 90 minutes. The protein of the slimy coating is somewhat denatured by hot water. The wound should then be cared for as for jellyfish and sea urchin stings. X-ray films may be useful because catfish barbs are radiopaque.

Stingrays

Stingrays constitute one of the largest and most important groups of venomous organisms. Nearly 1500 attacks occur yearly along our coasts.

The creatures usually swim just above the ocean floor in shallow coastal waters. Some are difficult to detect because of their habit of lying buried in mud or sand, with only a portion of their body exposed. Accidents usually occur when swimmers step on buried rays.

The stinger or envenomating apparatus is in the tail and consists of one or more venomous spines. The spine has a sharp arrow-like tip and backward pointing serrations along the sides, such that after penetration the barb is difficult to remove and lacerates the tissues as it is withdrawn. The venom apparatus consists of the spine, integumentary sheath, and associated venom glands. When the spine penetrates the flesh, the sheath is torn, the venom is released, and a violent tissue reaction is produced.

The venom is primarily protein and is one of the most powerful vasoconstrictors found among animal toxins. The venom is highly unstable and heat labile.

The majority of stings occur at the lower ankle or foot. The spine is very sharp, and it is common for a patient to receive a laceration rather than a puncture wound. The usual presenting complaint is severe shooting pain that increases in intensity over the first hour. Systemic symptoms, such as chest pain, syncope, atrioventricular block, arrhythmias, muscle weakness, paralysis, shock, and even death, have been reported.

Therapy

Treatment should be begun immediately with irrigation of the wound with salt water. The wound should be immersed in hot water (45–50°C) for 60 minutes to inactivate the venom and provide pain relief. The use of hot-water immersion is based on extensive clinical evidence and is standard care.

In the emergency department, hot-water immersion should be continued and pain relievers administered. The wound requires irrigation, debridement, and exploration for foreign bodies. Large lacerations should be sutured, and broad-spectrum antibiotics should be given.

Patients with systemic symptoms should be observed, and if the symptoms are persistent, the patient may require hospital admission.

Divers are sometimes stung in the chest or abdomen, and they may need surgical exploration.

References:
1. Haddad LM, Winchester JF. Toxic marine life. *In*: Clinical Management of Poisoning and Drug Overdose. Chapter 19. WB Saunders, Philadelphia: 1983.
2. Ratzan RM, Correia CJ, Cardoni AA. Poisoning by marine life, recognizing and treating water related stings and bites. Consultant, Aug. 1983; 29–41.
3. Podgorny, G. Bites, reptiles and marine fauna. *In:* A Study Guide in Emergency Medicine. Tintinalli J. (ed.). Dallas, Texas: ACEP, 1978.

MUSHROOM POISONING

Mushrooms are an unusual cause of acute poisonings, although recently there has been a nationwide increase in reports of acute mushroom toxicity. Because of the potential for fatalities in some mushroom poisonings, the emergency physician should be aware of the problem and its immediate management. Mushroom poisoning should be considered in any case of acute gastroenteritis or central nervous system dysfunction. Wild mushrooms grow best in the spring and fall so suspicion should be even greater during these seasons. The algorithm outlines the treatment approach once a positive history of ingestion of wild mushrooms has been attained from a patient with acute gastrointestinal or neurologic symptoms.

TREATMENT ALGORITHM FOR MUSHROOM POISONING

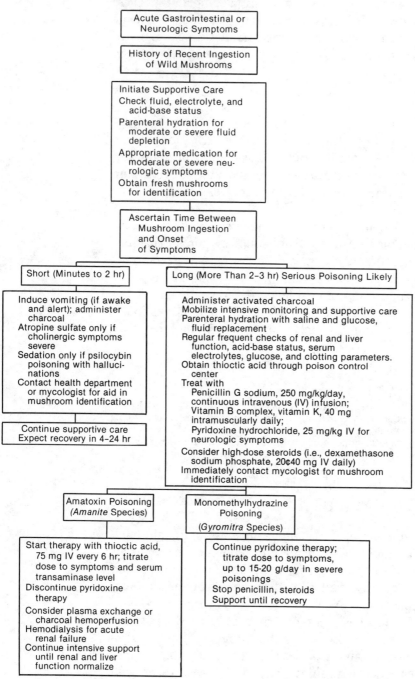

Acute Gastrointestinal or
Neurologic Symptoms

History of Recent Ingestion
of Wild Mushrooms

Initiate Supportive Care
Check fluid, electrolyte, and
acid-base status
Parenteral hydration for
moderate or severe fluid
depletion
Appropriate medication for
moderate or severe neu-
rologic symptoms
Obtain fresh mushrooms
for identification

Ascertain Time Between
Mushroom Ingestion
and Onset
of Symptoms

Short (Minutes to 2 hr)

Induce vomiting (if awake
and alert); administer
charcoal
Atropine sulfate only if
cholinergic symptoms
severe
Sedation only if psilocybin
poisoning with halluci-
nations
Contact health department
or mycologist for aid in
mushroom identification

Continue supportive care
Expect recovery in 4–24 hr

Long (More Than 2–3 hr) Serious Poisoning Likely

Administer activated charcoal
Mobilize intensive monitoring and supportive care
Parenteral hydration with saline and glucose,
fluid replacement
Regular frequent checks of renal and liver
function, acid-base status, serum
electrolytes, glucose, and clotting parameters.
Obtain thioctic acid through poison control
center
Treat with
Penicillin G sodium, 250 mg/kg/day,
continuous intravenous (IV) infusion;
Vitamin B complex, vitamin K, 40 mg
intramuscularly daily;
Pyridoxine hydrochloride, 25 mg/kg IV for
neurologic symptoms
Consider high-dose steroids (i.e., dexamethasone
sodium phosphate, 20¢40 mg IV daily)
Immediately contact mycologist for mushroom
identification

Amatoxin Poisoning
(Amanite Species)

Start therapy with thioctic acid,
75 mg IV every 6 hr; titrate
dose to symptoms and serum
transaminase level
Discontinue pyridoxine
therapy
Consider plasma exchange or
charcoal hemoperfusion
Hemodialysis for acute
renal failure
Continue intensive support
until renal and liver
function normalize

Monomethylhydrazine
Poisoning
(Gyromitra Species)

Continue pyridoxine therapy;
titrate dose to symptoms,
up to 15-20 g/day in severe
poisonings
Stop penicillin, steroids
Support until recovery

Therapy for a patient with acute mushroom poisoning hinges on identification of the offending mushrooms. The help of a skilled mycologist might be obtained from your state health department, a university botany department, or a state agricultural college. Mushrooms submitted for identification should be freshly picked and include cap, stem, and base, if possible. The specimen should be loosely wrapped in tissue paper and never placed in a plastic bag. If no fresh specimen remains, uncooked mushrooms that have been stored or cooked mushrooms can sometimes be successfully identified.

Thioctic acid is a Krebs cycle coenzyme that has been found to reduce mortality in amantadine poisoning in a number of clinical reports. It has not been tested in a well-designed clinical trial, and, therefore, its efficacy has been disputed by some workers. Thioctic acid is not generally available, but assistance in obtaining it may be provided by your regional Poison Control Center or State Health Department.

Reference:
1. Hanraham JP, Gordon MA. Mushroom poisoning. JAMA 1984;*251*:1057-1061. (Algorithm reproduced with permission.)

4

LICE – PEDICULOSIS

Pediculosis Capitis

Head lice eggs (nits) attach to the base of a hair shaft by a tenacious secretion, making it difficult to remove them by washing. Nits can survive off the host for ten days but do not hatch at room temperature. They look like small white fleas and hatch after one week's incubation at body temperature. The adult lice look blue-black and, when viewed under a microscope, crab-like.

Lice may be transmitted directly from person to person or through clothing, bed linens, combs and brushes. Lice can live off the host for 48 hours.

One treatment is lindane (gamma benzene hexachloride), a formula available by prescription, under the trade name Kwell. One tablespoon of the shampoo is massaged into the scalp hair for four minutes. The hair is then rinsed and dried. Combing removes nits. Treatment may be repeated in seven to ten days. The shampoo is a local irritant that is absorbed through the skin and can be neurotoxic. It is not recommended for infants or pregnant women.

An alternative treatment is pyrethrins with piperonyl butoxide, which is sold without prescription as RID. It should be used to wet the hair and scalp, then washed out after ten minutes. Nits and eggs are then combed out. Treatment can be repeated in one week. Although it is a local irritant, it is poorly absorbed through the skin.

Reinfestation from clothing and linens can be prevented by machine washing in hot water; machine drying at a high temperature (20 minutes); ironing; drycleaning; or storage in a plastic bag for two weeks.

Infested combs and brushes may be soaked in Lysol for one hour; soaked in a pediculocide for one hour; or heated in water at 150°F for five to ten minutes.

All household members should be examined carefully for signs of infestation and treated if necessary.

Pediculosis Palpebrarum

For lice in the eyelashes, have the patient apply petroleum to the lashes twice a day for eight days and remove the nits mechanically with a fine-toothed comb or nit picker.

Pediculosis Pubis

This type of pediculosis is diagnosed by identifying the eggs at the base of the pubic hair. It can be treated by applying lindane to the hairy areas of the body after bathing. The solution is washed off in 24 hours. Treatment may be repeated in one week. The patient's sexual contacts should also be treated.

Pediculosis Corporis

Infestation of the body is usually relieved by bathing and changing clothes. Clothing should be treated as described earlier to prevent reinfestation. Lindane may be required to treat hairy areas.

References:
1. Treatment of head lice. The Medical Letter 1980;*22*(16):66–68.
2. Orkin M, Epstein E, Maibach H. Treatment of today's scabies and pediculosis. JAMA 1976;*236*:1136–1139.

MANAGEMENT OF ANIMAL BITES

Mammalian bites are responsible for approximately 1 per cent of all emergency department visits. Most are dog bites; however, cat, rat, and human bites are commonly seen. The majority of bites are minor, with sutures required in only 10 per cent and hospital inpatient treatment required in only 1 per cent. Management includes wound care and when indicated, prophylaxis for rabies and tetanus. Risk factors associated with an increased incidence of bite wound infection are as follows:

1. Puncture wound
2. Location on hand or foot
3. Human or cat bite
4. Treatment delay greater than 12 hours
5. Patient's age less than 2 or more than 50 years
6. Steroid therapy or immune disorder
7. Diabetes, asplenia, alcoholism

The initial management of the wound depends on its severity. If the skin is unbroken, only antiseptic cleansing is necessary along with application of cold compresses to decrease swelling and administration of analgesia for pain. For more extensive injuries, i.e., broken skin, more aggressive management is required to prevent infection and to provide good cosmetic and functional results.

Cleansing should be done with irrigation and gentle sponging of visible dirt after adequate analgesia has been given. Scrubbing should be avoided, since this may delay healing and increase the likelihood of infection. Good wound irrigation has been shown in several studies to markedly decrease the incidence of wound infection. Adequate pressure can be obtained with a 19 gauge needle and a 20 cc syringe. The volume used depends on the size of the wound. A sterile electrolyte solution (usually 0.9 per cent saline) is recommended for irrigation, since it does not harm tissues.

Once irrigation is complete, good debridement is necessary. It has been shown to decrease the incidence of wound infection by 30 fold. One to 2 mm of tissue should be removed from the wound edges unless this would compromise wound closure in areas of little excess tissue, such as the face or hand.

The decision to suture the wound depends on cosmetic and functional considerations as well as location. It is recommended that (1) bites on the hand be left unsutured, to heal by secondary intention; (2) puncture wounds should not be sutured, and (3) facial wounds generally should be sutured, because cosmesis is important and risk of infection is low.

Treatment of Infected Bites

Established wound infections must be treated aggressively with open drainage, thorough irrigation, and debridement of the wound followed by antibiotic therapy. Hospitalization is required for administration of intravenous antibiotics in patients with severe, established infections or those with medically compromising diseases such as diabetes mellitus. Antibiotics recommended for prophylaxis are also effective for established infections. Patients who are not hospitalized should be given their first dose of antibiotics intravenously in the emergency department before they are discharged. Outpatients need to be seen daily to ensure that the infection is not progressing.

Hepatitis

The possibility of hepatitis transmission should be considered in cases of human bites. If the biter is a known carrier or a likely carrier, the patient should receive hepatitis B immune globulin and hepatitis vaccine (see Viral Hepatitis, page 260.)

Tetanus and Rabies

Tetanus and rabies prevention is an important consideration in bite wounds. Careful irrigation and debridement of the wound are major deterrents to subsequent rabies and tetanus infections. Additional guidelines for prophylaxis can be found in Tetanus Prophylaxis (page 204) and Rabies Prophylaxis (page 131).

The likelihood of rabies should be assessed in the animal responsible for the bite. If possible, the animal should be captured and observed for ten days or killed and sent to the appropriate health agency for testing. Rodents (squirrels, rats, mice, hamsters) are rarely infected with rabies and have not been known to cause rabies in humans in the United States. Wild carnivores (skunks, bats, raccoons, foxes, coyotes) are responsible for most cases of rabies. To initiate prophylaxis is no longer the major decision it once was because the human diploid cell vaccine now used has very few serious side effects.

Antibiotic Prophylaxis

Antibiotic prophylaxis is currently recommended for treating bites, especially those on the hand, inflicted by cats, primates (including humans), and dogs.

Prophylaxis should be based on suspected "bite bacteriology." No single organism accounts for more than 15 per cent of infections. The table gives a list of the most common infecting organisms found in bite wounds, the animal causing the bite, and the recommended treatment schedules.

Antibiotic Prophylaxis for Bite Wounds

ANIMAL	COMMON INFECTING ORGANISM	RECOMMENDED TREATMENT SCHEDULE
Dog	Staphylococcus Streptococcus* Pasteurella multocida† Gram-negative rods Anaerobes‡	Dicloxacillin, 500 mg qid for 5 days or Cephalexin, 500 mg qid for 5 days or Erythromycin, 500 mg qid for 5 days (for patients allergic to penicillin)
Cat	Staphylococcus Streptococcus* Pasteurella multocida† Gram-negative anaerobes‡	Same as treatment schedule for dog bite wounds
Human	Staphylococcus Streptococcus* Gram-negative anaerobes‡ Eikenella corrodens (unusual sensitivity pattern)	Dicloxacillin, 500 mg qid plus penicillin V, 500 mg qid, both for 5 days or Cephalexin 500 mg qid for 5 days

*Commonly isolated
†Relatively more important for cat bites
‡Variable frequency

E. corrodens is involved in 10 to 30 per cent of human bites and it is sensitive to penicillin, ampicillin, and some cephalosporins but resistant to synthetic penicillins.

References:

1. Callaham M. Prophylactic antibiotics in common dog bite wounds, a controlled study. Ann Emerg Med 1980;*9*:410–414.
2. Hawkins J, Paris P, Stewart RD. Mammalian bites, rational approach to management. Postgrad Med 1983;*73:*52–64. (Table reproduced with permission of the authors and publishers.)

RABIES PROPHYLAXIS

Rabies is a viral illness of many carnivore species. When transmitted to humans, it is almost always fatal if untreated. Rabies virus is transmitted to man through the saliva of an infected animal, which enters the skin at a bite. The virus replicates locally for a variable period, then moves along nerves to the central nervous system, at which point clinical illness is manifest. The incubation period usually lasts from 20 to 60 days but may take as long as a year. Once clinical disease is established, rabies is almost always fatal, with only supportive therapy available.

Because of the grave prognosis once clinical disease is present, preventive efforts have been the mainstay of medical intervention. Because of the long incubation period, post-exposure immunization has been an effective means of preventing clinical disease. The original approach to this problem was sequential inoculation with infected rabbit spinal cord tissue—a method developed by Pasteur in the 1880's. Other nerve tissue vaccines have since been developed; each has varying side effects, serious reactions, and effectiveness.

In the 1950's, a duck embryo vaccine (DEV) was developed and, until recently, was the vaccine of choice in the United States. It is administered subcutaneously for 23 doses; anaphylaxis occurs in 0.4 to 0.9 per cent of those so treated. Systemic reactions (fever, myalgias) occur in a third of treated patients and nearly all of them experience local irritation. In addition, 14 patients who received DEV have died of rabies. Ten per cent of patients receiving DEV do not develop adequate antibody titers after 16 to 23 doses.

In 1980, an inactive virus vaccine grown in tissue culture, the human diploid cell vaccine (HDCV), was released. This vaccine is given in five doses intramuscularly. Experience indicates that few local and systemic reactions occur, and that all patients given the vaccine intramuscularly develop adequate titers after immunization, with peak titers greater than ten times those seen with DEV. Following the death from rabies of a Peace Corps worker who had been immunized with HDCV intradermally, a review of others so immunized revealed many with inadequate titers. Therefore, HDCV should not be given by the intradermal route.

Post-exposure prophylaxis of individuals previously immunized with three 1.0 ml doses of HDCV intramuscularly or of individuals immunized with HDCV intradermally, who have a *documented* rabies titer of 1:16 or greater, is additional doses of 1.0 ml of HDCV on days 0 and 3. Individuals previously immunized with HDCV intradermally, who have not had documented rabies titers of 1:16 or greater, should be treated like non-immunized patients.

In addition to active immunization with rabies vaccine, passive immunization is started at the time of initial treatment. It was originally done with equine anti-rabies serum (ARS) and had a consequent risk of allergic reaction, with up to 40 per cent of patients experiencing serum sickness. Equine ARS has been replaced with human rabies immune globulin (RIG), with only rare adverse reactions. Whereas hypersensitivity to other serum globulins has rarely been reported, no such reactions have been reported for RIG.

In addition to knowledge of the prophylactic agents available for rabies, some knowledge of the epidemiology of the disease in animal populations is needed to make a rational decision when to treat patients. In the past, the largest reservoir for the disease was in domestic animals, especially dogs, but with adequate immunization programs, the incidence of rabies in this population is extremely low, and rabies prophylaxis for dog bites is usually not recommended unless there are exceptional circumstances. Local and state public health officials can give specific information about the regional incidence of the disease in domestic animals to aid in this decision. Certain wild animal populations—rodents and lagomorphs (rabbits and hares)—also have little risk of rabies and prophylaxis is almost never indicated.

On the other hand, skunks, bats, foxes, coyotes, raccoons, bobcats, and other carnivores are the major reservoir of the disease in the United States. They should be considered rabid unless proven otherwise by fluorescent-antibody study of brain tissue. If the animal cannot be found, treatment with RIG and HDCV should be initiated.

If the animal is found, it should be killed and its head transported, under refrigeration, to the appropriate state or local health department laboratory for analysis. Treatment with RIG and HDCV should be started and continued for the full course unless the animal's fluorescent-antibody test results are negative.

In addition to RIG and HDCV, local wound care, including thorough cleansing, can greatly improve the chance of not contracting the disease. Washing the wound with ethanol or benzalkonium chloride has also been recommended, but the importance of washing is to be thorough, regardless of the solution used. Indications for post-exposure rabies prophylaxis are summarized in the next table; treatment protocols are summarized in the table following it.

Rabies Post-exposure Prophylaxis Guide[1]

GENERAL MEASURES AND COMMENTS

All bites and wounds should immediately be thoroughly cleansed with soap and water.* If vaccine treatment is indicated, both rabies immune globulin (RIG) and human diploid cell rabies vaccine (HDCV) should be given as soon as possible, regardless of interval after exposure. (The administration of RIG is the more urgent procedure. If HDCV is not immediately available, start RIG and give HDCV as soon as it is obtained.) If RIG is unavailable, substitute antirabies serum equine (ARS). Do not exceed recommended RIG or ARS dose. Vaccine use should be discontinued if tests of animal tissues for rabies antigen, using fluorescent reagents, are negative.

Rabies Post-exposure Prophylaxis Guide (Continued)

Animal Species	Condition of Animal at Time of Attack	Treatment of Exposed Person
Household pets Dogs and cats	Healthy and available for 10 days of observation.	None unless animal develops rabies. At first sign of rabies in animal, treat patient with RIG and HDCV. Symptomatic animal should be killed and tested as soon as possible.
	Rabid or suspect Unknown (escaped)	RIG and HDCV Consult public health officials. If treatment indicated, give RIG and HDCV.
Wild animals Skunks, bats, foxes, coyotes, raccoons, bobcats, other carnivores	Regard as rabid unless proved negative by laboratory tests. If available, animal should be killed and tested as soon as possible.	RIG and HDCV
Other animals Livestock, rodents, lagomorphs (e.g., rabbits, hares)	Consider individually. Local and state public health officials should be consulted on the need for prophylaxis. Bites by the following almost never call for antirabies prophylaxis: squirrels, hamsters, guinea pigs, gerbils, chipmunks, rats, mice, and other rodents, rabbits, and hares.	

*Although copious washing is more important than the type of solution used, I recommend following soap and water with 70% alcohol, which is rabicidal **(S.A.P.)**

Rabies Immunization Regimen for Post-exposure Rabies Prophylaxis

AGENT	DOSE	ROUTE OF ADMINISTRATION	TIME OF DOSAGE
HDCV	1 ml	Intramuscular	Days 0,3,7,14,28. Additional dose if inadequate antibody response.
RIG (omit if pre-exposure immunization with adequate titers has been documented).	20 IU/kg	Half of dose infiltrated at wound site; half of dose intramuscularly in another location.	Given at time of initiation of prophylaxis.
ARS	40 IU/kg	Same as RIG.	Same as RIG.

References:
1. Plotkin SA. Rabies vaccination in the 1980's. Hosp Pract 1980; 65–72. (Table reproduced with permission).
2. Immunization Practices Advisory Committee. Rabies prevention. Morbidity and Mortality Rep 1980;*29*:265.

THE GENERAL APPROACH TO THE POISONED PATIENT

Making the diagnosis of poisoning is often simple in straightforward cases, such as witnessed ingestions. In other situations, it may be ascertained only after drug screening reports confirm the presence of a toxin, often days later. Poisoning should always be suspected in the following patients: (1) any psychiatric patient, (2) a victim of trauma (especially an infant), (3) any comatose patient, (4) a young patient with a cardiac arrhythmia, (5) a patient with metabolic acidosis, and (6) *any* pediatric patient with a puzzling clinical presentation.

The simplest way to attain an early diagnosis of poisoning is to maintain a high level of suspicion. Diagnosis and appropriate treatment are facilitated if a consistent approach is utilized. The following outline summarizes the major steps in management.

1. Provide basic life support.
2. Complete a careful history and physical examination.
3. Eliminate diagnoses of head and neck trauma, and neurologic and metabolic diseases.
4. Attempt to identify "toxidrome."
   a. Narcotics—pinpoint pupils, CNS depression, hypotension, shallow respirations.
   b. Anticholinergics—dilated pupils, dry skin, decreased bowel activity, cardiac arrhythmias.
   c. Cholinergics—pinpoint pupils, sweating, increased secretions, diarrhea, bradycardia.
   d. Phenothiazines—dystonia, oculogyric crisis.
   e. Salicylates—fever, hyperpnea, acidosis.
5. Collect biological specimens for toxin analysis.
   a. Gastric aspirate.
   b. Urine.
   c. Serum.
6. If indicated, provide appropriate antidote.
7. Decontaminate eyes, skin, and clothing.
8. Carry out gastrointestinal decontamination (see accompanying table).
9. Perform fluid diuresis.
   a. Reserve for drugs that are not protein bound or metabolized primarily by the liver.
   b. Utilize for phenobarbital, PCP, salicylates, and amphetamines.
10. Perform ionized diuresis.
    a. Acid diuresis for amphetamines and PCP (with ammonium chloride, or ascorbic acid or hydrochloric acid).
    b. Alkaline diuresis for salicylates and barbiturates (with sodium bicarbonate).

References:
1. McGuigan MA. Poisoning in childhood. Emerg Med Clin North Am 1983;*1*:187–200.

Gastrointestinal Decontamination

METHOD	INDICATIONS	TIME	DOSAGES	CONTRAINDICATIONS
Ipecac Syrup	Ingestion of a toxic or unknown substance	Within 4–6 hours of ingestion	< 6 months old = none 6–12 months old = 10 ml (once) 1–10 years old – 15 ml (can repeat once) > 10 years old = 30 ml (can repeat once)	Nontoxic substance Acid Alkali Camphor Coma or absence of gag reflex Convulsions Some hydrocarbons
Activated Charcoal	Ingestion of a toxic or unknown substance Interruption of enterohepatic recirculation Slowly absorbed substances	Continue q 6h until recovery	0.5–1 g/kg	Acid Alkali Boric acid Cyanide Ethanol Methanol
Saline Cathartics	Delayed-release formulations Decreased peristalsis Slowly absorbed formulations	Within 6 hours of ingestion	Sodium sulfate (10%) = 250 mg/kg (maximum 15 g) Magnesium sulfate (10%) = 250 mg/kg (maximum 15g) Magnesium citrate = 0.5 ml/kg (maximum 200 ml)	Acid and alkali Cyanide Ethanol and methanol Abdominal trauma Congestive heart failure GI obstruction Renal failure

4

THE ANTIDOTE, PLEASE

> "Trust not the physician;
> His antidotes are poison, and he slays
> More than you rob."
>
> Shakespeare

The problem of accidental or self-induced poisoning is frequently encountered by all emergency departments. In some cases, a specific antidote is indicated. The table provides a summary of the local and systemic antidotes that you may be called upon to utilize.

Summary of Local and Systemic Antidotes

POISON	LOCAL ANTIDOTE	SYSTEMIC ANTIDOTE
Acetaminophen	Activated charcoal (lavage stomach after use if N-acetylcysteine is to be given)	N-Acetylcysteine (Mucomyst) initial dose of 140 mg/kg orally in Coca-Cola, Pepsi, Fresca, grapefruit juice, or water; then, 70 mg/kg every 4 hr for 68 hr (17 doses)
Acids, corrosive	Dilute with water or milk	
Alkali, caustic	Dilute with water or milk, then give demulcent	
Alkaloids (coniine, quinine, strychnine, etc.)	Activated charcoal	
Amphetamines	Activated charcoal	Chlorpromazine, 0.5 mg/kg IM or IV (administer slowly if given IV); may repeat in 15 min; reduce to 0.25 mg/kg if other CNS depressants involved.
Anticholinergics	Activated charcoal	Physostigmine (adult: 2 mg; child: 0.5 mg) may be given IV, IM, or SC; may repeat in 15 min until desired effect is achieved; subsequent doses may be given every 2-3 hr p.r.n.
Anticholinesterases Organophosphates Neostigmine Physostigmine Pyridostigmine	Activated charcoal	Atropine, 1-2 mg (for children under 2 yr., 1 mg or 0.05-0.1 mg/kg) IM or IV repeated every 10-15 min until atropinization is evident; then give pralidoxime chloride 25-50 mg/kg (1 g in adults) IV; repeat in 8-12 hr p.r.n.
Carbamates		Atropine as above, but *do not* use pralidoxime
Antihistamines	(*see* Anticholinergics)	
Arsenic	(*see* Heavy metals)	
Atropine	(*see* Anticholinergics)	
Barium salts	Sodium sulfate, 300 mg/kg	Sodium or magnesium sulfate, 10 ml of 10% solution IV every 15 min until symptoms stop
Belladonna alkaloids	(*see* Anticholinergics)	
Bromides		Sodium or ammonium chloride, 6-12 gm/day p.o., or the equivalent as normal saline, every 6 hr IV
Cadmium	(*see* Heavy metals)	
Carbon monoxide		100% oxygen inhalation for no more than 2 hr followed by inhalation of room air
Cholinergic compounds	(*see* Anticholinesterases)	
Copper	(*see* Heavy metals)	

Summary of Local and Systemic Antidotes (Continued)

POISON	LOCAL ANTIDOTE	SYSTEMIC ANTIDOTE
Cyanide		*Adult:* Amyl nitrite inhalation (inhale for 15-30 sec every 60 sec) pending administration of 300 mg sodium nitrite (10 ml of a 3% solution) IV slowly (over 2-4 min); follow immediately with 12.5 g sodium thiosulfate (2.5-5 ml/min of 25% solution) IV slowly (over 10 min)

Child: (Na nitrite should not exceed recommended dose as fatal methemoglobinemia may result)

Hemoglobin (gm)	Initial dose 3% Na nitrite IV ml(mg)/kg	Initial dose 25% Na thiosulfate IV (ml/kg)
8	0.22 (6.6)	1.10
10	0.27 (8.7)	1.35
12 (nl)	0.33 (10)	1.65
14	0.39 (11.6)	1.95

POISON	LOCAL ANTIDOTE	SYSTEMIC ANTIDOTE
Detergents, cationic	Ordinary soap solution	
Ethylene glycol	(*see* Methanol)	
Fluoride	Calcium gluconate or lactate, 150 mg/kg, or milk	Calcium gluconate, 10 ml of 10% solution, given slowly IV until symptoms abate; may be repeated p.r.n.
Formaldehyde	Milk or egg whites; or 1% solution of ammonium acetate or carbonate, preferably with lavage	
Gold	(*see* Heavy metals)	
Heavy metals	Milk or egg whites	BAL (dimercaprol), 3-5 mg/kg dose deep IM every 4 hr for 2 days, every 4-6 hr for an additional 2 days, then every 4-12 hr for up to 7 additional days
	Usual chelators used:	EDTA, 75 mg/kg/24 hr deep IM or slow IV infusion given in 3-6 divided doses for up to 5 days; may be repeated for a second course after a minimum of 2 days; each course should not exceed a total of 500 mg/kg
Arsenic	BAL	
Cadmium	Satisfactory use not demonstrated	
Copper	BAL, penicillamine	
Gold	BAL	
Lead	BAL, EDTA, penicillamine	
Mercury	BAL, penicillamine	Penicillamine, 100 mg/kg daily (maximum 1 g) p.o. in divided doses for up to 5 days; for long-term therapy do not exceed 40 mg/kg daily
Silver	Satisfactory use not demonstrated	
Thallium	Satisfactory use not demonstrated	
Hypochlorites	(*see* Alkali, caustic)	
Iodine	Starch solution, 3-10%	

Table continued on following page

Summary of Local and Systemic Antidotes (Continued)

POISON	LOCAL ANTIDOTE	SYSTEMIC ANTIDOTE
Iron	Sodium bicarbonate, 1-5% solution, preferably by lavage (Deferoxamine, 2 g/L in 1-2% bicarbonate lavage, and as post-lavage intragastric bolus, 10 g/50 ml)	Deferoxamine, 20-40 mg/kg IV given as slow drip over 4-hr period not to exceed 15 mg/kg/hr; followed by 20 mg/kg every 4-8 hr until urine color normal or iron level normal (can give 20 mg/kg IM every 4-12 hr if no IV sites available)
Isoniazid	Activated charcoal	Pyridoxine (vitamin B_6) 1 g per g of INH ingested, 5-10% concentration in 5% dextrose in water, IV over 30-60 min
Lead	(*see* Heavy metals)	
Mercury	(*see* Heavy metals)	
Methanol		Ethanol, loading dose to achieve blood level of 100 mg/100 ml *Adult:* 0.6 g/kg + 7–10 g to be infused IV over 1 hr *Child:* 0.6 g/kg to be infused IV over 1 hr Maintenance doses should approximate 10 g/hr in adults and 100 mg/kg/hr in children, to be adjusted according to measured blood ethanol levels

Methemoglobinemic agents
  Nitrites
  Nitrobenzene
  Chlorates
		Methylene blue, 1-2 mg (0.1-0.2 ml/kg) of a 1% solution IV slowly over 5-10 min if cyanosis is severe (or methemoglobin level is greater than 40%)

Narcotics	Activated charcoal	Naloxone, 0.005-0.01 mg/kg (adult 0.4 mg) IV at 2-3 min intervals p.r.n.
Nitrites	(*see* Methemoglobinemic agents)	
Oxalate	Dilute with water or milk, then give calcium gluconate or lactate, 150 mg/kg	Calcium gluconate, 10 ml of 10% solution, given slowly IV until symptoms abate; may be repeated p.r.n.
Phenol	Dilute with water or milk, then give activated charcoal, castor oil, vegetable oil	

Summary of Local and Systemic Antidotes (Continued)

POISON	LOCAL ANTIDOTE	SYSTEMIC ANTIDOTE
Phenothiazines (neuro-muscular reaction only)		Diphenhydramine, 0.5-1.0 mg/kg IM or IV; or benztropine, 2 mg IM or IV
Phosgene		Methenamine, 20 ml of 20% solution (4 g) IV. Probably ineffective after full development of pulmonary edema
Quaternary ammonium compounds	(*see* Anticholinesterases and/or detergents, cationic)	
Silver	(Also *see* heavy metals) Normal saline (lavage)	
Thallium	(Also *see* heavy metals) Activated charcoal may be given continuously to remove metal excreted via enterohepatic circulation	
Tricyclic antidepressants	(*see* Anticholinergics)	
Warfarin	Fresh Frozen Plasma	Vitamin K, 0.5-1.0 mg/kg IM or IV *Adults:* 10 mg IM or IV *Child:* 1-5 mg IM or IV

FOR ENVENOMATION*

Animals	Antivenin†
Snake, Crotalidae (all North American rattlers and moccasins)	Antivenin (Crotalidae), polyvalent (Wyeth)
Snake, coral	Antivenin (*Micrurus fulvius*), monovalent (Wyeth)
Spider, black widow	Antivenin (*Latrodectus mactans*), (Merck, Sharp & Dohme)

Note: All patients should be tested for sensitivity to horse serum.
†See package insert for dosage and administration.

Reference:

1. Fleisher G, Ludwig S. Textbook of Pediatric Emergency Medicine. Baltimore: Williams & Wilkins Company, 1983: 494–496. (Reproduced with permission.)

ACETAMINOPHEN OVERDOSE

Acetaminophen has become an important agent in acute poisonings because of its ever-increasing inclusion in a variety of over-the-counter drug preparations. Acetaminophen in small doses is not likely to cause serious problems. Once absorbed, it is metabolized in the liver via several pathways. Most of these metabolites are non-toxic and are excreted into the urine. A small percentage, however, is metabolized by the P-450 enzyme system to a toxic metabolite. This metabolite is then detoxified with glutathione and excreted. With large ingestions glutathione stores are exhausted, and the toxic metabolite accumulates,

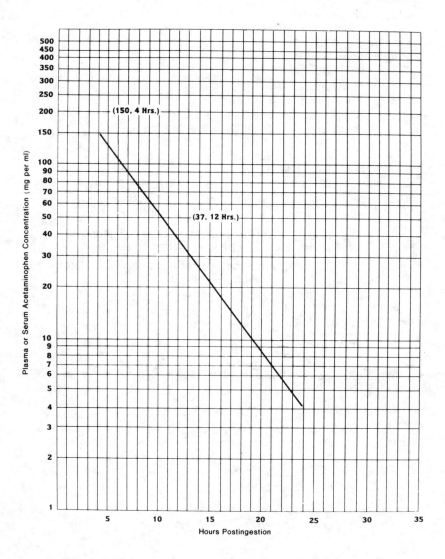

Fig. 4-1. Nomogram to establish acetaminophen hepatotoxicity. A high probability of serious hepatic damage exists if any level lies to the right of the solid line.

causing significant hepatotoxicity. This process depends on the dose ingested. Toxic doses are those greater than 140 mg/kg in children and greater than 10 g in adults. When acetaminophen levels are available, the accompanying nomogram may be used to establish the risk of hepatotoxicity. Several drugs induce the P-450 enzyme system and may lead to hepatotoxicity at lower doses. They include antihistamines, barbiturates, carbamazepine, glutethimide, griseofulvin, meprobamate, phenytoin, and rifampin.

Treatment of acetaminophen overdose is aimed at preventing hepatotoxicity. *N*-acetylcysteine (Mucomyst) enters the P-450 system to replace glutathione, so that the toxic metabolite can still be detoxified. Although this drug is widely used to treat acetaminophen overdose, it has not been specifically approved for this use at present. If acetaminophen levels are available, treatment may be initiated based on both the levels and the time after ingestion, using the nomogram. Treatment should begin within ten hours of ingestion. If levels are not readily available, treatment is based on the estimated dose ingested, with toxic levels as noted previously. If in doubt, it is best to begin treatment and continue until acetaminophen levels can be obtained. The dosage schedule is listed later. Treatment is given orally, and absorption of the antidote may be inhibited by administration of activated charcoal. If activated charcoal has been given, gastric lavage may be used to cleanse the stomach before *N*-acetylcysteine is given. Use of intravenous *N*-acetylcysteine has also been reported.[3]

N-Acetylcysteine Administration in Acetaminophen Overdose

	ENTERAL ROUTE	INTRAVENOUS ROUTE
Loading Dose	140 mg/kg	150 mg/kg
Maintenance Dosage	70 mg/kg q4h to a total of 17 doses	50 mg/kg over 4 hr (12.5 mg/kg/hr) *then* 100 mg/hr over 16 hr (6.25 mg/kg/hr)

References:
   1. Cilibert J. Acetaminophen overdose. *In:* Eisenberg MS, Copass MK, (eds.). Emergency Medical Therapy. Philadelphia: WB Saunders, 1982:197–199.
   2. Peterson RG, Rumack BH. Acetaminophen overdose: a high index of suspicion. Top Emerg Med 1979;*1*:43–49.
   3. Prescott LF, Park J, Ballantyne A, et al. Treatment of paracetamol (acetaminophen) poisoning with N-acetylcysteine. Lancet 1977;*2*:432–434.
   4. Rumack BH, Matthew H. Acetaminophen poisoning and toxicity. Pediatrics 1975;55: 871–78. (Nomogram reproduced with permission of the author and publisher; copyright American Academy of Pediatrics 1975.)

OVER-THE-COUNTER ACETAMINOPHEN PRODUCTS

The use of acetaminophen has risen dramatically in the United States over the past few years. Unfortunately, accidental and intentional ingestions parallel this increase in popularity. The abundance of acetaminophen-containing products available today is illustrated in the table.

Brand Names of Some Acetaminophen-Containing Products Available in the United States

Advanced Formula Dristan	Goody's Headache Powders	St. Joseph Aspirin-Free for Adults
Allerest	Headway	St. Joseph Aspirin - Free for Children
Aspirin-Free Arthritis Pain Formula	Liquiprin	Sinarest Tablets
Children's Anacin-3	Maximum Strength Anacin-3	Sine-Aid
Children's CoTylenol	Maximum Strength Panadol	Sine-Off
Comtrex	Novahistine	Sinutab
Congespirin	Nyquil	Sunril
Contac Jr.	Ornex	Teldrin
Contac	Pamprin	Tempra
Coricidin	Percogesic Analgesic Tablets	Trendar
Coryban-D	Pyrroxate	Tylenol
CoTylenol	Regular Strength Anacin-3	Vanquish
Daycare	Robitussin	Vicks Daycare
Dristan		Vicks Headway
Excedrin		Vicks Nyquil
Extra Strength Datril		

Reference:
    Physicians Desk Reference for Non-Prescription Drugs, 1983, 4th ed. Oradell, N.J.: Medical Economics Company, Inc.: 301. (With permission.)

ASPIRIN OVERDOSE

Aspirin overdose may be the result of an accidental ingestion in a child, a suicide attempt, or an accidental poisoning in an adult who is taking the drug for medical problems. Symptoms of an acute, single-dose ingestion are correlated with the serum salicylate level. The Done nomogram is helpful in determining the severity of the ingestion and is presented here (Fig. 4–2). To be meaningful, the serum salicylate level must be taken at least six hours after ingestion, and serial determinations are often helpful in monitoring the efficacy of treatment. The nomogram can not be used in chronic ingestions.

Mild intoxication is characterized by hyperventilation accompanied by some degree of lethargy and tinnitus. With moderate levels, nausea and vomiting, hyperpyrexia, and CNS changes, including agitation or lethargy increasing to stupor, are present. At severe levels, seizures, coma, and shock are common.

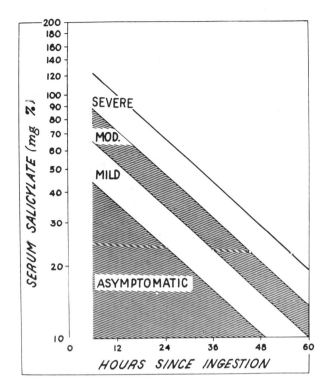

Fig. 4-2. The Done nomogram.

4

A variety of acid-base disturbances are noted. Salicylates have a direct stimulating effect on the respiratory center, causing respiratory alkalosis. Salicylates also interfere with Krebs cycle enzymes, leading to greater levels of lactic acid and metabolic acidosis. In association with ingestion of other drugs, resultant respiratory depression may lead to a respiratory acidosis. Attention to acid-base status is particularly important, because acidosis enhances CNS absorption of salicylate, worsening the severity of the intoxication. The accompanying table summarizes the acid-base disturbances noted in a series of salicylate poisoning cases.

Acid-Base Disturbances in Salicylate Poisoning

	SALICYLATES ALONE (%)	SALICYLATES PLUS OTHER DRUGS (%)*
Respiratory Alkalosis	22	27
Respiratory Alkalosis and Metabolic Acidosis	56	13
Metabolic Acidosis	20	36
Metabolic Acidosis and Respiratory Acidosis	2	18
Respiratory Acidosis	0	4

*Ethanol, benzodiazepines, tricylic antidepressants, barbiturates, LSD, acetaminophen, isopropyl alcohol, propoxyphene.

Fluid and electrolyte disturbances also occur. As previously mentioned, vomiting and hyperpyrexia may occur, leading to dehydration. In addition, salicylates enhance urinary sodium and potassium excretion.

Specific treatment of salicylate intoxication depends on the severity of the intoxication and the resultant acid-base, fluid, and electrolyte disturbances. Fluid therapy to maintain adequate blood pressure and urine output, sodium bicarbonate to correct acidosis or to alkalinize the serum and urine in severe intoxications, and KCl to correct hypokalemia are all indicated. In severe intoxications when such serious problems as continuing acidosis or renal failure are present despite these treatments, dialysis is useful. Hemodialysis is more effective than peritoneal dialysis, but, if unavailable, peritoneal dialysis with a solution containing albumin is effective.

References:
1. Done AK. Aspirin overdosage: incidence, diagnosis, and management. Pediatrics 1978; *62*:890–97. (Nomogram reproduced with permission.)
2. Eisenberg MS, Copass MK. Emergency Medical Therapy. Philadelphia: WB Saunders, 1982; 223. (Table reproduced with permission.)

IRON POISONING

Iron-containing preparations on the market today have come a long way from the vile-tasting elixirs and supplements of yesterday. They are now frequently found as ingredients in children's multivitamins, which have been carefully designed to appeal to the tastes of the pediatric age group. Unfortunately, however, if taken in sufficient quantity, those adorable, colorful, fruit-flavored "chewables" may provide a toxic amount of elemental iron. In fact, iron is the fourth most common toxic compound ingested by children and accounts for 3 per cent of all telephone calls to poison control centers annually.

How much iron is too much? Rough guidelines have been established that indicate an ingestion of greater than 60 mg/kg of elemental iron as potentially toxic. The lethal dose is estimated at 200 to 250 mg/kg of elemental iron. Most investigators agree, however, that any patient who ingests greater than 30 mg/kg should undergo hospital evaluation. The amount of *elemental iron* ingested can be calculated as follows: (1) ferrous sulfate contains 20 per cent elemental iron; (2) ferrous gluconate contains 12 per cent elemental iron; and (3) ferrous fumarate contains 33 per cent elemental iron.

The clinical features of acute iron poisoning are outlined.

Phase 1 (1–2 hours) Hemorrhagic gastroenteritis
Nausea, vomiting, abdominal pain
Hematemesis and melena

Phase 2 (2–12 hours) Latent period with transient improvement
Patient may appear well

Phase 3	(6–48 hours)	Shock and metabolic acidosis
		Fever, leukocytosis, hyperglycemia
Phase 4	(2–4 days)	Liver and renal failure
Phase 5	(2–4 weeks)	Pyloric stenosis, gastric strictures

One of the most challenging aspects of evaluating the patient who has ingested iron is that even in serious cases, the patient may appear clinically well when seen within the first 24 hours. The following guidelines should be utilized in treating all individuals who have ingested a potentially toxic dose of iron.

For All Patients with a History of Excessive Iron Ingestion

A. *Perform the following:*
1. Give deferoxamine (see The Antidote, Please, page 138 for dose)
2. Give ipecac (if patient is conscious and if gag reflex is present)
3. Lavage (after emesis) with deferoxamine (2 g in 1 liter of water containing enough $NaHCO_3$ to alkalinize the gastric contents [pH > 5])
4. Leave deferoxamine in the stomach (10 g in 50 ml of water with sufficient $NaHCO_3$ to alkalinize the gastric contents [pH > 5])
5. Provide IV fluids as necessary
6. Obtain a serum iron level
7. Obtain an abdominal roentgenogram

B. *Consider the following three conditions and initiate action as follows (C,D):*
1. Signs or symptoms by history or observation
2. Vin rosé-colored urine with good urine output
3. Evidence of iron tablets by abdominal roentgenogram

C. *If all three conditions are negative for six hours of observation, then discharge after six hours.*

D. *If any of the three conditions is positive, admit for further treatment as follows:*
1. Give deferoxamine by continuous IV infusion (15 mg/kg/hr)
2. Monitor and support intravascular volume and tissue perfusion
3. Continue therapy until urine is clear of vin rosé color and patient is asymptomatic for at least 24 hours
4. Discharge patient
5. Perform follow-up examination

References:
1. Bayer MJ, Rumack BH, Wanke LA. Toxicologic Emergencies. Bowie, Maryland: Robert J Brady Company, 1984.
2. Robotham JL, Leitman PS. Acute iron poisoning. Am J Dis Child 1980;*134*:875–880. (Guidelines reproduced with permission of the American Medical Association.)

THE DUST OF ANGELS

Phencyclidine (PCP or angel dust) is one of the most widely used and available hallucinogenic drugs in the United States today. It is easy and inexpensive to manufacture. PCP comes in various preparations, such as powders, tablets, crystals, and as a colorless solution. It can be added to marijuana and smoked, ingested, inhaled nasally, or taken parenterally. PCP is highly lipid soluble, weakly alkaline, and metabolized primarily through hepatic and renal mechanisms. The clinical effects of PCP abuse vary from person to person and, in some cases, are directly related to the amount ingested. PCP is rarely sold in its pure form and is often blended with other psychoactive chemicals. These additional agents may, in themselves, cause profound autonomic and central nervous system aberrations.

Clinical Findings

CNS. The patient is calm, unresponsive, or in coma. He may appear intoxicated, excited, or violent, or may exhibit bizarre behavior, or disordered thought processes. Amnesia, paranoia, dysphoria, dysarthria, and hallucinations (auditory and visual) are observed. Vomiting and status epilepticus may occur.

Ocular. There is a blank stare, disconjugate gaze, nystagmus (horizontal, vertical, or rotary), blurred vision, and miosis or mydriasis.

Sensory-Motor. Hyperactivity, tremor, myoclonus, dystonic movements (opisthotonos, facial grimacing, torticollis), and abnormal and variable deep tendon reflexes may be present.

Cardiovascular. Systolic and diastolic hypertension and sinus tachycardia are observed.

Muscle. Rhabdomyolysis is present.

Pulmonary. Tachypnea, irregular respiratory pattern, and rarely, apnea may be seen.

Laboratory Findings. Leukocytosis, muscle enzyme abnormalities (CPK, LDH, SGOT), ketonuria, and myoglobinuria may be found.

Diagnosis is confirmed on clinical and historical grounds and by qualitative identification of PCP in the blood, urine, or gastric contents. Therapy should include: (1) provision of a calm environment; (2) avoidance of restraints (if possible); (3) in cases of toxic psychotic episodes, haloperidol, 2 to 5 mg, IV; and (4) possible admission for observation to a controlled medical unit.

Most patients regain a normal state within several hours after ingestion of the drug. In cases of high-dose exposure, the recovery period may take days or even weeks.

References:
1. Cohen S. The angel dust states: phencyclidine toxicity. Pediatr Rev 1979;*1*:17–20.
2. Goldfrank L, Lewin N, Osborn H. Dusted (PCP). Hosp Phys 1982;May:62–73.

ORGANOPHOSPHATE POISONING

Now that DDT has been eliminated from general use as an insecticide, other compounds have been developed that are less hazardous to our environment. The two classes of insecticides that are most commonly employed today are organophosphates and carbamates. However, these agents are capable, in their own right, of provoking severe and sometimes fatal toxic reactions in exposed individuals. Exposure can occur by almost any route, including intact skin, conjunctiva, and respiratory and gastrointestinal mucosae. Both classes of compounds produce toxicity by inhibition of acetylcholinesterase, resulting in excess accumulation of acetylcholine at cholinergic synapses. The clinical manifestations of organophosphate poisoning are described in the following tables and discussions.

4

Muscarinic Effects

SYSTEM	SYMPTOMS
Bronchial tree	Bronchoconstriction, bronchorrhea, wheezing, dyspnea, cyanosis, pulmonary edema
Gastrointestinal tract	Anorexia, nausea, vomiting, cramps, diarrhea, fecal incontinence
Sweat glands	Increased sweating
Salivary glands	Increased salivation
Lacrimal glands	Increased lacrimation
Cardiovascular	Bradycardia, hypotension
Pupils	Constriction
Ciliary body	Blurred vision
Bladder	Urinary incontinence

Nicotinic Effects

SYSTEM	SYMPTOMS
Striated muscle	Fasciculations, cramps, weakness
Sympathetic ganglia	Hypertension, tachycardia, pallor

Restlessness, headache, tremor, confusion, slurred speech, ataxia, coma, convulsions, parkinsonism, or Bell's palsy are clinical manifestations of central nervous system toxicity.

A useful acronym that helps summarize the muscarinic manifestations is STUMBLED (salivation, tremor, urination, miosis, bradycardia, lacrimation, emesis, diarrhea). Carbamates do not penetrate the CNS to any great degree and therefore produce limited CNS manifestations; they do, however, mimic organophosphate toxicity clinically in almost every other way. Additional diagnostic criteria may include demonstration of inhibition of erythrocyte cholinesterase or plasma pseudocholinesterase activity; or positive results from urinary, gastric, and skin samples tested for organophosphates.

The treatment of organophosphate poisoning is summarized as follows:

Atropine
a. Blocks muscarinic and CNS effects.
b. Has no effect on skeletal muscle weakness.
c. Adult dose is 2 to 4 mg.
d. Pediatric dose is 0.05 mg/kg.
e. Administer by slow IV push.
f. Doses may be repeated every 15 minutes until signs of atropinization appear (clearing of bronchial secretions, mydriasis, dry mouth, and tachycardia).

Pralidoxime (PAM)
a. Restores acetylcholinesterase activity.
b. Reserved for acute organophosphate exposures only; effective only when instituted early in therapy.
c. Given intravenously over several minutes.
d. Adult dose is 1 g.
e. Pediatric dose is 10 to 12 mg/kg.
f. Relieves muscle weakness and fasciculations within 10 to 40 minutes.
g. May repeat dose in 1 to 2 hours.
h. Contraindicated in carbamate exposures.

Decontamination
a. Remove and dispose of contaminated clothing.
b. Thoroughly wash exposed skin surfaces.
c. Induce emesis in cases of ingestion.

Deaths from acute poisonings are usually caused by respiratory failure; fortunately, however, most cases are not serious and recovery is usually complete. Further information can be obtained from the National Pesticide Communications Network, Medical University of South Carolina (telephone 1-800-845-7633).

Reference:
1. Goldfrank L, Bresnitz E, Kirstein R, Weisman R. Organophosphates. Hosp Phys 1981; Dec:56–64.

MANAGEMENT OF CAUSTIC INGESTIONS

The patient who has ingested a caustic chemical requires careful physical examination and management. Anyone who has dealt with this problem is well aware of its serious nature and the importance of making correct therapeutic decisions. Caustic ingestions may result in severe tissue injury, both immediate and delayed, to all parts of the gastrointestinal tract. Keep these following facts in mind when evaluating patients who have ingested a caustic chemical:

	ALKALI	ACID
Frequency	Common	Rare
Type	Lye, Clorox	Toilet bowl cleaners
Mechanism of Injury	Liquefactive necrosis Local hyperthermia	Desiccant (dehydrating) action Local hyperthermia
Site of Injury	Oropharynx Esophagus Stomach	Oropharynx Stomach (pylorus, antrum)
Immediate Effect	Esophageal burn Esophageal perforation Upper airway edema	Gastric perforation Peritonitis Shock
Delayed Complication	Esophageal stricture	Pyloric stenosis

Important data that should be included in the patient's history are as follows:

1. Was the ingested material liquid or solid?
2. What was the pH of the corrosive involved?
3. Is there a sample available for testing?
4. How much was taken and did vomiting (re-injury) occur?
5. Was a diluent (milk, water) taken?
6. Is the patient drooling or complaining of dysphagia?
7. Is there pain (skin, lips, mouth, throat, chest, and abdomen)?

Considerable controversy surrounds the management options in caustic ingestions. Some of these options have been well investigated. Emesis and gastric lavage are currently *not* recommended for corrosive ingestions. The use of diluents should be restricted to milk and water only. Attempts to neutralize the exposure (i.e., giving mildly acidic substances to patients with alkali ingestions) should be avoided, since this mixture is exothermic in nature and may further injure the gastrointestinal tract. Activated charcoal, a mainstay in the early management of many overdoses, is contraindicated in caustic ingestions, since it poorly absorbs acids and alkalis and may limit the visualization of tissue injury at endoscopy.

A comprehensive management algorithm is provided. The reference provided is an excellent review of the problem.

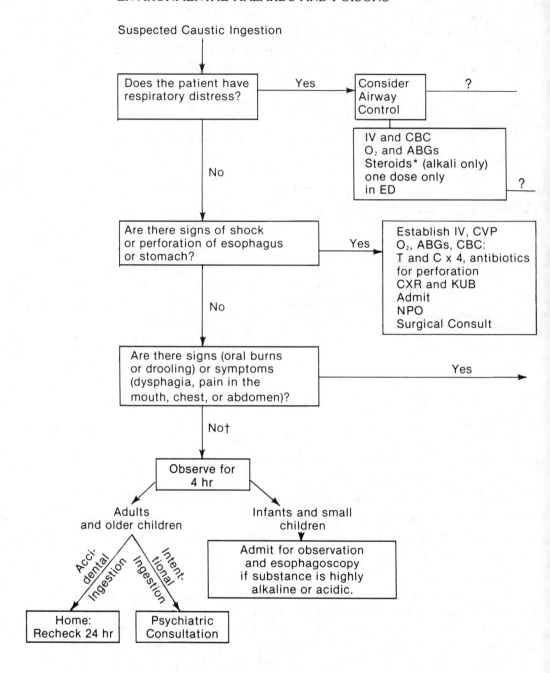

Fig. 4–3. Initial management of alkali and acid ingestions in the emergency room.

*Controversial; probably not beneficial unless given immediately after ingestion.
†Determine pH with pH paper — range 1–14.

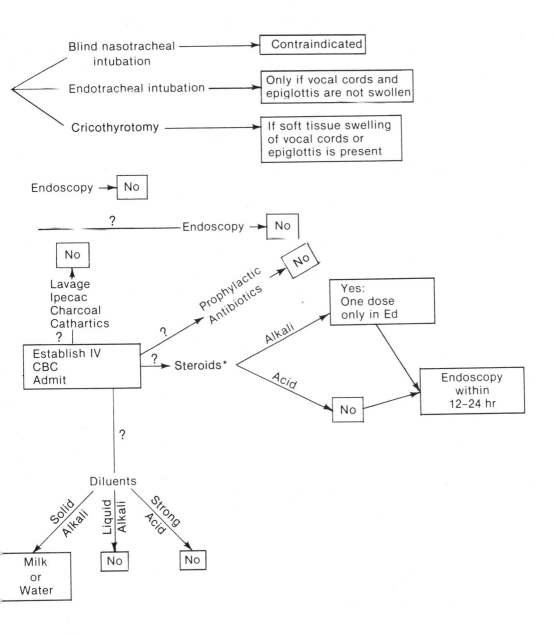

Reference:
1. Knopp R. Caustic ingestions. JACEP 1979;*8*:329–336. (Figure reproduced with permission.)

OVER-THE-COUNTER DRUG ABUSE

In our society today, losing weight seems to be the new American dream. We have all seen advertisements in which people claim: "I lost 20 pounds in 20 days"; and we've all seen smiling faces on television of happy, content dieters. The shelves of our supermarkets and drugstores are crowded with over-the-counter (OTC) medications that claim to help "lose weight fast without going hungry." These OTC appetite suppressants are, for the most part, combinations of phenylpropanolamine and caffeine, two agents that can induce serious side effects if taken in excessive amounts.

Phenylpropanolamine is similar to amphetamine in structure and is an alpha-adrenergic agonist. Overdoses (more than 100 mg in adults) produce tachycardia, hypertension, and, in severe cases, atrial and ventricular arrhythmias, anginal chest pain, and myocardial damage. Those who overdose are also subject to a spectrum of CNS derangements, including agitation, combativeness, muscle tremors, and seizures. An alpha-adrenergic blocker (i.e., phentolamine) has been utilized to counteract the untoward cardiovascular effects of phenylpropanolamine overdose. Most patients, however, require only close observation and monitoring, since phenylpropanolamine has a brief duration (1–2 hours) of action.

Caffeine overdose (lethal in adults at more than 150 mg/kg) manifests itself in ways similar to those of phenylpropanolamine overdose. The toxic dose in children is more than 30 mg/kg. Caffeine, like all methylxanthines, has both alpha- and beta-adrenergic cardiovascular and CNS effects. The half-life of caffeine is four to six hours in adults and greater than 40 hours in infants and young children. Treatment in severe cases has included propranolol for tachyarrhythmias and diazepam for seizures.

The table provides a formulary of the currently marketed OTC diet-aids.

BRAND NAME	PHENYLPROPANOLAMINE HYDROCHLORIDE (mg)	CAFFEINE (mg)
Anorexin capsules	25	100
Appedrine tablets	25	100
Appress	25	100
Ayds droplets	25	—
Coffee Break cubes	37.5	—
Coffee Tea + A New Me	25	—
Dex-A-Diet II	75	200
Dexatrim capsules	50	200
Diadax capsules	50	—
Diadax tablets	25	—
Odrinex tablets	25	50
Pro-Dax 21	75	—
Prolamine capsules	35	140
Spantrol capsules	75	150
Vitaslim capsules	50	—
Dexatrim capsules (timed release)	50	200
Dexatrim extra-strength capsules (timed release)	75	200

YOU'D BETTER WATCH OUT

The Christmas season is a time of excitement and merriment and, most of all, a time for children. It is also quite a busy period for parents, who, in the midst of all the frenzy, may be unaware that it is also a well-known time for childhood poisoning to occur. Even the safest home becomes a threatening environment when all the cooking, decorating, and celebrating are under way. The following table enumerates the holiday hazards to watch out for.

Hazard	Toxicant	Comment
Alcohol	Alcohol	Found in liquor, but also found in perfumes, colognes, aftershave lotions.
Angel hair	Spun glass	Can cause corneal abrasions.
Bubble lights	Methylene chloride	Can be ingested; toxic only if many bulbs are ingested.
Christmas tree ornaments	Lead	Antique ornaments may have been painted with lead.
Fireplace color crystals	Heavy metal salts	Can be alkaline and are corrosive to the GI tract.
Tinsel and glitter	Tin and lead	Non-toxic; lead nonabsorbable but pieces can be aspirated.
Snow scene globes	Calcium carbonate	Non-toxic.
Christmas berry	Cyanide	Leaves and unripe berries are poisonous.
Christmas berry tree	Safrole and saponins	Cause salivation, gastroenteritis, headache, fever, and muscle weakness.
Christmas cactus	None	Non-toxic.
Christmas rose	Veratrine	Burning in mouth and on the skin; nausea, vomiting, hypotension, convulsions.
Hollies	Ilicin (some species)	Berries cause gastroenteritis and narcosis.
American ivy	Oxalic acid	Leaves and berries cause local oral stinging, irritation, and swelling (usually preventing large intake). Large amounts can cause abdominal pain, headache, somnolence (can have a delayed onset of 24 hours), and renal damage.
English ivy	Saponins	Leaves and blackberries cause gastroenteritis and salivation.
Jerusalem cherry	Solanine (berries)	Gastroenteritis and stupor.
	Solanocapsine (leaves)	Cardiac depression.

Table continued on following page

Hazard	Toxicant	Comment
American mistletoe (all plant parts)	B-phenethylamine Tyramine	Smooth muscle stimulation, gastroenteritis, tachypnea, bradycardia, delirium, hypertension, and mydriasis.
European mistletoe	Histamine Tyramine	Hypertension, bradycardia.
Pines	Cone spurs	Pine cone spurs can be aspirated or cause contact dermatitis.
Rhododendrons	Andromedotoxins	All plant parts toxic; cause gastroenteritis, watery eyes, ataxia, bradycardia, hypotension, and weakness.
Poinsettia	None	Small amounts non-toxic.

Reference:
1. Poison Information Bulletin. vol. 4, no. 5 Available from the National Poison Center Network, 125 DeSoto St, Pittsburgh, Pennsylvania 15213

WORK MAY BE HAZARDOUS TO YOUR HEALTH

Environmental pollutants are well-known health hazards. Although they may seem nebulous and ubiquitous in their distribution, they pose a particular danger in a confined area, e.g., where one is employed or where one pursues hobbies. Unless a patient is overcome while on the job or in active pursuit of an avocation, the relationship is often overlooked. The major diagnostic problem is that these occupational disorders masquerade as other common medical diseases. As expected, a careful history will often uncover this connection. The following flow chart points the way. A table of common occupational poisons follows.

Some Occupational Hazards

OCCUPATION OR AVOCATION	TOXINS (The Most Important, Because of Either Severity or Frequency, Are Italicized)
Acid dipper	*Arsine; cyanogens;* hydrochloric, nitric, sulfuric acid fumes
Acid finishing worker (glass)	*Hydrochloric,* sulfuric acid; lead
Aircraft mechanic and pilot	Alcohols, *chlorinated and other solvents,* gasoline and other fuels, zinc chromate
Crop duster	Pesticides and their solvents
Aircraft worker	Cyanides, chromates, fiber glass and resin plastics, *solvents* (especially chlorinated), hydrofluoric acid

Table continued on following page

Systematic Approach to History Taking and Diagnosis of Toxic Occupational Illness

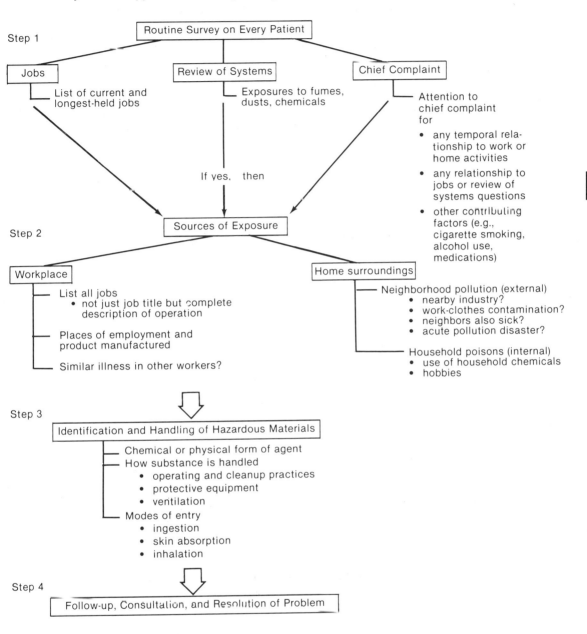

Fig. 4–4. Goldman RH, Peters JM. The occupational and environmental health history. JAMA 1981; *246*:2831. (Reproduced with permission.)

Fig. 4-4, Goldman RH, Peters JM. The occupational and environmental health history. JAMA 1981;*246*:2831–2836. (Reproduced with permission.)

Some Occupational Hazards (Continued)

OCCUPATION OR AVOCATION	TOXINS (The Most Important, Because of Either Severity or Frequency, Are Italicized)
Airplane hangar employee	As in other aircraft fields; and *carbon monoxide*
Alcohol distiller	Alcohols (including methanol), *amyl acetate, benzene,* mercury, toluene, xylene
Aluminum extraction worker	Aluminum, *hydrofluoric acid,* manganese
Amber worker	*Formaldehyde* (artificial amber), lead
Art-glass worker	Amyl acetate, copper, *hydrofluoric acid, lead,* methanol, volatile hydrocarbons (including benzine)
Asbestos products worker	*Asbestos,* benzene, formaldehyde, toluene, xylene
Automobile worker	Asbestos, chromates, *fiber glass and resin plastics,* gasoline, lead, *solvents*
Radiator cleaner	Borate, isopropanol, *oxalate,* sulfamic acid
Painter	Benzene, lead, *methanol,* zinc
Balloon operator	Arsine, *carbon monoxide*
Barber and beautician	Aliphatic solvents, alkyl sodium sulfates, borates, cadmium, cobalt, copper, detergents, *dyes,* essential oils, lead, oxalate (freckle remover), pyrogallol, resorcinol, salicylate, silver, *thioglycolate*
Barometer maker	Mercury
Battery worker	Acids, benzene, *mercury,* zinc, lead
Blacksmith	*Carbon monoxide* and dioxide, cyanogens, lead
Blast furnace worker	*Carbon dioxide* and monoxide, *cyanogens,* hydrogen sulfide, *phosphine,* sulfur dioxide
Bleacher	Caustic alkali, *chlorine,* chromium, *hydrochloric acid,* hydrofluoric acid, *peroxides,* nitric acid, oxalic acid, phosgene, sulfur oxides
Bookbinder	Acetate, arsenic, *formalin,* lead, methanol, *oxalate,* polyvinyl, solvents
Brass worker (founder)	*Antimony, arsenic,* carbon dioxide and monoxide, copper, lead, phosphorus, sulfur oxides
Brazer	*Lead,* zinc
Brewer	*Amyl alcohol, carbon dioxide* or monoxide, cobalt, formaldehyde, hydrofluoric acid, phenol, sulfuric acid
Brick worker	Carbon monoxide and dioxide, epoxy resins, *hydrofluoric acid, lead, lime,* magnesium, manganese, *silica,* sulfur oxides

Some Occupational Hazards (Continued)

OCCUPATION OR AVOCATION	TOXINS (The Most Important, Because of Either Severity or Frequency, Are Italicized)
Bronzer	*Acetone,* ammonia, amyl acetate, antimony, arsenic, benzene, benzine, cyanides, hydrochloric acid, hydrogen sulfide, lead, manganese, mercury, methanol, sulfur oxides, *zinc*
Burnisher	*Antimony, benzine,* carbon tetrachloride, sulfuric acid, trichloroethylene
Cabinetmaker, carpenter, woodworker (see also painter)	Acetone, *benzine,* bleaches, *methanol, methylene chloride,* resins, solvents, turpentine
Ironwood	*Arsenic*
Candle maker	*Aniline,* borates, chromates, potassium nitrate, sodium hydroxide
Cartridge maker	*Lead,* mercury, nitrites
Case hardener	*Cyanogens,* sodium dichromate or nitrite
Caster	See specific occupation
Cementer (rubber, plastic, etc.)	*Benzene, benzine,* butyl alcohol, *carbon disulfide,* carbon tetrachloride, methanol, naphtha, tetrachloroethane, trichloroethylene
Cement (Portland) worker	Arsenic, chromates, cobalt, lime, pitch, *silica*
Ceramist, glazer, pottery worker	Arsenic, *barium,* carbon monoxide, *chromium,* cobalt, *feldspars,* hydrochloric or hydrofluoric acid, *lead,* manganese, mercury, selenium, *silica,* sulfur oxides, tellurium
Charcoal cook	*Carbon monoxide* or dioxide
Chrome plater (see also electroplater)	*Chromium,* solvents, sulfuric acid
Coal tar worker	*Aniline, creosote, cresol,* cyanogens, naphtha, phenol, pitch
Cobbler	Amyl acetate, aniline, *benzene and related solvents,* benzine, carbon tetrachloride, methanol, plastics
Coke oven worker (see also coal tar worker)	*Ammonia, benzene, carbon monoxide,* hydrogen sulfide, sulfur oxides
Compositor	*Alkalis, aniline,* antimony, benzine, lead, *solvents*
Construction worker (see also brick worker, cabinetmaker, cement worker, ceramist, painter)	*Arsenic, creosote,* gasoline, glass fibers, paint products, *pitch, silica,* solvent
Cosmetic worker	Aniline, *arsenic, mercury,* nitrobenzene, solvents
Dentist	Anesthetics, clove oil, disinfectants, *mercury*

Table continued on following page

Some Occupational Hazards (Continued)

OCCUPATION OR AVOCATION	TOXINS (The Most Important, Because of Either Severity or Frequency, Are Italicized)
Dry cleaner	*Amyl acetate, benzine,* carbon tetrachloride, dichloroethylene, methanol, *naphtha,* oxalate, tetrachoroethane, tetrachorethylene, *trichloroethylene,* turpentine, waterproofing compounds
Dye maker	*Aniline,* antimony, arsenic, benzine, chlorates, chromates, coal tar products, cresol, *dimethyl sulfate,* ferrocyanides, formaldehyde, lead, manganese, mercury, methanol, nitrobenzene, phenol, titanium, *organotins*
Dyer	*Acetone, aniline,* other *aminobenzene derivatives,* bleaches, mercury, solvents, titanium, zinc
Electric apparatus maker	*Asbestos, epoxy and phenolic resins,* solvents
Electroplater	*Antimony, arsenic,* benzine, cadmium, *chromium,* copper, *cyanide,* gold, lead, lime, mercury, nickel, nitrous fumes, potassium hydroxide, silver, sulfuric acid, zinc
Enameler	*Amyl acetate,* antimony, arsenic, chromium, cobalt, lead, nickel, *silica*
Engraver	*Acids,* alkalis, *benzene, copper, cyanide,* solvents
Etcher	*Acids, alkalis, arsine, hydrofluoric acid,* nitrous fumes, picric acid
Explosive and firearms maker	Acetone, *ammonia, amyl acetate,* mercury, nitrites, *nitroglycerin,* picric acid, TNT
Farmer	Carbon monoxide, fertilizers, pesticides, plants with contact toxicity (poison ivy, sumac, oak, etc.), solvents, nitrogen dioxide (silo filler's disease), farmer's lung
Felt hat worker	*Carbon monoxide,* hydrogen peroxide, hydrogen sulfide, *mercury,* methanol, nitrous fumes, oxalic acid, sulfuric acid
Fertilizer producer and user	*Ammonia,* arsenic, *calcium cyanamide,* carbon dioxide, castor bean pomace, cyanogens, fluoride, hydrogen sulfide, lime, magnesium, manganese, nitrates, nitric acid, phosphates, sulfur oxides, sulfuric acid
Fire extinguisher maker	*Carbon dioxide,* chlorobromomethane, *ethyl bromide, ethyl chloride,* ethylene dibromide, methyl bromide, sodium dichromate
Fireworks maker (see also explosives maker)	*Antimony, arsenic,* barium, bismuth, mercury, phosphorus, picric acid, thallium

Some Occupational Hazards (Continued)

OCCUPATION OR AVOCATION	TOXINS (The Most Important, Because of Either Severity or Frequency, Are Italicized)
Fish-meal processor	*Hydrogen sulfide, triethylamine*
Foundry worker (see also particular occupation)	*Acids, carbon dioxide and monoxide, lime, resins, silica*
Furniture polisher	*Amyl acetate, benzine,* chromium, methanol, naphtha, petroleum hydrocarbons, pyridine, rosin, turpentine
Fur processor	*Alum, bleaches,* chromates, dyes, formaldehyde, hydrogen sulfide, lime, mercury, nitrous fumes
Galvanizer	Acids, *ammonia,* arsenic, *arsine,* benzine, nitrous fumes, sulfur oxides, trichloroethylene, *zinc*
Garage worker	*Benzine, carbon monoxide,* detergents, *epoxy resins,* gasoline, glass fibers, lead, paints, solvents
Gardener	Arsenic, calcium cyanamide, *fertilizers, fungicides, herbicides, insecticides,* lead, *pesticides,* poisonous plants, venomous insects
Gem/lapidary/ jewelry maker	*Arsenic,* asbestos, benzene, bisulfate, borates, cadmium, *cyanide,* epoxy resins, hydrochloric acid, *hydrofluoric acid,* lead, *mercury* (gold extraction), methanol, methyl salicylate, nitric acid, selenium, silica, sulfur oxides, sulfuric acid, trisodium phosphate, zinc
Glass worker (see also art-glass worker)	Acids, *arsenic, borates,* carbon monoxide, chlorine, *glass fibers,* hydrofluoric acid, lead, nitrogen oxides, sulfur
Gold and silver extractor	*Arsenic, arsine,* bromides, *cyanide,* formaldehyde, hydrofluoric acid, lead, *mercury*
Gunsmith/hunter/ marksman (see also explosives maker)	Cyanide, *kerosene, lead,* magnesium, mercury, nickel, *nitrites, nitrobenzene, solvents*
Bluing	*Chlorate, mercury,* methanol, nitrite, selenium
Browning	Benzine, *cyanide, lead,* petroleum hydrocarbons
Ice cream maker	*Ammonia,* carbon dioxide
Ink maker	*Ammonia, arsenic,* benzene, benzine, *chromates, cobalt,* formaldehyde, lead, mercury, *nitrites,* other solvents, *silver*
Insecticide maker and applier	Solvents as well as specific insecticides
Insulation maker and applier	*Asbestos,* formaldehyde, glass fibers, *silica*

Table continued on following page

Some Occupational Hazards (Continued)

OCCUPATION OR AVOCATION	TOXINS (The Most Important, Because of Either Severity or Frequency, Are Italicized)
Iron and steel worker	*Arsenic,* cadmium, *carbon monoxide,* hydrofluoric acid, nitrogen oxides, sulfur oxides, *titanium*
Jeweler (see also gem worker)	*Acids, amyl acetate,* chromates, *cyanide,* mercury, nickel, nitric acid, nitrous fumes, solder fluxes
Lacquer maker and applier	Acetaldehyde, *acetone,* alcohols, *amyl acetate,* benzine, butanone, cresyl phosphate, methylene chloride, solvents
Laundry worker	*Alkaline caustics, bleaches,* chloride, chlorine, detergents, formaldehyde, lime, ozone
Lead smelter	Antimony, *arsenic,* cadmium, carbon monoxide, *lead,* selenium, sulfur oxides, tellurium
Leather worker	Acids, *amyl acetate, barium,* carbon tetrachloride, methanol, trichloroethylene
Tanner	*Acetates,* acids, *aniline,* arsenic, benzene, carbon dioxide, chromates, cyanide, diethylamine, dyes, formaldehyde, hydrogen sulfide, mercury, *nitrites,* oxalate, picric acid, sodium sulfide, tannin
Linoleum worker	*Amyl acetate, asphalt,* benzene, benzine, carbon tetrachloride, chromates, *dyes,* methanol, resins, solvents
Linotyper	*Antimony,* carbon monoxide, lead
Lithographer	Acids, *aniline,* arsenic, benzene, benzine, chromates, lead, mercury, methanol, nitric acid, *nitrites,* oxalate, tetrachloroethane, turpentine
Longshoreman	Manganese, *various chemicals and fumigants* (depending on cargo), venomous insects and snakes
Match worker	Alkalis, antimony, carbon disulfide, *chlorates, chromates,* hydrogen sulfide, manganese, *phosphorus*
Metal polisher	Acids, *ammonia, benzine, cyanide,* methanol, *naphtha,* oxalates, solvents, trichloroethylene, triethanolamine
Miner (varies with type)	*Asbestos,* carbon dioxide and monoxide, hydrogen sulfide, manganese, nitrogen oxides, *silica, talc*
Mirror maker	*Acetaldehyde, ammonia,* benzene, *cyanide,* lead, *mercury,* silver, solvents
Painter	*Acetone, acids,* alkalis, aniline, arsenic, barium, *benzine,* carbon disulfide, carbon tetrachloride, chromates, *lead,* manganese, mercury, methanol, methylene chloride, nitrogen oxides, *solvents,* trichloroethylene, turpentine

Some Occupational Hazards (Continued)

OCCUPATION OR AVOCATION	TOXINS (The Most Important, Because of Either Severity or Frequency, Are Italicized)
Paintmaker	*Cadmium, chlorinated diphenyls,* petroleum distillates, titanium, zinc
Paper maker	*Acids,* acrylamide, *alkalis,* ammonia, amyl acetate, bisulfide, calcium chloride, chromates, *DMSO,* formaldehyde, hydrofluoric acid, hydrogen sulfide, lead, resins, sulfur oxides, titanium
Petroleum refiner	Acetone, ammonia, arsenic, *benzene, benzine,* gasoline and other petroleum distillates, hydrofluoric acid, *hydrogen sulfide,* nitrites, solvents, sulfur oxides
Photoengraver	Acids, alkalis, *ammonia,* ammonium bichromate, *amyl acetate,* methanol, nitrous fumes, solvents
Photographer	*Acids, alkalis,* aminophenols, *amyl acetate, benzene,* borates, bromides, chromates, cyanide, ethylene glycol, formaldehyde, hydroquinone, iodine, lead, mercury, methanol, oxalate, pyrogallic acid, silver, *sodium bisulfide,* sodium hypochlorite, sodium sulfite, sodium thiosulfate, tellurium, trichloroethylene, uranium, vanadium
Plastics and resin maker or user	None with finished plastics but unreacted resins are toxic
Plumber	Acids, alkalis, *arsine, carbon monoxide, lead,* solvents, zinc
Printer	*Alkalis, aniline, benzine,* carbon tetrachloride, chromates, cyanide, lead, mercury, methanol, tetrachloroethylene, other solvents
Railroad shop and track worker	*Chromates,* contact plant poisons (poison ivy, etc.), *creosote,* detergents, dichlorobenzenes, diesel fuel oil, fungicides, herbicides, insecticides, paint, paint strippers, solvents, venomous insects and snakes
Rayon worker	*Acetic anhydride,* acids, ammonia, benzine, bleaches, butyl alcohol, *calcium bisulfite,* carbon disulfide, chlorinated diphenyls, cyanogens, *dioxane,* formaldehyde, hydrogen sulfide, methanol, nitrous fumes, solvents, sulfide, sodium sulfite, tetrachloroethane
Refrigeration worker	*Acrolein, ammonia,* carbon dioxide, carbon monoxide, *ethyl bromide, ethyl chloride,* glass fiber, *methyl bromide, methyl chloride,* methyl formate, ozone, sulfur oxides

Table continued on following page

Some Occupational Hazards (Continued)

OCCUPATION OR AVOCATION	TOXINS (The Most Important, Because of Either Severity or Frequency, Are Italicized)
Rubber worker	*Acetaldehyde, acetone,* amyl alcohol, aniline, antimony, arsenic, barium, benzene, benzine, carbon disulfide, carbon tetrachloride, *chloroprene,* chromates, cresol, ethylene dichloride, formaldehyde, lead, magnesium, methanol, nitrogen oxides, *plasticizers, pyridine, silica,* solvents, tellurium, zinc
Sewage worker	*Ammonia,* carbon dioxide, chlorine, *hydrogen sulfide,* methane
Shoemaker (see also leather worker)	*Acetone, adhesives,* ammonia, amyl acetate, amyl alcohol, *aniline and dyes,* benzene, benzine, carbon tetrachloride, methanol, naphtha, plastics, tetrachloroethane, trichloro-ethylene, waxes
Solderer	*Acids,* antimony, arsenic, *arsine,* borates, cadmium, cyanide, *hydrazine salts,* lead, potassium bifluoride, rosin, zinc
Stone worker	*Lime, silica*
Sugar refiner	*Acids, ammonia, bagasse,* barium, burlap, carbon dioxide, hydrogen sulfide, sulfur oxides
Tannery worker	Acetic acid, acids, alum, ammonia, *amyl acetate, aniline and dyes,* arsenic, benzene, ben-zine, calcium hydrosulfide, chromates, cyanide, dimethylamine, dyes, formaldehyde, hydrogen sulfide, lead, lime, mercury, oxalate, sodium sulfide, solvents, sulfur oxides, tannin
Tar worker	*Arsenic, cresols,* pitch, tar
Taxidermist	*Arsenic,* calcined alum, *mercury,* solvents, tannin, zinc
Upholsterer (see also lacquer maker)	*Glues, lacquer,* lacquer solvents, methanol
Waterproofer	*Alum,* benzene, *benzine,* carbon tetrachloride, chromates, formaldehyde, melamine, pitch, resins, solvents, tar
Welder	*Arsenic,* benzene, cadmium, chromates, fluoride, lead, manganese, mercury, nitrous fumes, ozone, phosphorus, selenium, *zinc*
Wood preserver	*Arsenic, chlorophenols,* chromates, copper compounds, creosote, cresols, dinitrophenols, mercury, pitch, resins, tar, zinc

Reference:
1. Done, AK. Work can be hazardous to your health. Emerg Med 1982;Nov:191–217. (Reproduced with permission from the author and publisher.)

RADIATION DOSE EFFECTS

The standard unit of radiation is the rem (*r*oentgen *e*quivalent *m*an), which takes into account the effects of the three different types of radiation. Approximate estimates of the long-term effects of some of the doses are shown in the table. The dose is calculated for whole-body exposure, not for exposure of a small localized area of the body.

DOSE (rem)	COMMENT
0.03	Average dose from one chest x-ray.
0.2	Average annual dose for New York area residents from environmental and medical sources.
0.5	Exposure limit set by the Nuclear Regulatory Commission for pregnant workers in the nuclear industry throughout pregnancy.
1.0	Average dose from one lumbosacral spine x-ray.
1–5	Federal guidelines call for action to protect public if it is anticipated that a nuclear accident would result in a dose of this amount.
5	Annual exposure limit for most nuclear workers.
10	The 30-year cancer incidence rises by about 1193 cases per million in persons exposed to this level in addition to the 170,000 fatal cancer cases that would be expected without the exposure.
10–25	Small short-term changes in the blood of some of those exposed.
25	Limit for most emergency workers.
25–50	Nearly all those exposed show low white and red blood cell counts in 24 hours.
50–100	Nausea within 12 hours for 5 per cent of those exposed.
75	Limit for emergency workers in lifesaving activities.
100–200	Vomiting in 5 to 50 per cent of those exposed within three hours; hair loss in up to 10 per cent of population in 5 to 10 days.
225	Death within 60 days for 5 per cent of those exposed, without medical care.
400	Death within 60 days for 50 per cent of those exposed, without medical care.
500–600	Death within 60 days for 90 per cent of those exposed, without medical care.

INITIAL MANAGEMENT OF RADIATION INJURY

Irradiation vs. Radioactive Contamination

A person may be irradiated by gamma rays or x-rays, may be contaminated with radioactive material, or may incorporate radioactive material into his body. Just as a person who has been burned does not give off heat, a person who has only been irradiated without contamination or incorporation does not give off radioactivity.

Get Help

In the event of a radiation emergency, don't panic: help is only a phone call away. Many hospital staffs have a specialist in nuclear medicine or radiation physics who can give technical advice. Industries using radioactive material employ physicists to help with problems. Regional hospitals may specialize in managing radiation problems. The Department of Energy offers assistance and can be contacted through the following phone numbers.

Department of Energy
Regional Coordinating Offices for Radiologic Assistance

Brookhaven Area Operations Office
    Conn, Del, Maine, Md, Mass, NH,
    NJ, NY, Pa, PR, RI, Vt, VI
	516-282-2200

Oak Ridge Operations Office
    Ark, Ky, La, Miss, Mo, Tenn, Va,
    WVa
	615-576-1005

Savannah River Operations Office Ala, CZ, Ga, Fla, NC, SC	803-726-3333
Albuquerque Operations Office Ariz, Kans, NMex, Okla, Tex	505-844-4667

Chicago Operations Office
    Ill, Ind, Iowa, Mich, Minn, Nebr,
    NDak, Ohio, SDak, Wis
	312-972-4800 (duty hours)
	    972-5731 (off duty hours)

Idaho Operations Office Colo, Idaho, Mont, Utah, Wyo	208-526-1515
San Francisco Operations Office Calif, Hawaii, Nev	415-273-4237
Richland Operations Office Alaska, Oreg, Wash	509-373-3800

Reference:

1. Department of Energy, 1978. Information updated and verified March, 1985.

Get the Facts

Establish whether a patient is actually contaminated, using a Geiger-Müller counter or dosimeter. Special instruments are needed to measure alpha and neutron particles. *Remember*—background radio-activity of approximately 100 counts/min will be included in the measurement. Compare the count recorded 2 inches from the patient's skin with the background count.

Truckers carrying radioactive materials are required to carry papers describing the contents of the truck. Radioactive packages are labeled according to their output.

Labeling of Radioactive Packages

LABEL	DOSE RATE AT SURFACE (mR/hr)	DOSE RATE AT 3 FEET (mR/hr)
White I	< 0.5	—
Yellow II	0.5–50	< 1
Yellow III	50–200	1–10

Adapted from Richter.

Procedures for Treatment of Radioactive Contamination or Incorporation

Decontamination uses principles of care with which we are familiar, i.e., they are the same as those for sepsis. A contaminated patient's linens and body fluids are considered "dirty" and are discarded carefully to avoid spreading contamination. The attendant protects himself from contamination. He does not leave the contaminated area until all of his protective clothing has been left in the "dirty" area, making the attendant "clean." "Clean" items can be passed into the "dirty" area by a "clean" person. Decontamination is simply a formalized bath.

I. In the field
   1. Ambulance personnel should wear protective clothing.
   2. Remove the patient's clothes and leave them at the site of exposure. Cover open wounds to avoid contaminating them while disrobing the patient.
   3. Wrap the patient in sheets to avoid contaminating the ambulance.

II. Prepare the emergency department (ED)
   1. Open the decontamination room. It should be a room not essential to the rest of the ED, with a separate outside

entrance. It should be equipped with a draining table, a collection system for effluent, and hot and cold running water. Protect the room by covering switches and handles with tape, and by covering the floor with paper or plastic. Turn off the ventilation system or cover the exhaust duct with a particle filter if the room is vented to the outside.

2. Notify the hospital operator, security, administration, public relations, and environmental services.

3. Appoint a monitor, who will restrict access to and from the decontamination area, enforce the use of protective clothing, and record dosimeter readings. Also appoint a "circulator" who will pass equipment into the decontamination room.

III. Prepare personnel

1. All personnel should use the bathroom before entering the decontamination area.

2. Wear dosimeters under protective clothing; take initial readings.

3. Wear two sets of scrub suits, masks, caps, shoe covers, gloves as well as plastic apron. Wear lead shields if exposure is more than 5 R/h.

4. Minimize physical proximity and duration of exposure to patient. Estimate exposure as radiation dose rate (measured 6 inches above patient) times the duration of exposure. Attendants are permitted up to 5 R for routine treatment and decontamination; up to 25 R for emergency treatment; and up to 75 R for lifesaving procedures.

IV. Document contamination

1. Measure with a Geiger counter, holding the probe 2 inches from the patient's skin.

2. Record levels on an anatomic diagram.

V. Take samples

1. Begin 24-hour urine and 72-hour fecal collections.

2. Collect sputum, vomit, debrided tissue and exudate.

3. Sample nares, wounds, and skin with cotton swabs or commercial pads.

4. Obtain a whole-body count if indicated.

5. Obtain a radioiodide count if indicated.

VI. Bathe the patient

1. Wash from the areas of highest to lowest contamination.

2. Use pHisoHex®, detergents, Clorox®, and peroxide, progressing from milder to harsher agents.

3. Use lukewarm water and gentle technique. Abrading, vigorous scrubbing, and hot water irritate the skin and cause

vasodilation, increasing the chance for transcutaneous incorporation.

4. Rinse.

VII. Problem areas

1. Wounds—irrigate and remove devitalized tissue.
2. Puncture wound—let it bleed; may need excision.
3. Ears, eyes, and mouth—irrigate.
4. Hair—shampoo. Hair retains some isotopes and in such cases it must be cut. (Shaving scalp wounds injures the skin and increases incorporation.)
5. Inhalation—half of the contaminated material that has been inhaled is returned to the pharynx by ciliary action and is swallowed. Use treatment for ingestion; lung lavage may be of benefit.
6. Ingestion—use emetics, gastric lavage, and cathartics.

VIII. Check for contamination and record levels on an anatomic diagram

1. Repeat bathing and checking until background levels of radioactivity are reached.

IX. If contamination persists Surgical debridement may be necessary—but don't mutilate just to decontaminate. Cover the area with plastic. Sweating and exfoliation will reduce contamination. Recheck levels in 24 hours.

X. When decontamination is complete

1. Apply an emollient to the patient's skin.
2. Transfer the patient to a "clean" area.
3. Clean the room; gather all materials including effluent, light-switch coverings, and floor coverings into plastic containers. Label the containers, and give them to those responsible at the site of origin of the radioactive material for disposal.
4. Attendants can now remove outer garments. Everyone must be checked and found free of contamination before he can leave the area.
5. Record final dosimeter readings.

Specific Antidotes

Certain radioactive isotopes require specific therapy. It ranges from blocking agents (e.g., iodine for radioiodine), to dilution (e.g., water for tritium), to displacement (e.g., calcium for radiostrontium), to chelation. These therapies should be given under the direction of a radiation specialist.

Management of Radiation Injury

TEST	MANAGEMENT	LONG-TERM CARE	REASON
—	Do lifesaving measures first; avoid mouth-to-mouth ventilation.	—	Radiation damage is rarely imminently life-threatening. Protect personnel from contamination.
—	Document prodromal symptoms: Anorexia, nausea, vomiting, diarrhea, fatigue, apathy, prostration, perspiration, erythema, conjunctivitis, fever, shortness of breath, excitability, ataxia.	—	Incidence of prodromal symptoms peaks 6–7 hours after exposure. Higher levels of radiation increase the number of people developing symptoms but don't affect the severity of symptoms in an individual. (These symptoms are nonspecific and could be induced by the suggestion of radiation exposure.)
CBC with differential, platelet count, initially and q4–6h	—	Protective isolation. Transfusions for support. May benefit from bone-marrow transplant.	Hematopoietic tissue is the most sensitive to radiation injury. The rate of change and absolute values of lymphocyte and granulocyte counts reflect the severity of injury and have prognostic value.
Serum electrolytes and blood chemistry	—	May need total parenteral nutrition for support.	Intestinal mucosa is sensitive to radiation injury, becoming denuded and ulcerated. Severity of symptoms peaks 10–12 days after exposure.
Chromosomal analysis: 10 ml heparinized blood on ice	—	Patient should use contraception for "several months" after exposure. Sperm analysis or amniocentesis for karyotyping recommended.	Gonadal tissue is sensitive to radiation damage.
	Photograph affected areas for best documentation of initial appearance.	Give sedative and analgesics.	The physical signs of radiation injury may be minimal initially. Signs vary from erythema to exudative dermatitis and depilation.

4

	—	Radiation burns are more painful than third-degree thermal burns, because the nerve endings remain intact.
	Palpate thyroid for pre-existing nodules.	Endocrine tissue is the second most sensitive to radiation injury. Thyroid cancer can be induced (after several years latency) at less than 10 rads of exposure.
EEG (if head was irradiated)	Thorough neurologic examination.	Nerve tissue is the most resistant to radiation injury. High doses can cause tremors, ataxia, convulsions, and rapid death.
X-rays of extremities (if irradiated)	—	Baseline for subsequent radiation necrosis.
Chest x-ray (if irradiated)	—	Baseline for subsequent radiation pneumonitis.
Ophthalmoscopy with slit lamp (if eyes were irradiated)	—	Baseline for subsequent radiation cataracts.
ECG (if thorax was irradiated)	—	Baseline for subsequent radiation myocarditis.
Collect rings, glasses, and samples of hair and nails.		Neutrons activate metal.

Suggested Reading

1. International Atomic Energy Agency. Manual on Early Medical Treatment of Possible Radiation Injury. Safety series no. 47. Vienna, Austria, 1978.
2. International Commission on Radiological Protection. 1978. The Principles and General Procedure for Handling Emergency and Accidental Exposures of Workers. ICRP publication no. 28. Oxford: Pergamon Press, 1978.
3. Leonard RB, Ricks RC. Emergency department radiation accidental protocol. Ann Emerg Med 1980;9:462–470.
4. Lincoln TA. Importance of initial management of persons internally contaminated with radionuclides. Am Ind Hyg Assoc J 1976;37:16–21.
5. Mettler FA Jr. Emergency management of radiation accidents. JACEP 1978;7:302–305.
6. Mettler FA Jr, Kelsey CA, Baram MS. Medical and legal implications of a large release of radioiodine. Nuclear Safety 1978;19:741–747.
7. Richter LL, Berk HW, Teates CD, et al. A systems approach to the management of radiation accidents. Ann Emerg Med 1980;9:303–309.

DISASTER MANAGEMENT: EVACUATION

A reference librarian pointed out the paradox in the term "disaster management." "If it were manageable, it wouldn't be a disaster." Nonetheless, the usual definition describes a situation that overwhelms the normal capacity of facilities.

One technique of disaster management, which may be used for toxic spills, flooding, fires, radiation exposure, and close encounters of the third kind, is evacuation. The scenario presented by the media is one of mass panic, confusion, breakdown of organization, pillaging, and poor morale. A study of 64 evacuations involving 1,142,336 people, however, showed that human nature is at its best during such a challenge. There were only ten deaths (one by a heart attack, two by drowning when a car was mistakenly driven into high water, and seven by a helicopter crash) and two injuries (one broken arm and one nonfatal heart attack). Vehicular traffic moved at an orderly 35 mph; there were no drunk drivers. Few people used public shelter or transport; most found their own accommodations and used private transportation. Though looting was reported frequently, it was rarely verified. The enthusiastic over-response of volunteer help actually caused logistic problems.

Reference:

1. Hans JM Jr, Sell TC. Evacuation risks — an evaluation. US Environmental Protection Agency PB-235-344, Las Vegas, 1974.

HOW HOT IT FEELS

When the apparent temperature (see table) rises above 130°F, the Weather Service warns that it is becoming extremely dangerous—heat stroke or sunstroke may be imminent. Between 105 and 130°F, sunstroke, heat cramps, and heat exhaustion are possible, and heat

Relative Humidity	Air Temperature										
	70	75	80	85	90	95	100	105	110	115	120
	Apparent Temperature*										
0%	64	69	73	78	83	87	91	95	99	103	107
10%	65	70	75	80	85	90	95	100	105	111	116
20%	66	72	77	82	87	93	99	105	112	120	130
30%	67	73	78	84	90	96	104	113	123	135	148
40%	68	74	79	86	93	101	110	123	137	151	
50%	69	75	81	88	96	107	120	135	150		
60%	70	76	82	90	100	114	132	149			
70%	70	77	85	93	106	124	144				
80%	71	78	86	97	113	136					
90%	71	79	88	102	122						
100%	72	80	91	108							

*Degrees Fahrenheit.

stroke is possible with prolonged exposure or physical activity. Of course, severity of heat stress will vary with age, health, and body conditions.

Reference:
    1. Reprinted from "U.S. News & World Report". Copyright, 1981, U S. News & World Reports, Inc. August 17, 1981:69. With permission.

HEAT INJURY IN LONG-DISTANCE RUNNING

Current interest in long-distance running and long-distance racing has contributed to an increasing number of heat injuries associated with such events, especially during the summer. The American College of Sports Medicine gives the following recommendations to reduce the risk of heat injury during racing events.

1. Distance races (16 km or 10 mi) should not be conducted when the wet-bulb temperature—globe temperature exceeds 28°C (82.4°F).

2. During periods of the year when the daylight dry-bulb temperature often exceeds 27°C (80°F), distance races should be conducted before 9:00 A.M. or after 4:00 P.M.

3. It is the responsibility of the race sponsors to provide fluids that contain small amounts of sugar (< 2.5 g glucose/100 ml of water) and electrolytes (< 10 mEq of sodium and 5 mEq of potassium per liter of solution).

4. Runners should be encouraged to ingest fluids frequently during competition and to consume 400 to 500 ml (13–17 oz) of fluid 10 to 15 minutes before competition.

5. Rules prohibiting the administration of fluids during the first 10 kilometers (6.2 mi) of a marathon should be amended to permit fluid ingestion at frequent intervals along the race course. In light of the high sweat rates and body temperatures produced during distance running in the heat, race sponsors should provide "water stations" at 3 to 4 kilometer (2–2.5 mi) intervals for all races of 16 kilometers (10 mi) or more.

6. Runners should be instructed in how to recognize the early warning symptoms that precede heat injury. Recognition of symptoms, cessation of running, and proper treatment can prevent heat injury. Early warning symptoms include the following: piloerection on chest and upper arms, chilling, throbbing pressure in the head, unsteadiness, nausea, and dry skin.

7. Race sponsors should make prior arrangements with medical personnel for the care of cases of heat injury. Responsible and informed personnel should supervise each "water station." Organization personnel should reserve the right to stop runners who exhibit clear signs of heat stroke or heat exhaustion.

An in-depth look at this problem was conducted during the 1979 Peachtree Road Race, held on July 4, in Atlanta, Georgia. England and coworkers found that greater levels of pre-race training, use of sprinklers during the race, and lower levels of exertion during the race were the significant factors that protected runners from the development of heat injury. In addition, the runners who suffered heat injury were taller than their matched controls. In contrast to the previous recommendations, there was no difference between groups with respect to fluid intake before or during the race. In addition, 91 per cent of runners who had heat injury experienced either no, or only one, warning symptom. And of 59 per cent of these runners who had any symptoms, nearly all reported weakness, tiredness, or dizziness as their only "warning" symptom.

References:
1. Gary J. Prevention of heat injuries during distance running: a position statement from the American College of Sports Medicine. J Sports Med 1975;*3*:194.
2. England AC 3d, Fraser DW, Hightower AW. Preventing severe heat injury in runners: suggestions from the 1979 Peachtree Road Race experience. Ann Intern Med 1982;*97*:196–201.

HYPERTHERMIA

Nonseasonal heat stroke is the final common pathway of a diverse group of disorders varying in cause, all of which are characterized by agitation and hyperthermia. Delirium tremens is the prototype of these disorders, and its treatment serves as a guide to proper management of the patient with hyperthermia and agitation of any cause. Figure 4–5 lists the disorders that may be associated with hyperthermia and the mechanism involved. Notice that a variety of prescribed drugs are implicated in these reactions.

Thermoregulatory Interference

DRUG	STIMULATION	UNCOUPLED OXIDATIVE PHOSPHOR-YLATION	MUSCULAR HEAT PRODUCTION	DECREASED SWEATING
Amphetamine	X		X	
Cocaine	X		X*	
Salicylates	X	X		
Antihistamines				X
Atropine				X
Phenothiazines	X		X	X
Lithium	X		X	
Phencyclidine	X		X	
Ethanol withdrawal	X		X	
Inhalation anesthesia			X*	
Succinylcholine			X*	
Pancuronium bromide			X*	
Tricyclic anti-depressant	X		X	X

*Malignant hyperthermia

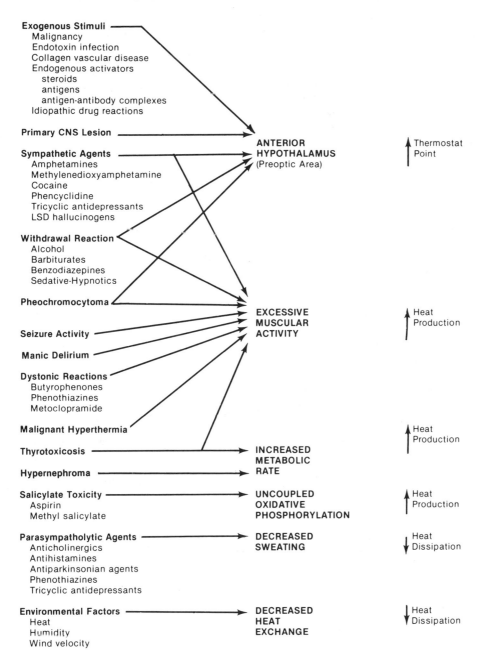

Fig. 4-5. The disorders associated with hyperthermia and their mechanisms.

Drugs Associated with Hyperthermia

HYPERSENSITIVITY, IDIOSYNCRATIC REACTIONS

Penicillin	Isoniazid
Methyldopa	Nitrofurantoin
Procainamide	Rifampin
Quinidine	Streptomycin
Sulfonamides	Mithramycin
Allopurinol	Phenytoin
Cephalosporins	Barbiturates
Hydralazine	Cimetidine
Iodides	

PYROGENIC STIMULATION

Bleomycin
Streptokinase
BCG

DRUG-DRUG INTERACTIONS

Lithium—haloperidol
MAOI—sympathomimetic amine
MAOI—tricyclic antidepressants

The initial treatment of any type of life-threatening hyperthermia involves hydration, sedation, avoidance of physical activity, and immediate cooling. Temperature reduction is especially important, and effective methods include sponging or splashing the entire skin surface with cool or iced water followed by fanning to promote evaporative cooling, application of hypothermic blankets, and the use of ice packs to the groin and axillae.

Iced water baths are not recommended for several reasons. It is more difficult to handle your patient, peripheral vasoconstriction may decrease heat transfer to the skin surface, and intense shivering may result that actually increases endogenous heat production. Infection should be searched for carefully.

Benzodiazepines are useful to control agitation. Dantrolene sodium is specifically indicated for malignant hyperthermia. All other medications must be discontinued if possible, particularly when a drug-related cause is suspected.

References:

1. Goldfrank L, Flomenbaum N, Lewin N, Weismann RS. Nonseasonal heatstroke. Hosp Phys 1982;*18*:50–70. (Figure and tables reproduced with permission.)

2. Vance M. Heat emergencies. *In*: Tintinalli J, ed. A Study Guide in Emergency Medicine: Dallas: American College of Emergency Physicians, 1978:5–25–5–30.

FROSTBITE

Frostbite is an injury caused by exposure to freezing temperatures. Injury is caused by freezing of the tissue or by anoxia secondary to vasospasm, or by both. The extent of injury is related to the amount of heat loss, and factors that increase heat loss, such as wind, wetness, and contact with metal or a volatile liquid, such as gasoline, will increase the risk of frostbite. Other factors that contribute to the development of frostbite include ethanol use, fatigue, immersion in water, and injury.

Ideally, prevention is the best way to decrease morbidity from frostbite, but when frostbite has occurred the most important principle of treatment is to avoid further injury to the affected part after rewarming. Thawed tissue is especially sensitive to such insults as additional thermal injury (both heat and cold), abrasion, and pressure. Rewarming should be delayed if further cold exposure is anticipated; some of the worst tissue damage occurs with refreezing. Rapid rewarming by immersion in a water bath maintained at 40°–42°C is the treatment of choice. At temperatures more than 45°C, thermal injury occurs. Rubbing of the affected part is contraindicated.

When the fingers and toes are involved, after rewarming, mechanical injury is avoided by placing cotton between them. Infection is prevented by keeping the injured part clean, ideally in a whirlpool bath with an antiseptic. Blisters should be left intact. If there is no infection, dead skin should be allowed to separate spontaneously. Maximum tissue preservation occurs when surgical debridement is delayed as long as possible, a period that may extend to months after the injury.

5

ORTHOPEDICS

ORTHOPEDIC INJURIES AND ASSOCIATED INJURIES 177

COMPLICATIONS OF FRACTURES 177

BLOOD LOSS FROM FRACTURES 178

CERVICAL SPINE INJURIES 179

LUMBAR SPINE X-RAYS 180

FRACTURES INVOLVING THE EPIPHYSEAL PLATE 180

GLASS IN THE HAND OR FOOT: TO X-RAY OR NOT? 182

ASSESSMENT OF HAND INJURIES 182

THE ADOLESCENT KNEE 187

ANKLE FRACTURES—MORE THAN MEETS THE EYE 192

THE 6 P'S OF COMPARTMENT SYNDROMES 195

IT'S AS EASY AS 1,2,3 (REFLEXES) 195

TWO FOR THE PRICE OF ONE (SENSORY) 196

ORTHOPEDIC INJURIES AND ASSOCIATED INJURIES

When one is evaluating injured extremities, the tendency is to look at the most obvious injury. By taking into consideration the mechanism of injury and by examining for associated injuries, other less apparent ones might be detected. The table lists the associated injuries to look for in patients with a specific injury.

SPECIFIC INJURY	ASSOCIATED INJURY
Knee	Hip fracture or dislocation
Hip	Opposite hip
Femur fracture	Hip dislocation
Calcaneus fracture	Lumbar spine (L1 and L2 most common)
Wrist	Elbow or shoulder

COMPLICATIONS OF FRACTURES

Definition of a fracture. A soft tissue injury that also includes bone.

In addition to examination of the fracture, the physical examination of the injured extremity must include a thorough search for associated injuries to adjacent structures, especially arteries and nerves. The following is a list of complications associated with various fractures and dislocations.

INJURY	COMPLICATION	INCIDENCE OF COMPLICATION
Fracture, medial two thirds of clavicle	Subclavian artery or vein or brachial plexus injury	Unusual
First rib fracture	Subclavian artery or vein or brachial plexus injury; may have severe chest injury	3% subclavian artery laceration 9% brachial plexus injury 47–64% severe chest injury (pneumothorax, hemothorax, pulmonary contusion, flail chest, hypoxemia)
Shoulder dislocation	Axillary nerve injury Axillary artery injury	2–35% Rare, only 200 cases reported
Humeral fracture	Radial nerve injury	5–10%, especially associated with spiral, distal third fractures
	Brachial artery injury	1%

Table continued on following page

INJURY	COMPLICATION	INCIDENCE OF COMPLICATION
Elbow fracture or dislocation	Ulnar nerve injury Brachial artery injury	10–15% 1–4%
Wrist fracture	Median nerve injury	Common, especially with displaced fractures
Posterior hip dislocation	Sciatic nerve injury	6–13%
Knee dislocation	Popliteal artery injury Tibial and common peroneal nerve injury	20–35% 17%
Ankle dislocation	Anterior and posterior tibial artery injury	Infrequent, unless displacement is great

Reference:
   Chipman C, Strangeland RG. Basic Principles of Emergency Orthopedics. *In*: Chipman C, (ed). Emergency Department Orthopedics. Rockville, Md.:Aspen Systems Corp., 1982:3. (Reproduced with permission.)

BLOOD LOSS FROM FRACTURES

Hemorrhage is the predominant cause of shock in trauma, and physicians are well attuned to seeking its source in the chest and abdomen. Scalp lacerations can also be the source of major bleeding. Finally, fractures, whether open or closed, can be a source of considerable blood loss, especially when multiple sites are involved. The degree of blood loss from fractures is not often appreciated, however. The following list summarizes the potential hemorrhage in liters of blood for various fracture sites.

FRACTURE SITE	LITERS OF BLOOD
Humerus	1–2
Elbow	0.5–1.5
Forearm	0.5–1
Pelvis	1.5–4.5
Hip	1.5–2.5
Femur	1–2
Knee	1–1.5
Ankle	0.5–1.5

Reference:
   Iverson I.D., Clawson DK. Manual of Acute Orthopedic Therapeutics. Boston: Little, Brown & Co., 1982:3. (Reproduced with permission).

CERVICAL SPINE INJURIES

"The radiologists' national flower is the hedge."
Bernstein's Precept

INJURY	MECHANISM OF INJURY	STABILITY	COMMENTS
Anterior subluxation	Flexion	Stable	Disruption of posterior ligament complex; 20% delayed instability.
Bilateral interfacetal dislocation	Flexion	Unstable	Disruption of anterior and posterior longitudinal ligaments and disc.
Wedge fracture	Flexion	Stable	
Clay shoveler's fracture	Flexion	Stable	Fracture of spinous process of C7, T1, or C6, in that order of frequency.
Flexion tear-drop fracture	Flexion	Unstable	Associated with acute anterior spinal cord syndrome: quadriplegia, loss of pain sensation and touch. Preserved vibration and position.
Hyperextension dislocation	Extension	Unstable	Transient or permanent neurologic deficit. Only finding on lateral x-ray may be soft tissue swelling.
Extension tear-drop fracture	Extension	Stable in flexion; unstable in extension	Triangular shaped fracture of the anterior, inferior aspect of vertebral body of C2.
C1 posterior neural arch fracture	Extension	Stable	
Hangman's fracture	Extension	Unstable	Bilateral pedicle fracture of C2.
Hyperextension fracture-dislocation	Extension	Unstable	Body of vertebra is displaced anteriorly.
Unilateral interfacetal dislocation	Flexion-rotation	Stable	Inferior facet of affected vertebra becomes wedged in intervertebral foramen.
Pillar fracture	Extension-rotation	Stable	Loss of superimposition of lateral masses on lateral x-ray: the double outline sign.
Bursting fracture	Vertical compression	Stable	Variable transient or permanent neurologic deficit.
Jefferson fracture	Vertical compression	Unstable	Bilateral fracture of anterior and posterior neural arch of C1.

Reference:
1. Harris JH, Harris WH. The Radiology of Emergency Medicine. 2nd ed. Baltimore: Williams & Wilkins Co., 1981:114–134.

5

LUMBAR SPINE X-RAYS

Signs and symptoms were correlated with radiographic findings in 552 patients who had lumbar spine x-rays in emergency departments. There was no significant association of x-ray findings with any historical data or symptoms. The results for the particular physical findings are shown in the next table. Group I includes those with normal radiographic findings and those with radiographic findings that might be significant etiologically, but wouldn't influence therapy. Group II includes those with definite bone injury.

Patient Totals and the Frequency of Physical Findings of the Combined Negative and Possibly Significant Groups (Group I) and the Positive Group (Group II)

PHYSICAL FINDINGS	GROUP I (NEGATIVE AND POSSIBLY SIGNIFICANT GROUPS %)		GROUP II (POSITIVE GROUP %)	
Normal*	197	(38.5)	4	(10)
Contusion/abrasion*	14	(2.7)	6	(15)
Tenderness*	211	(41.2)	29	(72.5)
Spasm	87	(17.0)	10	(25)
Sensory deficit	9	(1.8)	1	(2.5)
Motor deficit	4	(0.8)	0	(0)
DTR (deep tendon reflex) abnormality	25	(4.9)	3	(7.5)
Positive SLR (straight leg raising)	88	(17.2)	7	(17.5)
Multiple signs*	106	(20.7)	17	(42.5)
Total Patients	512	(100.0)	40	(100.0)

*Those occurring with statistically different ($P < .01$) frequencies between the two groups.

Note that 2 per cent of those with normal physical examination findings had x-rays showing bone injury. Those with contusions, abrasions, or tenderness, or with two or more physical findings, had a statistically greater frequency of x-rays showing bone injury than those with other physical findings. If a history of trauma and the three positively correlating physical findings had been used as the criteria for obtaining lumbar spine x-rays, only three cases of bone injury would have been overlooked.

Reference:
1. Patrick JD, Doris PE, Mills ML, et al. Lumbar spine x-rays: a multihospital study. Ann Emerg Med 1983;*12*:84–87. (Table reprinted with permission of the author and publisher.)

FRACTURES INVOLVING THE EPIPHYSEAL PLATE

Fifteen per cent of all fractures in children involve the epiphyseal plate. Correct diagnosis and treatment may prevent the growth disturbances that occur following 15 per cent of such injuries.

In Salter's textbook on musculoskeletal disorders, he classified fractures involving the epiphyseal plate as illustrated in the table.

Fractures Involving the Epiphyseal Plate

SALTER TYPE	DIAGRAM	DESCRIPTION	RADIOGRAPHIC FINDINGS	USUAL TREATMENT	PROGNOSIS FOR GROWTH*
I		Separation of the epiphysis	Soft tissue swelling by the epiphyseal line; widening of the epiphyseal line; displacement of the epiphysis from the metaphysis (may have bony avulsion at periosteal attachment)	Closed reduction	Excellent
II		Separation of the epiphyseal plate, with fracture extending into the metaphysis	Triangular fragment of the metaphysis attached to displaced epiphysis	Closed reduction	Excellent
III		Separation of the epiphyseal plate, with fracture extending through the epiphysis into the joint space	Vertical fracture through the epiphysis, to the epiphyseal plate	Open reduction	Good
IV		Fracture extending from the joint surface, across the epiphysis and epiphyseal plate, through the meta-physis	Fracture line through the epiphysis, epiphyseal plate, and metaphysis	Open reduction, internal fixation	Poor, unless perfect reduction is attained
V		Crush injury to the epiphyseal plate	Very difficult to diagnose (because epiphysis is not displaced)	Avoid Weight-bearing	Poor

*A good prognosis requires that the blood supply to the epiphysis be intact. This is usually the case, since the blood supply to the epiphysis typically enters from the epiphyseal surface. However, the blood supplies to the proximal femoral epiphysis and the proximal radial epiphysis cross the epiphyseal plate: as the plate is separated, the blood supply may also be interrupted, and avascular necrosis results.

References:
1. Harris JH Jr, Harris WH. The Radiology of Emergency Medicine. 2nd ed. Baltimore: Williams & Wilkins Co., 1981:604-613. (Line drawings reproduced with permission of the author and the Williams & Wilkins Co.)
2. Salter RB. Textbook of Disorders and Injuries of the Musculoskeletal System. Baltimore: Williams & Wilkins Co., 1970:417-422.

5

GLASS IN THE HAND OR FOOT: TO X-RAY OR NOT?

*"All foreign bodies are presumed opaque until an
x-ray is taken."*

Marshall B. Segal, M.D., J.D.

The presence or absence of a glass fragment in an injured hand or foot is an important factor in clinical management. Most of us have been taught that only leaded or pigmented glass will be evident on standard x-ray films. A study was undertaken to test this traditional clinical adage. Sixty-six common varieties of glass were embedded into the leg muscles of chicken cadavers. The fragments ranged from 0.5 to 14 mm in dimension. Standard soft tissue x-rays were taken in order to investigate the incidence of false-negative findings. The results demonstrated that:

1. All 66 varieties tested were clearly seen, including fragments as small as 0.5 mm.

2. The presence or absence of pigment did not noticeably affect their detectability.

3. Windshield glass particles from old (1930) and new car models were equally radiopaque.

The investigators concluded that fragments of glass embedded in an injured patient's hand or foot should be easily visible on standard x-rays.

Reference:
  1. Tandberg D. Glass in the hand and foot. JAMA 1982;*248*:1872.

ASSESSMENT OF HAND INJURIES

A large percentage of acute hand injuries can be cared for by the emergency physician. The most important responsibility of the primary care physician is to properly evaluate the injury and to determine if immediate consultation with an experienced surgeon is necessary.

Vascular supply, sensation, and motor and tendon function must all be tested. When you describe injuries to the hand, remember that there are five digits, but only four are called fingers (i.e., the index, long, ring, and small). The use of these terms avoids confusion.

Vascular Supply

The blood supply to the hand is via the ulnar and radial arteries. Patency of these vessels can be tested by using the Allen test. Press the radial artery firmly while the patient clenches his fist several times to clear blood from the palm and fingers. Then have the patient relax his hand. The skin should turn pink within a few seconds if the ulnar artery is patent. Repeat the test with pressure over the ulnar artery to test patency of the radial artery. You can also test the blood supply to individual digits by checking capillary filling at the nail bed or by pressing on the skin surface of the digit distal to the injury.

Sensation

This portion of the examination should be done prior to administration of anesthetic. Be sure to test ulnar, median, and radial nerve sensation. Two-point discrimination is the best test. Using calipers or tweezers, touch the patient lightly with both tips, then slowly move them closer together until the patient can no longer identify two points. This test should also be done on the non-injured hand for a normal control, usually 3–5 mm on the digits.

Motor Function

A complete evaluation of motor function includes that of the tendons and nerves. The following table lists the tendons and the appropriate maneuvers for testing them.

TENDON	TEST
Profundus flexor tendon	Flex distal phalanx while PIP (proximal interphalangeal) joint is held in extension
Flexor pollicis longus	Same as above (no PIP joint in thumb)
Superficialis flexor tendon	Holding all but finger to be tested in extension, flex finger to be tested at PIP joint. (Test ring and small finger together since superficialis may not function well independently in these digits.)
Extensor tendon	Patient may be able to extend digit even though extensor tendon is completely divided. The remaining fibrous bands allow extension; these bands will weaken over days to weeks, causing loss of extension. Explore these wounds carefully.

The next table lists the nerves, the muscles they innervate, and the maneuvers to test them.

NERVE	MUSCLE	FUNCTION
Median	Flexor pollicis brevis Abductor pollicis brevis Opponens pollicis	Abduction and opposition of the thumb to touch the small finger
Ulnar	Adductor pollicis	Adduction toward the first finger; test by holding a piece of paper between thumb and first finger.
	Interossei of hand	Test by spreading the fingers, i.e. adduction and abduction of the digits
Radial	Abductor pollicis longus Extensor pollicis brevis	Test by extending the thumb straight up
	Extensor digitorum	Test by extending the fingers with the wrist extended

Types of Injuries

Most lacerations, fingertip amputations, small areas of skin loss, and some extensor tendon lacerations or avulsions can be handled in the emergency department. Cleansing techniques and nerve blocks are discussed in other portions of this manual. (See Closing the Wound, page 198 and Regional Anesthesia, page 368.)

The accompanying table lists the injuries requiring immediate consultation and treatment by a hand surgeon. It also includes those injuries that can be managed with primary wound care in the ED and later referral to a hand surgeon and those that can be cared for entirely by the primary care physician.

Appropriate Care According to Type of Hand Injury

IMMEDIATE CONSULTATION WITH HAND SURGEON
Amputations other than fingertips
Heavily contaminated injuries (including human bites)
Injection injuries (with grease gun or paint gun)
Crush injuries
Joint injuries
Open fractures
PRIMARY WOUND CARE AND LATER REFERRAL
Nerve injuries
Injuries requiring skin flaps
Flexor tendon lacerations
Multiple extensor tendon lacerations
TREATMENT BY PRIMARY CARE PHYSICIAN
Most lacerations
Isolated extensor tendon avulsions or lacerations
Nail bed injuries
Small areas of skin loss
Multiple fingertip amputations

Nail Bed Injuries

Hematomas beneath the nail should be drained. A heated paper clip or battery-operated drill will work well, producing immediate pain relief.

If injury to the nail has occurred, you must evaluate the nail bed for laceration. If present, it requires closure with 6-0 ophthalmic chromic sutures. Adequate closure may necessitate removal of part or all of the nail. If the laceration extends into the nail bed skinfold, a nonadherent dressing should be placed in the sulcus to prevent skin adhesion to the bed. The nail will regenerate in three months.

Extensor Tendon Injuries

Injuries to extensor tendons are quite common because of the close proximity of these structures to the skin surface. Avulsion fractures of the attachment of the extensor tendon to the distal phalanx often result from blunt trauma. If the fractures are not treated appropriately a mallet finger results that is very difficult to repair at a later date (Fig. 5-1). Generally, splinting straight or in extension for six weeks gives excellent results. Dorsal splinting of the distal interphalangeal joint alone is adequate and allows normal use of the hand.

Another common injury is damage to the complicated extensor apparatus at the level of the proximal interphalangeal joint, resulting from lacerations. This wound can be repaired with 3-0 polypropylene suture and splinted in extension with good results. Failure to do so may lead to development of a boutonnière deformity (Fig. 5-2).

Extensor tendons at the metacarpal-phalangeal joints or over the dorsum of the hand will not retract; therefore, both ends are readily available for primary repair. Use 4-0 nylon and a figure-eight suture followed by splinting in extension. Isolated extensor tendon injuries will generally heal in three weeks.

INJURY	CLUES TO DIAGNOSIS
Mallet finger	Avulsion of extensor tendon attachment to the distal phalanx, creating a dropped tip or mallet finger (see Fig. 5-1).
Buttonhole (boutonnière) deformity	Laceration of extensor tendon attachment to the middle phalanx, causing eventual splitting of lateral bands allowing protrusion of joint through defect (see Fig. 5-2).
Gamekeeper's or skier's thumb	Complete tear of the ulnar collateral ligament, allowing more than 40 degrees of lateral motion at the metacarpal-phalangeal joint (normal up to 20°)

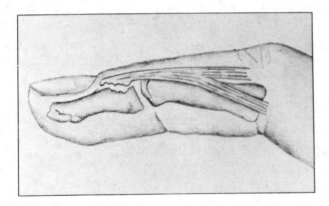

Fig. 5-1. Mallet finger. The distal insertion of the extensor tendon is avulsed. Closed treatment by immobilization is usually adequate.

Fig. 5-2. Buttonhole or boutonnière deformity with disruption of the extensor tendon over the proximal interphalangeal joint. The lateral bands spread the central slip defect, allowing the bone to protrude.

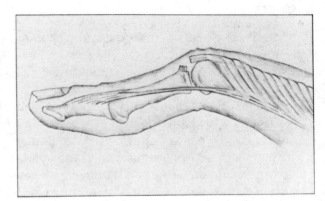

Thumb Injuries

Trauma to the thumb is of critical significance because of the thumb's role in 50 per cent of the hand's total function. With the amount of dependence on this digit, it is often held in full extension and abduction during trauma in the attempt to prevent or break a fall. As a result, injuries to the thumb occur more frequently than to any other digit. The preceeding table of this section contains a description of gamekeeper's thumb and gives clues to its detection. Tears of the radial collateral ligament of the metacarpal-phalangeal joint may occur, but they are less common and much less severe than a complete tear of the ulnar collateral ligament. Figure 5-3 shows the different motions of the thumb, and the second table of this section lists the nerves and muscles involved and their respective functions.

Dorsal and lateral dislocations caused by disruption of the radial collateral ligament respond well to closed reduction and splinting at 30 to 40 degrees of flexion for two to three weeks. If a lateral dislocation secondary to ulnar collateral ligament damage shows less than 40 degrees of instability, it may respond to splinting. Otherwise, these dislocations should be immobilized for five weeks in a spica cast. If there is greater than 40 degrees of instability or if there is a displaced fracture, surgical repair is necessary.

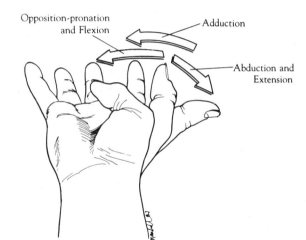

Opposition-pronation
and Flexion

Adduction

Abduction and
Extension

Fig. 5-3. Diagram of thumb motions.

References:
1. Achauer BM. Treating hand injuries in the emergency department. Hosp Physician 1983; 19(12):56-64. (Figs. 5-1 and 5-2 reproduced with permission.)
2. Carter P. Hand injuries and infections. *In:* Tintinalli J (ed.). A Study Guide in Emergency Medicine. Dallas: American College of Emergency Physicians, 1978:101-113.
3. Hay EL. Detecting and managing thumb injuries: a specialized approach. Emerg Med Rep 1983;4:42-47. (Fig. 5-3 reprinted courtesy of American Medical Reports.)

5

THE ADOLESCENT KNEE

The current emphasis on fitness and health, along with early institution of organized sports in our schools, has resulted in a greater number of orthopedic injuries related to these endeavors. The knee is the most commonly injured joint in sports and recreational activities; it is also the anatomic site that most often requires surgical intervention. There are four conditions that warrant immediate orthopedic referral: (1) intra-articular fractures, (2) complete ligamental tears, (3) complete muscle or tendon tears, and (4) mechanical blockage of normal knee motion.

The majority of the remaining complaints require nonoperative initial care, however, they do merit follow-up evaluation by an orthopedist to assure resolution and proper prevention of recurrence.

A complete history of the events surrounding the knee injury can immensely aid diagnosis. The following points are helpful:

1. "Straight-ahead" walking/and running rarely produce injury. If one occurs, it is usually caused by a recurring dislocation of the patella or dislodgement of a bony fragment (osteochondritis dissecans).

2. Deceleration with cutting (turning) maneuvers is apt to injure a meniscus or the anterior cruciate ligament.

3. Stepping in a hole or slipping on a wet surface can tear ligaments, menisci, or tendons.

4. Jumping or leaping usually injures the patellar tendon or dislocates it entirely.

5. Complete medial collateral ligamental tears are rare without a history of either a direct lateral blow (from a football helmet) or lever action (when ski-boot release fails).

6. Dashboard injuries can result in patellar fracture, or if more distal, posterior cru iate ligament involvement.

7. A "pop" or "snap" heard during deceleration or twisting indicates an anterior cruciate injury until proven otherwise.

8. The patient's own description of where the pain occurred at the time of injury is quite reliable; hours later, however, findings and complaints become more diffuse.

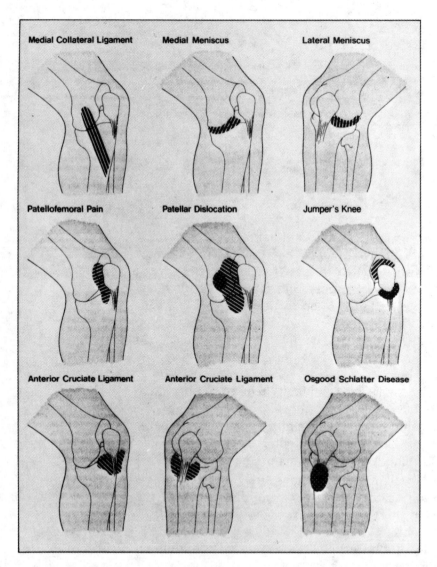

Fig. 5–4. Adolescent knee. Surface anatomy and landmarks.

9. If heat was applied to the knee after the injury (an unwise procedure), the joint will appear more swollen and, indeed, more tender than if heat was not applied.

Proper examination of the patient with a knee injury is facilitated if one is familiar with the surface anatomy and landmarks as shown in Figure 5–4.

The more commonly encountered acute knee syndromes are summarized in the following tables:

Medial Collateral Ligament Injury

HISTORY
   Direct blow to lateral part of knee
   "Outward twisting" stress to knee in a fall while skiing in
      which binding does not release
   Sensation of "tearing" or "letting go"
   Instability with ambulation usually means complete tear
   May be relatively painless (especially with complete tear)
   Diffuse swelling at 24 hours

EXAMINATION
   Swelling and tenderness over ligament
   Pain at full extension or flexion
   Medial instability: present with knee fully extended indicates a
      complete tear; present at 20 degrees of flexion with no firm
      end point indicates a complete tear

SPECIAL TESTS
   Stress roentgenograms if epiphyses open and complete tear
   suspected (to rule out epiphyseal fracture)

Anterior Cruciate Ligament Injury

HISTORY
   Weight-bearing
   Usually no direct blow to knee with cutting, deceleration, or
   jumping
   Feels a "pop" or "snap"
   Swelling within 24 hours
   Vague sense of Instability
   Modest discomfort

EXAMINATION
   Hemarthrosis (mild to moderate)
   Tenderness of anterior tibia
   Lachman test positive: lax with firm end point indicates
      a partial tear; no firm end point indicates a complete tear
   Drawer test: if positive, complete tear; if negative, no tear

SPECIAL TESTS:
   None

Patellar Dislocation (First Episode)

HISTORY
Usually weight-bearing
External rotation of foot
Partially bent knee
"Ripping" or "tearing" sound, which may be heard by others
Immediate disability, unwilling to bear weight
Immediate, severe swelling
Increasing pain with increasing swelling

EXAMINATION
Tense, large hemarthrosis
Tenderness medial to patella (occasionally lateral)
Knee held flexed 10–15°
Unwilling to contract (tighten) quadriceps

SPECIAL TESTS
Sunset roentgenographic view of patella may reveal intra-articular fracture
Fat floating in bloody aspirate indicates intra-articular fracture

Meniscus Injuries

HISTORY
Abrupt onset
Weight-bearing
Rotation of foot (internal or external)
Locking, inability to extend knee fully (occasional inability to flex fully)
Unlocking occurs abruptly, usually as result of manipulation ("shaking" or "twisting" knee)

EXAMINATION
If "locked," anteromedial or anterolateral joint line pain with attempts at extension
Tenderness over joint line (medial or lateral)
Effusion may or may not be present

SPECIAL TESTS
Arthrogram (ordered only with clinical evidence of impingement)

Finally, one must not forget knee problems that are caused by chronic abuse or overuse. While these are not dramatic injuries, they can lead to long-term problems if not recognized. The next table lists and describes the more pertinent overuse syndromes.

Overuse Injuries

PATELLOFEMORAL PAIN (CHONDROMALACIA OF PATELLA, QUADRICEPS INSUFFICIENCY SYNDROME, OR PATELLAR COMPRESSION SYNDROME)
HISTORY
Gradual onset
Diffuse pain (most likely medial)
Aching or "stiffness" after sitting with knee flexed
"Swelling"
Pain while climbing hills or stairs, and squatting
"Giving way"

Overuse Injuries (Continued)

EXAMINATION
    Atrophy and loss of tone in vastus medialis
    Tender behind patella-medial more often than lateral
    Effusion minimal if present
    Crepitation may be present

SPECIAL TESTS
    Clinical examination for femoral anteversion and/or external
      tibial torsion

JUMPER'S KNEE—PATELLAR TENDON TENDONITIS

HISTORY
    Participation in running/or jumping sport activity
    Recent growth spurt
    Pain with or after activity
    Pain at inferior pole of patella

EXAMINATION
    Point tenderness at inferior pole of patella deep in tendon
    Quadriceps tightness
    No effusion

SPECIAL TESTS
    None

OSGOOD-SCHLATTER DISEASE (TIBIAL TUBEROSITY APOPHYSITIS)

HISTORY
    Gradual onset
    Pain and swelling at tibial tuberosity
    Pain with or after running, jumping, or squatting
    May include patellofemoral pain symptoms

EXAMINATION
    Swollen, tender tibial tuberosity
    Pain with hyperflexion of knee
    Tight quadriceps

SPECIAL TESTS
    None

OSTEOCHONDRITIS DISSECANS

HISTORY
    If fragment is detached in knee: momentary locking, loose
      body sensation, recurrent effusions
    If fragment is not detached in knee: vague pain or aching,
      activity-related, no typical history (complaints that fit no pattern
      and are accompanied by essentially normal examination
      suggest osteochondritis dissecans until proven otherwise)

EXAMINATION
    If fragment detached: palpable loose body, often effusion
    If fragment not detached: may be effusion, may have femoral
      condyle tenderness, examination often normal

SPECIAL TESTS
    Knee roentgenograms should include notch view

5

Reference:
    1. Garrick V. Knee problems in adolescents. Pediatr Rev 1983:*4*:235–243. (Figure and tables reproduced with permission.)

ANKLE FRACTURES – MORE THAN MEETS THE EYE

Ankles are not just "broken": the type of fracture suggests the mechanism of injury, ligamentous damage, and methods for reduction.

In the 1940's, the Danish physician Lauge-Hansen took amputated legs, nailed the feet onto boards, and secured the boards in a vise. He maneuvered the limbs by hand to induce fractures, simulating various motions. The ankles were then x-rayed and dissected. He correlated the direction of injury with the resultant damage. His work forms the basis for the classifications of ankle fractures listed here, although his descriptions have been simplified.

The types of injuries are listed for each motion. Generally, impacting forces cause oblique or spiral fractures and avulsing forces cause transverse or horizontal fractures.

Inversion Injuries (Fig.5 - 5)

Laterally — a sprain, rupture, or avulsion (from the malleolus) of the lateral collateral ligaments, or a horizontal, tranverse fracture of the malleolus.

Medially — an oblique or spiral fracture of the malleolus; the deltoid ligament is rarely sprained.

Posteriorly — Fractures of the posterior tibia may be caused by inversion injuries or by posterior dislocations of the talus.

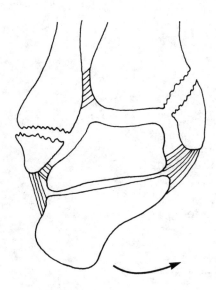

Fig. 5-5. Fractures typical of inversion injuries.[1]

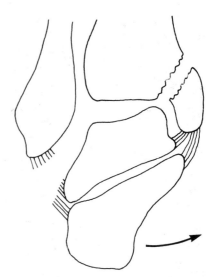

Fig. 5-6. Oblique medial malleolar fracture with rupture of the lateral collateral ligament.

Pearl. If an oblique fracture of the medial malleolus is present, and there is no fracture of the tibia, a rupture of the lateral collateral ligament must be present. It is evidenced clinically by increased movement of the foot around the leg during forced inversion (Fig. 5-6).

Pearl. When inversion fractures the posterior part of the tibia, the ankle mortise is widened. If there is no fracture of the lateral malleolus, the tibiofibular ligaments must be torn. To demonstrate the tear, move calcaneus and talus side-to-side, without inversion or eversion. The talus will bump against the malleoli (Fig. 5-7). (Posterior tibial fractures caused by compression need not have associated mortise widening and the lateral malleolus and tibiofibular ligaments may be intact.)

Fig. 5-7. Side-to-side motion of the talus with torn tibiofibular ligament and interosseous membrane.

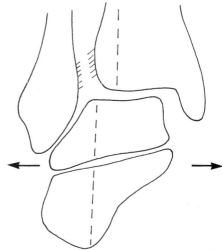
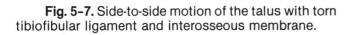

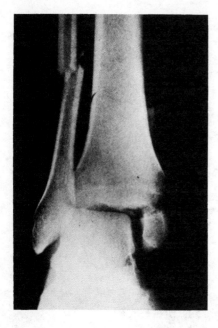
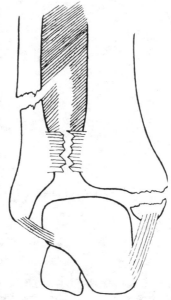

Fig. 5-8. Fractures typical of eversion injuries.[1]

Eversion Injuries (Fig. 5 - 8)

Laterally — an oblique or spiral fracture of the malleolus, or rupture of the tibiofibular ligaments (may occur with or without fracture of the fibula).

Medially — a sprain, avulsion (from the malleolus), or rupture of the deltoid ligament, or a transverse fracture of the medial malleolus.

Posteriorly — no involvement.

Pearls. If there is a spiral or oblique fracture of the distal fibula or diastasis of the tibiofibular joint and no evidence of tibial fracture, the deltoid ligament must be ruptured. It is evident clinically by excess movement of the foot around the leg with forced eversion (Fig. 5-9). If there is a transverse fracture of the medial malleolus and no evidence of a fibular fracture, there must be a tear of the tibiofibular ligament.

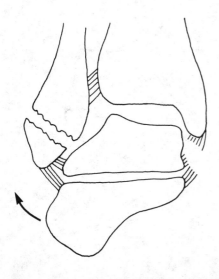

Fig. 5-9. Deltoid ligament rupture.

There can be complete rupture of the deltoid and tibiofibular ligaments without a fracture. Again, deltoid injury is tested by forced eversion, and injury of the tibiofibular ligament is tested by side-to-side movement. The injury may be seen as talar dislocation or tibiofibular diastasis on x-rays taken without stress. If the index of suspicion for ligamentous injury is very high, stress views may be used.

The Maisonneuve fracture is a special case, with disruption of the deltoid and distal tibiofibular ligaments and interosseous membrane, tibiofibular diastasis, and a fracture of the proximal third of the fibula. The fracture won't be seen on routine ankle films—the entire fibula must be shown.

References:
1. Edeiken J, Cotler JM. Ankle trauma. Semi Roentgenol 1978;13:145–155. (Figures reproduced with permission.)
2. Harris JH Jr., Harris WH. The Radiology of Emergency Medicine. 2nd ed. Baltimore: Williams & Wilkins Co., 1981:613–628.
3. Lauge-Hansen N. Fractures of the ankle. II. Combined experimental-surgical and experimental-roentgenologic investigations. Arch Surg 1950:60:957–985.
4. Roy SP. Sports medicine for emergency clinicians. *In:* Chipman C. (ed.). Emergency Department Orthopaedics. Rockville, Maryland: Aspen Systems Corp., 1982:144–145.

5

THE 6 P'S OF COMPARTMENT SYNDROMES

Pain — greatest when involved muscles are stretched.

Paresis

Paralysis

Puffiness

Pallor — check capillary refill.

Pulselessness — variable; compartment syndrome may exist in presence of pulses.

IT'S AS EASY AS 1,2,3 (REFLEXES)

To remember the nerve roots that are tested by the reflexes, all you have to do is start at the ankles and count to eight:

S1–2	Ankle jerk
L3–4	Knee jerk
C5	Brachioradialis
C6	Biceps
C7–8	Triceps

TWO FOR THE PRICE OF ONE (SENSORY)

By testing the appropriate areas of the upper and lower extremities, the sensory function of both peripheral nerves and spinal cord segments can be evaluated at the same time. These areas and the nerve and cord segments that they test are listed in the following table.

AREA TESTED	PERIPHERAL NERVE	CORD SEGMENT
Upper Extremity		
Shoulder (over deltoid)	Axillary	C4
Lateral forearm	Musculocutaneous	C5
Hand, dorsally, at base of thumb	Radial	C6
Tip of index finger	Median	C7
Tip of little finger	Ulnar	C8
Lower Extremity		
Proximal, anterior area of thigh	Genitofemoral	L2
Medial area of the thigh, above the knee	Obturator	L3
Anterior area of the thigh, above the knee	Femoral	L3
Medial area of the calf	Saphenous	L4
Web space between first and second toe	Deep peroneal	L5
Lateral area of the foot	Sural	S1
Posterior area of the thigh	Posterior femoral cutaneous	S2

6

SURGERY AND ITS SUBSPECIALTIES

SURGERY
CLOSING THE WOUND 198
ALL ABOUT SUTURES 202
TATTOOS TWO 204
TETANUS PROPHYLAXIS 204
THORACIC AORTIC DISSECTION 206
INTESTINAL OBSTRUCTION 208
ACUTE CHOLECYSTITIS 209
ACUTE PANCREATITIS............................ 210
TORSION OF THE TESTIS 214

OBSTETRICS AND GYNECOLOGY
PREGNANCY TESTS.............................. 215
VAGINAL BLEEDING DURING PREGNANCY 217
MATERNAL MEDICATION DURING PREGNANCY
AND BREAST-FEEDING 220

EAR, NOSE, AND THROAT
EVALUATING FOR FACIAL TRAUMA.................. 224
MANAGEMENT OF EPISTAXIS....................... 225
TINNITUS 228
FOOD OBSTRUCTION OF THE ESOPHAGUS 229
MISSING TEETH DEPARTMENT 230
ACUTE EPIGLOTTITIS IN ADULTS.................. 231

OPHTHALMOLOGY
THE RED EYE 232
CHEMICAL INJURY TO THE EYE.................... 232
FLASH BURNS TO THE EYE 233
TONOMETRY 234

CLOSING THE WOUND

"He that relieves pain is blessed, but he that causes none is doubly so."

Anonymous

1. Did you check both distal *sensation* and *motor function* before you anesthetized the patient?

2. Have you ordered *x-rays* for suspected fractures or foreign bodies? Ask for a soft tissue x-ray if there is any likelihood of metal, glass, stone, or wood foreign body. All types of glass give an x-ray shadow (see page 182). Retained foreign bodies greatly increase the risk of tetanus and infection.

3. *Clean the skin* with care but don't make it hurt. The best cleansing and the least pain are obtained by using pluronic F–68 (Shur-Clens®) a detergent solution that is not an antiseptic. Detailed wound cleansing should be postponed until the wound is anesthetized.

4. Local anesthetic *can* be injected painlessly. Since its purpose is to avoid pain, don't cause pain when injecting.

   a. Inject deep to the dermis through the cut edge of the wound where the pain fibers have already been divided. You should not inject through the intact skin because that hurts most. Infection risk is not increased by injecting through the cut. Wait two minutes for anesthesia to develop.

   b. Inject *slowly* and move the tip of the needle slowly to-and-fro while injecting. Rapid distention of tissues hurts a lot, especially if injection is made into dermis or into tight fibrous tissue. A small syringe (3 or 5 ml) and a fine needle (25 G or finer) both help to prevent a too rapid injection. A large syringe (10 ml or larger) and a large needle (21 G) make a too rapid injection easy to do, and you also lose the sensation of feeling a pressure that is too high.

   c. A warm solution (near body temperature) hurts less than a cold solution.

   d. Use 0.5 or 1 per cent lidocaine (maximum 7 mg/kg) or mepivacaine (maximum 7 mg/kg). Stronger solutions (2 per cent) inhibit healing, as does epinephrine, so avoid both.

   e. Aqueous 4 per cent lidocaine is an effective topical anesthestic when applied to abrasions. Soak a small (2″ × 2″) square of gauze and apply it to the abrasion for five minutes before scrubbing. Clean with a nailbrush or toothbrush.

      Viscous 2 per cent lidocaine adheres to mucous membranes and is useful in the mouth and nose and on abrasions.

      Lidocaine cream, 30 per cent, can be applied to the intact skin to anesthetize the skin.

5. *Irrigate effectively.* Don't assume that the wound is clean. *You* must

ensure that every wound is clean. You must look into each wound and irrigate any that are deep, or any that could possibly be contaminated. The irrigating fluid must be under high pressure and flowing fast to dislodge small foreign bodies, dirt particles, and bacteria. Recent studies have shown that low-pressure irrigation (e.g., bulb syringe or an IV bag and tube flowing with gravity only) is almost useless, even though it is traditional. You must use a large syringe (30 to 35 ml) that is compressed firmly and a small cannula or needle (19 G or smaller in diameter). Good irrigation sprays the surroundings, so a scrub suit is advisable. Use a nonirritant fluid such as pluronic F-68 (Shur-Clens) or lactated Ringer's solution.

6   *Debride precisely.* Good irrigation makes debridement much easier, because loosely attached nonviable tissue fragments (especially fat) are seen floating in the fluid. These fragments and any dirt-bearing areas are usually better excised, unless they are near to a neurovascular bundle; then you must depend on high-pressure irrigation and friction to dislodge foreign bodies. Magnifying lenses and loupes are especially helpful in recognizing hair and small particles in the wound.

If tissue is of doubtful viability, excision is wise so that only clean tissue with a good blood supply is left in the wound. Primary healing is then assured.

Record on the patient's chart the absence or presence of foreign bodies.

Puncture wounds (e.g., nail punctures, cat bites) are dangerous because effective irrigation and debridement are not possible unless the wound is opened.

Even dog bites have been closed primarily with an infection rate of less than 1 per cent when high-pressure irrigation and careful debridement were performed.

Human bites, when they create puncture wounds, especially of the hands, are irrigated, debrided, and left open initially. These patients are mostly treated as inpatients.

Delayed primary closure about five (± 1) days after injury is recommended for a wound in which effective debridement has not been achieved.

7. *Hemostasis* is best achieved by local pressure for both venous and arterial bleeding. Temporary use of a hemostat may help, but apply a hemostat only when there is visibility. Never grope blindly in a bleeding wound with a hemostat, or you may damage a main nerve. Superficial bleeding can nearly always be controlled by appropriately placed skin sutures. Ligation of bleeding vessels is not often needed in wounds seen in the emergency department, and buried sutures increase the chance of infection. Vasoconstricting drugs inhibit wound healing to some degree and it is better to avoid them. Tourniquets may cause nerve damage and are almost never advised.

8. *Close the skin* with monofilament, nonabsorbable sutures. Braided sutures have a capillary action and increase the infection rate. Silk

is the worst offender and should not be used. Nylon or polypropylene (Prolene) are preferred. Deep sutures should be placed only if a tissue plane needs to be closed; use the least number necessary. Use the finest absorbable suture that will hold the tissues together, i.e., polyglactin 910 (Vicryl) and polyglycolic acid (Dexon). The more buried sutures, the more risk of infection. Natural catgut may be useful for closing mucous membranes in the mouth, but has little place elsewhere. Fat layers should not be sutured.

Suggested suture sizes for the face are 6-0 suture on a fine needle (P-1) and for the fingers, 5-0. Limbs would be 4-0 and the scalp, 3-0 on a large needle.

A continuous suture (simple continuous with no locking) is much quicker to use for long wounds and heals as well as interrupted sutures.

Staples give excellent healing and are worth using on long wounds of limbs or trunk because they are quicker to use, and wounds heal better than with sutures.

Wound healing has been shown to be better when *adhesive tape closure* was used than when sutures were used; so tape closure is preferred when it gives a good closure. It is not practical on hair-bearing scalp areas or over moving joints. It is useful on facial wounds after early suture removal.

9. *Technical points* include the following:
   a. Sit comfortably on a stool with wheels, so you can position yourself as needed.
   b. A good light source is critical.
   c. Good instruments make a real difference. Use a needle holder; a hemostat used as a needle holder gives poor control. Use fine-toothed tissue forceps in your other hand (e.g., Adsons), so you can pull the tissue into the wound and thus place the stitch in the desired place.

      If you use your finger or thumb for counterpressure, be sure to have been vaccinated with hepatitis B vaccine or, better still, preserve your liver by using a forceps or a gauze swab in your other hand rather than your finger or thumb.

      Consider buying your own loupes. You will improve greatly your technical performance for finer work. They will last for 30 years, so their cost per year is not that high.

      Learn to use regional nerve blocks for the sole of the foot, for the palm, and for the digits. Start with a 27 G needle if you have not anesthetized the skin with 30 per cent lidocaine cream (see Regional Anesthesia, page 000).

      Record the wound's appearance on the chart with a simple diagram (= 10^3 words).

      Infection rates of 1 per cent or less have been reported from many centers, so higher infection rates are now quite unacceptable.

      Antiseptic solutions are not the secret of good wound care —mechanical cleaning of the wound is the common denominator of success. Using antiseptic solutions that cause pain and have been shown to inhibit wound healing is neither scientific nor humane.

The observations of Lister and Halstead are still very pertinent but surprisingly often misquoted. Dead space is not always evil, a hematoma is not always infected, and buried sutures and drain tubes are often better avoided.

Two questions concerning *prophylactic antibiotics* must be addressed. What is the effect of *systemic prophylactic antibiotics*, and what is the effect of *topical prophylactic antibiotics* flooded into the wound just before closure?

Systemic prophylactic antibiotics do not reduce the infection rate of clean wounds—indeed a higher infection rate, and growth of resistant bacteria, may result. Systemic antibiotic prophylaxis does not substitute for good local wound cleaning. However, for contaminated wounds, the advantage of systemic antibiotic prophylaxis is clearly evident. Human bites of the hand are about the most challenging of bites to treat. The cultures grow mixed organisms of which three quarters are usually resistant to penicillin, so a wide-spectrum antibiotic (e.g., cephalosporin) is mandatory in these cases, and careful wound debridement and delayed wound closure are usual. Call the hand surgeon for each knuckle bite.

The reported results after using *topical prophylactic antibiotics* are quite different from those after using systemic prophylactic anti-biotics. This fact seems to be a strange hiatus in the knowledge of most surgeons. Every reported study using randomized controls has shown a large advantage to the group receiving an antibiotic wound rinse before closure. Halasz, in 1977, identified 19 randomized and nonrandomized trials; all but one showed a much lower wound infection rate when topical antibiotics were used. The value of topical prophylactic antibiotics in surgical wounds seems to be established beyond scientific challenge. The only question remaining is what is the antibiotic of choice. One study showed that 10 ml of 5 per cent sodium benzyl penicillin was highly effective. Other investigators have used various wide-spectrum antibiotics, but later studies support Halasz's conclusion. Obviously, this question must be studied repeatedly, as antibiotics and current nosocomial bacteria change; but not to use topical prophylactic antibiotics is to ignore a mass of medical information.

0. Do you have a routine that ensures that no patient needing *tetanus prophylaxis* leaves the emergency department without receiving adsorbed tetanus toxoid and tetanus immune globulin (human)? Tetanus prophylaxis is so effective, and tetanus is such an awful disease to allow to develop (see Tetanus Prophylaxis, page 204).

Contributed by Eoin Aberdeen, M.D.

eferences:
1. Halasz NA. Wound infection and topical antibiotics: the surgeon's dilemma. Arch. Surg. 977;*112*:1240–1244.
2. Additional extensive reference list available on request.

ALL ABOUT SUTURES

"Never do an elective procedure in the ED."
          Marshall B. Segal, M.D., J.D.

Many types of sutures are available today. The emergency department physician would do well to learn the characteristics of but a few and to understand the setting in which each is used.

All suture material produces a foreign body reaction, but using the most appropriate and finest gauge suture that will do the job lessens the chance of infection and improves the cosmetic results.

Absorbable sutures are made of various materials including catgut, polyglycolic acid (Dexon), and Vicryl, a copolymer of glycolic acid and lactic acid in a ratio of 90:10. Catgut is digested by the proteolytic enzymes of inflammatory cells, a process that occurs at a variable rate of two weeks to two years. Polyglactin (Vicryl) and polyglycolic acid disappear at a more predictable rate, 80 days and 100 to 120 days, respectively. Absorbable sutures lose their strength more rapidly than they disappear. At 14 to 21 days both polyglactin and polyglycolic acid have lost all of their tensile strength; however, both of these synthetic sutures are stronger and produce less inflammatory reactions than catgut at all stages of healing in normal and infected tissue, because they break down by hydrolysis.

Nonabsorbable sutures are made of silk, cotton, nylon, polyester (Dacron), polypropylene (Prolene), and steel. They are classified as monofilament (nylon, steel, polypropylene) and multifilament (steel, nylon, silk, cotton, polyester). Silk is classified as nonabsorbable, but it has been clearly shown to lose all of its tensile strength after one year and usually disappears after two years. All nonabsorbable sutures produce an inflammatory reaction, silk and cotton the greatest, nylon, polypropylene, and steel the least. Because of their construction, multifilaments have a greater likelihood of infection; therefore, monofilament sutures are suggested for use when the chance of infection is high.

Nonabsorbable sutures should be used in the closure of skin and fascia and in the repair of lacerated tendons. Absorbable sutures are used to close periosteum, muscle, and subcutaneous tissue, and to ligate small blood vessels.

The *Guide to Suturing* lists types of sutures, techniques of suturing, and sizes used in various locations. It also includes a guide to skin suture removal. The numbers of square knots necessary to prevent slippage for each type of suture material are also listed.

Guide to Suturing

SKIN	SIZE OF SUTURE (NYLON OR POLYPROPYLENE)	TIME OF SUTURE REMOVAL (DAYS)	SUBCUTANEOUS TISSUE AND MUSCLE	STITCH USED
Face	6-0	3-5	4-0, 5-0 Dexon or Vicryl	Simple, simple running or subcuticular
Scalp	4-0	5-8	3-0, 4-0 Dexon or Vicryl	Simple, simple running
Trunk	4-0	7-10	3-0, 4-0 Dexon or Vicryl	Simple, vertical mattress, running simple or vertical mattress
Extremities	4-0	7-10	4-0 Dexon or Vicryl	Simple, vertical mattress, running simple or vertical mattress
Hands and feet	4-0, 5-0	10-14	4-0, 5-0 Dexon or Vicryl	Simple, vertical mattress
Mucous membranes	—	—	4-0, 5-0 Dexon or Vicryl	Inverted simple
Tendons	—	—	4-0 nylon or wire	Figure eight

Number of Square Knots

TYPE OF SUTURE	THROWS
Wire	2
Silk, cotton, and other braided multifilaments	3
Nylon, Vicryl, Dexon, and catgut	4

6

Linear skin wounds subject to low, static skin tensions can be closed with tape. Taped wounds clearly have superior resistance to infection when compared with sutured wounds. Not all wounds, however, can be closed with surgical tapes. Secretions in areas such as the palm, the soles of the feet, and the axillae limit the tape's adhesiveness. Wounds subjected to high skin tensions and those perpendicular to wrinkle lines or across joints will dislodge the tapes when underlying muscles contract or when the joint is flexed and extended.

References:
1. Cracroft D. Minor lacerations and abrasions. *In*:Kravis TC, Warner CG, (eds.) Emergency Medicine, A Comprehensive Review. Aspen Systems Corporation, Rockville, Maryland: 1983;137–154.
2. Edlich RF, Rodheaver GT. Scientific basis for emergency wound management. *In*:Rund DA, Wolcott BW. (eds.). Emergency Medicine Annual: 1983. Appleton-Century-Crofts, New York: 1983;1–31.
3. Van Winkle W, Hastings JC. Considerations in the choice of suture material for various tissues. Surg Gynecol Obstet 1972;*135*:113–126.

TATTOOS TWO

Tattoos One contains descriptions of tattoos that are acquired for body ornamentation. Tattoos that are the result of trauma are a different kind of problem for the emergency physician. These tattoos are undesirable, and proper wound care at the time of the patient's initial presentation is necessary to avoid them.

Typically the patient has fallen on dirty pavement or gravel, abrading the skin with tiny particles of sand or grit embedded in the wound. If these particles are not removed, they will remain in the skin and form an unsightly mark.

The key to management of this type of injury is adequate anesthesia. Occasionally, the patient has had enough ethanol before the injury so that no further anesthesia is required. Most of the time, however, a topical anesthetic will be necessary. Remember that a significant amount of anesthetic may be absorbed through the injured skin, so that the total amount used should be limited to nontoxic levels. This precaution is especially important for use on large areas, or for use in children. Sedation will also help, and general anesthesia will rarely be necessary.

Scrubbing the wound with an antiseptic soap and scrub brush removes most of the dirt. A toothbrush is also useful. For deeper particles, dermabrasion—scraping the skin with the sharp edge of a scalpel blade—will be necessary. Afterwards, antibiotic ointment is applied to the wound and a sterile dressing is applied. On the face, where bandaging may be difficult, frequent application of the antibiotic ointment will suffice.

TETANUS PROPHYLAXIS

"When in doubt, treat."
Marshall B. Segal, M.D., J.D.

In addition to appropriate local wound care, including irrigation and debridement of devitalized tissue, prevention of tetanus depends on proper immunoprophylaxis. It, in turn, is determined by the prior immunization history of the patient and the specific wound factors that increase the risk of tetanus. In a recent study of antitetanus treatment, Brand and coworkers found improper tetanus prophylaxis in 23 per cent of patients, with 6 per cent undertreated and 17 per cent overtreated. The accompanying tables outline appropriate tetanus prophylaxis, including recommendations for primary immunization. In addition, wound factors that predict tetanus risk are identified.

Primary Immunization Against Tetanus

Children	DPT at age 2 months, 4 months, and 6 months
	DPT at age 18 months
	DPT at age 4–6 years
	dT at age 16 years (and every 10 years following)
Adults	dT initially and one month later, then
	dT one year later and every 10 years following

Note: dT contains less diphtheria toxoid than DT and should be used for adults and children over age 7 years. DT is used for children less than 7 years of age.

Tetanus Prophylaxis for Open Wounds

PRIOR IMMUNIZATION	CLEAN WOUNDS		DIRTY WOUNDS	
	Tetanus Toxoid*	*Tetanus Antitoxin†*	*Tetanus Toxoid**	*Tetanus Antitoxin†*
None or incomplete	Yes‡	No	Yes‡	Yes
Complete and				
Last booster within 5 years	No	No	No	No
Last booster within 5-10 years	No	No	Yes	No
Last booster > 10 years previously	Yes	No	Yes	No

* If < 7 years old, DT 0.5 ml IM; otherwise, dT 0.5 ml IM

† Dose schedule:

Age	*Moderately Tetanus-prone (units)*	*Very Tetanus-prone (units)*
< 5 years	75	150
5–10 years	125	250
> 10 years	250	500

‡Complete primary immunization

Wounds and Tetanus Risk

NOT TETANUS-PRONE	MODERATELY TETANUS-PRONE	VERY TETANUS-PRONE
Exposed to low level of bacteria (household objects) Wound does not satisfy criteria for moderately or very tetanus-prone	Exposed to moderate level of bacteria (wood, pavement, industrial areas, and non-abdominal bullet wounds) Crush injury Puncture wound Wound extending into muscle	Exposed to high level of bacteria (barnyard, sewer, meat-packing plant, and bullet wounds to the colon) Wound more than 24 hours old Wound with devitalized tissue that cannot be debrided

References:
1. Brand DA, Acampora D, Gottlieb LD, et al. Adequacy of antitetanus prophylaxis in six hospital emergency rooms. N Engl J Med 1983;*309*:636–640.
2. Diphtheria and tetanus toxoids and pertussis vaccine. MMWR 1981;*30*:392–96, 401–407, 420.

THORACIC AORTIC DISSECTION

Thoracic aortic dissection is a hematoma that develops in the wall of the aorta as a result of an intimal tear. Although the pathology is similar, the clinical presentations and treatments of patients with thoracic aortic dissection vary depending on the site of the dissection. Most clinicians distinguish between dissections that include the ascending aorta—proximal, Type A, or Types I and II—and those that do not—distal, Type B, or Type III. Hypertension and aortic atherosclerosis are common with distal dissections, whereas Marfan's syndrome and cystic medial necrosis are more common in proximal dissections. Proximal lesions are more commonly associated with complications, such as congestive heart failure, which is usually secondary to acute aortic insufficiency; cerebral vascular accident secondary to occlusion of the carotid arteries by the hematoma; and acute cardiac tamponade secondary to rupture of the hematoma into the pericardial sac. Complications of distal dissections include rupture and organ ischemia when the dissection extends distally into the abdomen, occluding major branches of the aorta. The clinical presentations of 124 patients with aortic dissections were reviewed by Slater and DeSanctis,[1] and are summarized in the accompanying table.

Emergency treatment is geared toward reducing the chance of further dissection. Thus, in the hypertensive patient, nitroprusside or trimethaphan infusion is used to lower the systolic blood pressure to 100 to 120 mmHg. In addition, intravenous propranolol can be used to decrease the force of cardiac contraction and reduce the shearing forces acting on the aorta. Analgesics are indicated for patients who experience pain after these measures have been instituted. Of course, if life-threatening complications, such as tamponade or rupture, develop, immediate surgical intervention is undertaken. Otherwise, after medical therapy has been initiated, the patient should have aortography to determine the site of the dissection. Generally, proximal dissections are repaired surgically, whereas distal dissections are sometimes treated medically. The decision should be made by an experienced cardiothoracic surgeon. If one is not available, early transfer of the patient to an appropriate hospital for treatment should be arranged.

Reference:
1. Slater EF, DeSanctis RW. The clinical recognition of dissecting aortic aneurysm. Am J Med 1976;*60*:625–633.

Clinical Presentation and X-ray Findings in Patients
with Thoracic Aortic Dissections

	PROXIMAL	DISTAL
Male	36	54
Female	17	17
Age [years] Mean (range)	55(19-75)	62(42-81)
Predisposition	Total = 53	Total = 71
Hypertension*	34	68
Marfan's syndrome†	5	1
Cystic medial necrosis*	16	4
Arteriosclerotic aorta*	0	9
Presenting Symptom	Total = 53	Total = 71
Pain	47	69
alone	37	66
with syncope	4	2
with CHF	4	1
with CVA	2	0
CHF without pain	4	0
CVA without pain	2	0
Abnormal chest x-ray findings without pain	0	2
Site of major pain	Total = 47	Total = 69
Anterior area of chest*	31	19
Posterior area of chest*	5	39
Both	4	8
Site of any pain	Total = 47	Total = 69
Anterior*	23	4
Posterior*	5	25
Both	19	20
Back pain*	23	65
Jaw and throat†	12	7
Physical Findings	Total = 53	Total = 71
Hypertension*	5	40
Hypotension*	12	1
Pulse deficit*	27	11
Aortic regurgitation*	36	4
Neurologic manifestations*	19	4
X-ray Findings	Total = 45	Total = 71
Abnormal aortic contour	34	64
Possible abnormal aortic contour	8	5
Normal	3	2
"Calcium sign" (aortic calcification separated from wall of the aorta)	0	10
Pleural effusion	2	9

*p: < 0.01.
†p: < 0.05.

The astute reader will notice that the totals given and sums of the columns are not equal. This is because small numbers of patients with atypical findings were not included in this summary but can be found in the original reference.

INTESTINAL OBSTRUCTION

Intestinal obstruction is a serious emergency that leads to a fatal outcome in most cases without surgical intervention. In order to prevent serious morbidity or mortality, early diagnosis and definitive treatment are mandatory. Diagnosis depends on the history and the physical examination. The cardinal symptoms and signs of intestinal obstruction include pain, nausea, vomiting, constipation or obstipation, distension, tenderness, visible peristalsis, and shock. These symptoms and signs may be present or absent in variable patterns, depending on the location of the obstruction, the delay between onset of symptoms and the patient's presentation to the emergency department, involvement of the mesentery and its vessels, and the completeness of the obstruction.

In general, three syndromes of obstruction can be identified, although overlap occurs. These syndromes are characterized by the anatomic site of obstruction, and the findings of each are compared in the accompanying table. If the mesentery and its vessels are involved, the symptoms and signs are more severe. Greater severity is also found with complete, as opposed to partial, obstruction. When compression of the mesentery and its vessels is present, the situation is urgent and requires early operative intervention. There is a rapid onset of symptoms with early vomiting and severe pain. The severity of these symptoms usually leads to the early presentation of the patient and thus, distension is not usually present. Signs of peritonitis also may be present.

The common causes of obstructions differ with age. Hernia is the most frequent reason for obstruction for all ages. In adults, other usual conditions, in order of occurrence, are adhesions, intussusception, cancer, and volvulus. In children, the common problems are pyloric stenosis, ileocecal intussusception, congenital anomalies, such as atresia or annular pancreas and adhesions.

Emergency management includes resuscitation using crystalloid. Often, a central venous line will be necessary. A nasogastric tube and Foley catheter should be placed. Laboratory evaluation includes CBC and serum electrolytes. X-rays of the abdomen, including supine and upright films, and a chest x-ray should be obtained.

Syndromes of Intestinal Obstruction

		UPPER SMALL BOWEL OBSTRUCTION	LOWER SMALL BOWEL OBSTRUCTION	COLON OBSTRUCTION
Symptom	Pain	Acute, severe, frequent (every 3-5 min)	Less severe, less frequent (every 6-10 min)	May be minimal
or	Vomiting	Early, violent, frequent, bilious, not feculent	Late, progressing to feculent vomiting	Late and infrequent
Sign	Distension	Minimal (in epigastrium) Greater with strangulation	Progressive and generalized	Early and remarkable (except with intussusception, when it may be absent)

ACUTE CHOLECYSTITIS

Acute cholecystitis is an inflammatory process of the gallbladder usually caused by the impaction of a gallstone in the cystic duct. Patients present with acute abdominal pain in the right upper quadrant, which often radiates to the infrascapular region. There is usually fever, nausea, vomiting, and anorexia. On physical examination, tenderness is found in the right upper quadrant, with guarding and rebound tenderness. There may be a mass palpated in the right subcostal region. Murphy's sign (midinspiratory arrest during palpation in the right subcostal region) is usually present. Laboratory findings include leukocytosis, mildly elevated levels of liver transaminases, alkaline phosphatase, and often bilirubin. The bilirubin level may be as high as 5 mg/100 ml, but higher levels usually indicate obstruction of the common bile duct.

Diagnosis of acute cholecystitis can usually be made on the basis of the history and physical examination. There are a variety of acute processes that must be considered in the differential diagnosis, however, and they are listed in the accompanying table. In addition to the history, physical examination, and laboratory findings, further studies are warranted to confirm the diagnosis. Abdominal and chest x-rays should be obtained. Some 15 per cent of patients will have calcified gallstones. In addition, air in the biliary tree, as a result of cholecystoenteric fistula, may be identified.

Other methods of visualizing the gallbladder include oral cholecystography, intravenous cholangiography, ultrasonography, and radionuclide cholescintigraphy (HIDA scan). The HIDA scan is most useful. Within 30 to 60 minutes after injection of labeled HIDA, radionuclide will normally be detected in the common bile duct, gallbladder, and intestine. Nonvisualization of the gallbladder with visualization of the common bile duct and duodenum suggests acute cholecystitis with a sensitivity and specificity of approximately 95 per cent. HIDA scan is less useful when the bilirubin level exceeds 5 mg/100 ml.

Ultrasonography of the gallbladder is also helpful in diagnosing acute cholecystitis. The presence of gallstones in a patient with the clinical findings of acute cholecystitis strongly supports the diagnosis. In addition, ultrasonography provides some extra information about other organs in the region. Evidence of common bile duct dilatation, pancreatitis, and kidney disease may be obtained. Its disadvantage is that bowel gas, secondary to an ileus that is often present in these patients, or excessive adipose tissue, may make ultrasonic imaging difficult, limiting its usefulness.

Oral cholecystography is an extremely useful study for patients with chronic cholecystitis, but not for patients with acute cholecystitis. It may take 24 to 48 hours to complete, and factors that lead to nonvisualization of the gallbladder are common in patients with suspected acute cholecystitis. These factors include difficulty ingesting the dye because of nausea and vomiting, ileus or intestinal obstruction preventing the dye from being absorbed, and upper biliary tract

6

obstruction preventing the dye from entering the gallbladder. Likewise, with the availability of much better tests, intravenous cholangiography is not useful in diagnosing acute cholecystitis. It cannot be done with a bilirubin level greater than 3 mg/100 ml and carries a high false-negative rate.

Thus, patients with acute right upper quadrant pain and a clinical diagnosis of acute cholecystitis should have either HIDA scanning or ultrasound examination to confirm the diagnosis. The treatment of choice is cholecystectomy.

Differential Diagnosis of Acute Cholecystitis

Peptic ulcer disease
Acute pancreatitis
Viral hepatitis
Alcoholic hepatitis
Hepatic abscess
Renal calculus
Acute pyelonephritis
Acute appendicitis
Fitz-Hugh–Curtis syndrome
Salpingitis
Acute myocardial infarction
Right lower lobe pneumonia

Reference:
1. Matolo NM, LaMorte WW, Wolfe BM. Acute and chronic cholecystitis. Surg Clin North Am 1981;*61*:875–83.

ACUTE PANCREATITIS

Pancreatitis is a term that describes a spectrum of diseases involving inflammation of the pancreas. The process may be one of chronic, low-grade symptoms to rapidly progressive deterioration and death within hours. Pathologically, peripancreatic edema may be the only finding. Extensive hemorrhage or fat necrosis sometimes may be present.

More than 95 per cent of patients with pancreatitis will present with abdominal pain, and most will also have nausea and vomiting. The pain is usually epigastric and often is described as radiating to the back. Physical examination reveals upper abdominal tenderness, guarding, and frequently fever and tachycardia. The problem is that a variety of acute abdominal processes also have a similar constellation of signs and symptoms. The differential diagnosis is presented in the accompanying table.

Three fourths of acute pancreatitis cases are associated either with gallstones or with heavy alcohol intake. In addition, a variety of causative factors have been implicated in acute pancreatitis and are listed in the accompanying table. However, in approximately 20 per cent of cases, no etiologic factor can be identified.

When history, physical examination, and the presence of etiologic factors suggest a diagnosis of acute pancreatitis, serum amylase level determination may help confirm it. More than 90 per cent of patients will have an elevated serum amylase level, but it is not specific for acute pancreatitis. Many of the diseases included in the differential diagnosis are associated with elevated serum amylase levels to varying degrees. Measurement of the ratio of amylase clearance to creatinine clearance has also been used to help confirm the diagnosis, with variable results.

Treatment of acute pancreatitis is generally medical, with careful monitoring of fluid and respiratory status. Whereas no single clinical factor correlates with outcome, Ranson[1] has identified several factors that have prognostic significance. These factors are listed and the presence of three or more of them is associated with a major increase in morbidity and mortality, as indicated.

In summary, pancreatitis is a disease of variable severity, with a differential diagnosis that includes many processes that require early surgical intervention. Diagnosis is clinical on the basis of history, physical examination, and the presence of etiologic factors. Laboratory confirmation adds to the clinical diagnostic impression.

6

> "The majority of abdominal pains which ensue in patients who have been previously fairly well, and which last longer than six hours, are of surgical import."
>
> SIR ZACHARY COPE

Differential Diagnosis of Acute Pancreatitis

Perforated peptic ulcer
Acute cholecystitis
Perforated gastric carcinoma
Acute appendicitis
Ruptured spleen
Liver abscess
Alcoholic hepatitis
Acute porphyria
Perinephric abscess
Myocardial infarction
Mesenteric thrombosis or embolism
Ischemic colitis

Early Prognostic Signs of Risk of Major Complications in Patients with Acute Pancreatitis

At admission or diagnosis
    Age over 55 years
    WBC > 16,000/mm^3
    Blood glucose > 200 mg/100 ml
    Serum LDH > 350 IU/I
    SGOT > 250 units
During initial 48 hours
    Hematocrit drop > 10 points
    BUN rises > 5 mg/100 ml
    Serum calcium < 8 mg/100 ml
    Arterial Po$_2$ < 60 mmHg on room air
    Base deficit > 4 mEq/I
    Estimated fluid sequestration > 6000 ml

Number of Positive Early Prognostic Signs Correlated with Morbidity and Mortality in 450 Patients with Acute Pancreatitis

Number of Positive Signs

	0–2	3–4	5–6	7–8
Number of patients	347	67	30	6
Number who died (%)	3(0.9)	11(16)	12(40)	6(100)
Number who survived more than 7 days of intensive care (%)	10(2.9)	16(24)	16(53)	
Number who died or needed more than 7 days of intensive care (%)	13(3.7)	28(40)	28(93)	6(100)

Etiologic Factors in Acute Pancreatitis

Alcohol abuse
Gallstones
Abdominal trauma

Viral infections
  Mumps
  Coxsackie virus, Group B
  Infectious mononucleosis
  Viral hepatitis
Metabolic problems
  Types I, IV, or V hyperlipoproteinemia
  Diabetic ketoacidosis
  Kwashiorkor
  Hypercalcemia associated with hyperparathyroidism, sarcoidosis,
    multiple myeloma, or hypervitaminosis D
Drugs
  Steroids
  Diuretics
  Immunosuppressants
  Oral contraceptives
  Isoniazid
  Salicylates
Duodenal disease
  Periampullary diverticula
  Crohn's disease
Postoperative complications
Pregnancy
Cancer of the pancreas
Scorpion bite
Toxins
  Methanol
  Zinc oxide
  Cobaltous chloride
Hereditary
Vascular disease
  Atheromatous embolization
  Polyarteritis nodosa
  Systemic lupus erythematosus
Endoscopic retrograde choledochopancreatography (ERCP)
Hypothermia

Reference:
  1. Ranson JHC. Acute pancreatitis—where are we? Surg Clin North Am 1981;*61*:55-70.
(Tables reproduced with permission.)

6

TORSION OF THE TESTIS

"Surgery is advisable in every instance in which there is doubt. In our experience there is always a doubt."

THOMAS A,
Testicular torsion. JACEP
1979;*828*:31.

"Torsion of the testis remains unrivaled among surgical emergencies for the frequency with which it is misdiagnosed."

BAILEY.
Hamilton Bailey's
Demonstration of Physical
Signs in Clinical Surgery.

Testicular torsion is one of the more difficult problems of differential diagnosis for the emergency physician. Differential diagnosis includes incarcerated hernia, epididymo-orchitis, and scrotal trauma. One approach is to consider acute scrotal problems as testicular torsion until proved otherwise by surgical exploration. This approach is based on several factors. First, testicular salvage is inversely proportional to the time delay between onset of symptoms and surgical correction. Second, many of the clinical findings, both the history and the physical examination, are confusing or unreliable, leading to the wrong initial diagnosis and thus a delay in treatment. Finally, whereas most cases of testicular torsion occur during puberty, as many as 25 per cent of cases occur in adults more than 20 years of age.

Doppler ultrasonography and testicular scanning have been employed to increase the diagnostic accuracy of the acute scrotum. An ultrasonic stethoscope is placed over the affected scrotum. The absence of pulsations represents a loss of blood flow to the testis. The presence of pulsations, which are lost with pressure on the spermatic cord, indicates adequate blood flow. Pulsations that do not disappear with spermatic cord pressure are due to increased scrotal wall blood flow, and this results in an indeterminate test. The procedure is accurate to approximately 80 per cent.[1] Testicular scanning, using 99^m technetium pertechnetate is much more accurate, approaching 100 per cent in some series.[2]

Despite the accuracy of these newer techniques, they are not infallible. When, after careful evaluation that includes history, physical examination, and laboratory and diagnostic studies, the diagnosis of torsion remains a possibility, early operation remains the gold standard for the diagnosis and treatment of this problem.

References:
    1. Rodriguez DD, Rodriguez WC, Rivera JJ, et al. Doppler ultrasound versus testicular scanning in the evaluation of the acute scrotum. J Urol 1981;*125*:343–46.
    2. Stage KH, Schoenvogel R, Lewis S. Testicular scanning: clinical experience with 72 patients. J Urol 1981;*125*:334–337.

PREGNANCY TESTS

Knowledge of the presence of pregnancy can be medically critical. It prevents the administration of potentially teratogenic x-rays or drugs. It assists in excluding or including diagnoses, especially that serious but elusive condition, ectopic pregnancy. If the pregnancy test is understood, its results will not be given undeserved significance. The charts show the sensitivities of urine and serum pregnancy tests of various manufacturers. Note that the units of urine tests are IUs (international units), whereas those of serum tests are mIUs (*milli-international units*).

Protein, blood, drugs (such as methadone), bacteria, and detergent may interfere with urine test results. Thus, a patient with a urinary tract infection may show a false-positive test for pregnancy. IUDs and tubo-ovarian abscesses have also caused false-positive test results.

The graph (Fig. 6–1) shows typical levels of serum hCG. Urine concentrations of hCG correlate with serum levels but are altered by

6

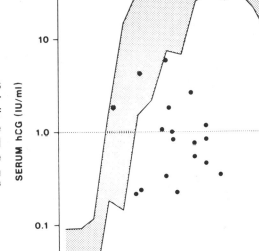

Fig. 6-1. Serum hCG levels in early pregnancy. The upper line (···) indicates the level of detection of urine tests, the lower line (---) indicates the level of detection of serum tests. The dots represent the levels found in patients with ectopic pregnancy.[3]

urine volume. Generally, the amount of hCG in 1 liter of serum equals the amount in a 24-hour urine collection. If urine production is 1 liter per 24 hours, serum and urine hCG concentrations are roughly equivalent. The upper line indicates the level of detection of typical urine tests; the lower line indicates the level of detection of typical serum tests. The graph also illustrates that patients with ectopic pregnancy have lower levels of hCG than normal; therefore, urine pregnancy tests are even less likely to be positive. This finding also occurs in patients with a "blighted ovum" and an inevitable abortion. Serum tests detect most patients with ectopic pregnancy, except for those with chronic conditions (about 2 per cent).

Ask your hospital's laboratory staff what kit they use for pregnancy tests. Find the level of sensitivity from these charts. Mark the level on the graph to get an idea of how soon after the last menstrual period you might expect a pregnant patient to show a positive result.

Slide Tests (Urine)

KIT	SENSITIVITY (IU hCG/ml)	EARLIEST DETECTION
Pregnosis	1.5–2.5	5 days FMP*
UCG-Slide Test	2	5 days FMP
Dap Test Macro	2	4 days FMP
Pregnosticon Dri-Dot	1–2	5–7 days FMP
Pregnosticon Slide Test	1–2	5 days FMP
Gravindex 90	3.5	No claim (~7–10 days FMP)
Pregnate	2–4	No claim (~7–10 days FMP)
Pregna β-Slide	2	No claim
Sensi-Tex	0.25	At or before missed period
Placentex	1.0	4 days FMP
UCG-Test	0.5 (undiluted; 1.3 (diluted)	4 days FMP
UCG-Quik-Tube	1.0	4 days FMP
UCG-Lypho-Test	0.5–1.0	4 days FMP
Neocept	0.2	At or before missed period
Pregnosticon Accuspheres	0.75–0.85	4 days FMP
Gravindex 90	0.5	4–7 days FMP
Pregna-β	0.4–0.8	4 days FMP

*Following Missed Period.

Radioassays –

KIT	SENSITIVITY (mIU hCG/ml)
Roche β-hCG RIA	6 (50 cutoff)
Beta-Tec	30 (range 3–50)
Preg-CG Assay	40
Radioimmunoassay of hCG beta subunit specific	0.4 (range 2–1000)
Concept-7-βHCG	30 (serum) 100 (urine)
Chorlo-Shure	40
RIA-Nate	25
β-hCG Radioimmunoassay Kit	30 (serum) 100 (urine)
HCG-β Radioimmunoassay Kit	< 6
HCG-β Radioimmunoassay Kit	< 20
Beta-hCG RIA	5
Beta-hCG Pregnancy Assay Monitor	40
Preg-Stat	25
RSL hCG β-subunit kit	not stated (< 0.5 ng hCG/ml; 2.5 mIU hCG/ml is stated as negative for hCG)
Biocept-G	200

6

References:
1. Derman R, Corson SL, Horwitz CA, et al. Early diagnosis of pregnancy. A symposium, J Reprod Med 1981;*26*(suppl 4):149–178. (Tables adapted with permission.)
2. Pritchard JA, MacDonald PC. William's Obstetrics. 15th ed. New York: Appleton-Century-Crofts, 1976: 209.
3. Rasor JL, Braunstein GD. A rapid modification of the beta-hCG radioimmunoassay. Use as an aid in the diagnosis of ectopic pregnancy. Obstet Gynecol 1977;*50*:557. (Figure adapted with permission.)

VAGINAL BLEEDING DURING PREGNANCY

Abnormalities during pregnancy threaten both mother and fetus. The emergency physician must be able to rapidly assess these patients, make the correct diagnosis, and begin appropriate therapy to minimize morbidity and mortality. Vaginal bleeding is a common problem encountered both in women who are aware of their pregnancy and in those who are not. Ectopic pregnancy, spontaneous abortion, and hydatidiform mole are the three most common complications of early pregnancy causing vaginal bleeding. *Placenta previa* and *abruptio placentae* are the most serious causes of vaginal bleeding in late pregnancy.

When a patient complains of vaginal bleeding and is admitted to the emergency department, it should first be determined whether or not she is pregnant. Several methods are available for measurement of human chorionic gonadotropin (hCG) in urine and serum. In general, urine tests that are readily available are positive in about 50 per cent of those tested at 6 weeks gestation. Serum tests are much better indicators, with 95 per cent of those pregnant for one to two weeks showing positive results (see Pregnancy Tests, page 215).

Bleeding during pregnancy is commonly described according to the gestational stage in which it occurs. The following table contains clues found in the history and physical examination to help decide on the approximate gestational age. Alternatively, Nagele's rule (subtract 3 months from the first day of the last normal menstrual period and add 7 days) can be used to estimate delivery date.

CLUE	GESTATIONAL AGE (WEEKS)
Uterus first palpable as abdominal organ	12–13
Uterus palpable at level of umbilicus	20
Measurement from top of symphysis pubis to top of uterus is 28 cm	28
Fetal movement	16–17
Fetal heart tones (Doppler)	9–11
Fetal heart tones (fetoscope)	19–21

The symptoms, physical findings, methods of diagnosis, and treatment of these early complications of pregnancy are outlined next. Numerous incidental causes of vaginal bleeding occur during pregnancy, including cervical polyps, acute or chronic cervicitis, vaginal trauma, and nonuterine bleeding from the urethra or rectum. They are easily discovered with a careful history and physical examination. Treatment is specific for the condition.

The most serious causes of bleeding in late pregnancy are abruptio placentae and placenta previa. A vaginal or rectal examination of the cervix is contraindicated in vaginal bleeding in late pregnancy. You may precipitate fatal hemorrhage. All examinations should be done by a skilled obstetrician with a "double set-up." This procedure involves the surgical preparation and draping of the patient on the operating room table so that vaginal delivery or cesarean section may be done if necessary.

Placenta previa

This disorder's hallmark is painless vaginal bleeding after 20 weeks gestation. These patients often tell the physician that they were awakened by a feeling of wetness, only to find themselves lying in a pool of blood. On physical examination the uterus is soft and nontender, and fetal heart tones are normal (120–160 beats/min). If the patient is stable, ultrasound examination for location of the

	SYMPTOMS	PHYSICAL FINDINGS	METHODS OF DIAGNOSIS	TREATMENT
Hydatidiform mole	Vaginal bleeding > 90% Hyperemesis or toxemia before 24 weeks. Passing of grapelike clusters of tissue.	Uterus larger than normal in 50%, smaller than normal in 38%. Lack of fetal heart tones at appropriate age. Molar tissue in vagina.	Molar tissue seen in vagina on examination. Ultrasonography shows homogenous echo pattern filling the uterine cavity, absence of fetal parts. False positive and negative ~4%. Amniogram—inject dye into uterine cavity; see "moth-eaten or honeycomb" appearance. Analysis of any tissue passed.	Stabilize patient for evacuation of uterus or hysterectomy. Enter patient in trophoblastic disease registry, follow hCG every 1–2 weeks until negative then every 2 months for 1 yr. Persistent levels mean continued trophoblastic disease. Treat with birth control to avoid confusion in follow-up of hCG.
Abortion threatened		Closed cervix, no tissue loss.	Physical examination and positive pregnancy test; ultrasonography to confirm status of fetus.	Bedrest, avoid coitus, remove IUD if present. Return if there is fever, increased bleeding, pain, or passage of tissue.
inevitable		Dilated cervix or ruptured membranes.	Physical examination and pregnancy test.	Immediate evacuation, IV oxytocin.
incomplete	Cramps and bleeding in all.	Dilated cervix and some tissue loss.	History, physical examination; may have positive or negative pregnancy test.	Immediate evacuation, IV oxytocin
complete		History of tissue loss, closed cervix, and minimal bleeding.	History and physical examination.	Oxytocin and evacuation of uterus, may require D & C.
missed	None.	Failure of uterine growth, no bleeding or tissue loss.	Conversion of positive pregnancy test to negative; no uterine growth; loss of heart tones; death confirmed by ultrasound.	Uterine curettage as soon as practical.
Ectopic pregnancy	Abdominal or pelvic pain~95%.* Vaginal bleeding, Abnormal menses in 50%	Palpable adnexal mass.* Scant vaginal bleeding.*	High index of suspicion; positive pregnancy test and physical findings. Ultrasonography may show adnexal mass, fluid in cul-de-sac, or extrauterine gestational sac. Culdocentesis—nonclotting blood, (Hct > 15%, 95% are ectopic). Laparoscopy or laparotomy.	Surgery Partial or complete salpingectomy. Salpingostomy with partial salpingectomy and later anastomosis.

6

*Triad for ectopic pregnancy.

placenta can be done. However, if she is bleeding profusely or is in labor, a double set-up examination should be done. If placental tissue is palpated on pelvic examination the infant is delivered immediately by cesarean section.

Abruptio placentae

The hallmark of abruptio placentae is "painful" uterine bleeding. The pain may be mild to severe, the bleeding overt or occult, slight or massive. On physical examination, the uterus is quite tender, rigid, and very irritable. When mild, abruptio placentae is difficult to differentiate from placenta previa. It can be differentiated safely using the double set-up examination. In the emergency department, IV lines should be established and blood obtained for an immediate type and crossmatch, CBC with differential, platelet count, coagulation studies, and fibrinogen determination. Fetal heart tones should be frequently auscultated. In cases of obvious severe abruptio placentae, the placental membranes should be immediately ruptured, thereby reducing uterine size, decreasing bleeding, and, hopefully, allowing the more efficient progression of labor. Delivery must be accomplished as quickly as possible.

Further complications of this disorder include disseminated intravascular coagulation resulting from release of tissue thromboplastins into the maternal circulation, consumptive coagulopathy secondary to an expanding clot that consumes fibrinogen faster than it can be produced by the liver, and renal failure.

Fetal outcome is directly related to the amount of placental separation and the time from abruptio placentae to delivery. Mild cases can be treated expectantly, especially if the fetus is immature. Systemic complications are rare. If the fetus is mature, oxytocin induction is indicated.

References:
1. Cucco CD, Moawad AH. Obstetric and gynecologic emergencies. *In:*Kravis TC, Warner CG, (eds.). Emergency Medicine, A Comprehensive Review. Rockville, Maryland: Aspen Systems Corporation, 1983:943–958.
2. Meier P, Clewell W. Obstetrical emergencies. *In:*Tintinalli J, (ed.). A Study Guide in Emergency Medicine. ACEP: Dallas, 1978:8–9 to 8–20.
3. Weiss B. Diagnosing and treating selected abnormalities of pregnancy. Emerg Med Rep 1983,*4*(16):95–102.

MATERNAL MEDICATION DURING PREGNANCY AND BREAST-FEEDING

When drug therapy is considered for a woman who is pregnant or breast-feeding, the risks and benefits for her, as well as for the fetus or infant, must be considered. Because controlled trials in humans are unethical, studies only note an association between maternal use of a drug and adverse effects in the offspring. Such an association does not constitute a causal relationship. For example, the use of insulin is associated with congenital defects in offspring. However, poorly controlled diabetes may do more to cause abnormalities than the insulin itself.

The table lists associations between drugs used during pregnancy and congenital malformations in infants. Note is made as to whether a drug is excreted into breast milk when such information is available. The degree of excretion is taken from the ratio of the drug concentrations in the breast milk and in the maternal serum. Only drugs that are likely to be prescribed independently by an emergency physician have been included.

Maternal Medication Use During Pregnancy and Breast-feeding: Effects on Offspring

DRUG	USE DURING PREGNANCY: ASSOCIATION WITH CONGENITAL MALFORMATIONS	USE DURING BREAST-FEEDING: EFFECT ON BREAST MILK
Antihistamines	Possible; particularly significant for brompheniramine	No data available
*Anti-infectives**		
Penicillins, ampicillins, amoxicillin, methicillin, oxacillin, dicloxacillin, and nafcillin	None; except for possible association with methicillin	Excreted in moderate amounts; no particular adverse effects (data not available for dicloxacillin, methicillin, or nafcillin)
Cephalosporins	None reported; crosses placenta	Excreted in small amounts; no particular adverse effects
Chloramphenicol	No anomalies noted; gray baby syndrome if given near term	Excreted in moderate amounts; theoretical risk of bone marrow depression
Clindamycin	None reported	Excreted; infant had bloody stools in one case
Erythromycin	None reported; estolate causes hepatotoxicity in 10% of pregnant women	Excreted in moderate amounts; no particular adverse effects
Lincomycin	None reported	Excreted in large amounts; no particular adverse effects
Mandelic acid	None reported	Excreted; the significance is unknown
Methenamine	None reported	Excreted; no adverse effects reported
Aminoglycosides	Possible damage to cranial nerve VIII	Excreted in small amounts; because oral absorption is poor, ototoxicity is not expected
Nitrofurantoin	None reported; possible anemia if infant is deficient in glucose-6-phosphate dehydrogenase (G-6-PD)	Excreted in small amounts; possible anemia if infant is deficient in G-6-PD

*All anti-infectives that are excreted into breast milk may modify the nursing infant's normal flora, cause an allergic reaction in the infant, or interfere with culture results if the infant is investigated for sepsis.

Table continued on following page

Maternal Medication Use During Pregnancy and Breast-feeding: Effects on Offspring (Continued)

DRUG	USE DURING PREGNANCY: ASSOCIATION WITH CONGENITAL MALFORMATIONS	USE DURING BREAST-FEEDING: EFFECT ON BREAST MILK
Anti-infectives* (Continued)		
Sulfonamides	Not reported but jaundice, hemolytic anemia, and kernicterus possible	Excreted in moderate amounts; infant rarely develops rash or diarrhea; avoid use if infant is premature, has hyper-bilirubinemia or G-6-PD deficiency
Tetracyclines	Effects on teeth and bones; possible hepatotoxicity in pregnant women	Excreted in moderate amounts; infant may have dental staining and inhibition of bone growth
Spectinomycin	None reported	No data available
Miconazole	None reported; small amounts are absorbed from the vagina	No data available
Nystatin	Only association attributed to simul-taneous tetracycline use	None appears in maternal serum or breast milk
Anticoagulants		
Coumarin	Bone malformations, low-set ears, palatal defects, and hemorrhagic diathesis	Warfarin not excreted; metabolites of other coumarins may be excreted causing bleeding diathesis
Heparin	None reported; does not cross placenta	Not excreted
Analgesics		
Acetaminophen	Apparently safe for short-term use in therapeutic doses; in toxic doses, possible renal or hepatic toxicity	Excreted in large amounts; no adverse effects reported
Codeine	Respiratory and other malformations; use in labor may cause withdrawal or respiratory depression in infant	Excreted in small, probably insignificant, amounts
Meperidine	None; use in labor may cause respiratory depression in infant	Excreted in large amounts; adverse effects reported
Morphine	None; use in labor may cause respiratory depression in infant	Excreted in small amounts; unknown significance
Pentazocine	Withdrawal in infant possible	No data available
Propoxyphene	Some reported; withdrawal in infant possible	Excreted; unknown significance
Salicylates	Possible with cleft palate; may prolong gestation and labor; ductus arteriosus may close *in utero;* bleeding diathesis and displacement of bilirubin in infant	Excreted in small amounts; no adverse effects reported, but platelet inhibition possible
Anticonvulsants		
Phenytoin	Multiple physical anomalies; mental retardation; coagulation abnormalities	Excreted in small amounts; may cause anemia, drowsi-ness, poor sucking reflex

Maternal Medication Use During Pregnancy and
Breast-feeding: Effects on Offspring (Continued)

DRUG	USE DURING PREGNANCY: ASSOCIATION WITH CONGENITAL MALFORMATIONS	USE DURING BREAST-FEEDING: EFFECT ON BREAST MILK
Anticonvulsants, (Continued)		
Phenobarbital	Possible association with neonatal withdrawal; coagulopathy	Excreted in moderate amounts; sedation possible
Trimethadione	Cardiac and facial	No data available
Anti-asthma Drugs		
Epinephrine	Statistically significant association	Degraded in infant's GI tract with no effect on infant
Theophylline	None reported; crosses placenta	Excreted in moderate amounts; irritability possible
Cardiovascular Drugs		
Diazoxide	Alopecia (four cases)	No data available
Digoxin	None reported	Excreted in large amounts; no adverse effects reported
Propranolol	Growth retardation; hypoglycemia; bradycardia; heart block; small placenta	Excreted; no adverse effects reported
Diuretics		
Thiazides	Some risk if used in first trimester; possible reactive hypoglycemia; thrombocytopenia; electrolye imbalance	Excreted in small amounts (chlorothiazide); possible thrombocytopenia; used to suppress lactation
Furosemide	None reported	Excreted; no adverse effects reported
Hormones		
Corticosteroids	Some malformations associated with cortisone and prednisone; dexamethasone used to stimulate maturation of fetal lung	Prednisone excreted in small, probably insignificant amounts; no data for cortisone or dexamethasone
Insulin	Association; may be due to poorly controlled maternal diabetes; does not cross placenta	Not excreted
Psychotherapeutics		
Amitriptyline	Skeletal	Excreted in small amounts; no apparent clinical effects
Chlordiazepoxide	Some association; possible hypotonia or hypothermia if used at term; possible neonatal withdrawal	No data available
Diazepam	Cleft palate; possible apnea, hypothermia, hypotonia, or poor feeding if used at term	Excreted; may cause lethargy and weight loss
Ethchlorvynol	Neonatal lethargy; hypotonia, irritability, and jitteriness	No data available
Haloperidol	Limb anomalies if used in early pregnancy	Excreted in moderate amounts; no adverse effects reported
Imipramine	Limb defects and facial clefts	Excreted in large amounts; significance unknown

6

Table continued on following page

Maternal Medication Use During Pregnancy and
Breast-feeding: Effects on Offspring (Continued)

DRUG	USE DURING PREGNANCY: ASSOCIATION WITH CONGENITAL MALFORMATIONS	USE DURING BREAST-FEEDING: EFFECT ON BREAST MILK
Psychotherapeutics (Continued)		
Lithium	Ear, heart, and CNS; neonatal hypotonia, cyanosis, hypothermia possible	Excreted in moderate amounts; no adverse effects reported
Meprobamate	Some, if used in early pregnancy	Excreted in large amounts; effect on infant unknown
Naloxone	Crosses placenta; possible respiratory failure if used just before delivery; drug of choice to reverse opioid effects after delivery	No data available
Miscellaneous		
Caffeine	Possible musculoskeletal defects, hydronephrosis, hemangiomas and granulomas	Excreted in moderate amounts; no adverse effects reported
Guaifenesin	Possible inguinal hernia if used in the first trimester	No data available
Magnesium sulfate	None reported	Excreted in large amounts; no apparent effect on infant's stool
Probenecid	None reported	No data available
Simethicone	None reported	No data available

References:
   1. Briggs GG, Bodendorfer TW, Freeman RK, Yaffe SJ. Drugs in Pregnancy and Lactation. A Reference Guide to Fetal and Neonatal Risk. Baltimore: Williams & Wilkins Company, 1983.
   2. Gottlieb AJ, Zamkoff KW, Jastremski MS, et al. The Whole Internist Catalog. Philadelphia: WB Saunders, 1980:534–542.

EVALUATING FOR FACIAL TRAUMA

Figure 6–2 provides a helpful outline for the proper examination of the patient who has sustained facial injuries.

Sequential steps in examination for facial fractures are as follows: *(A)* The supraorbital ridges are palpated while steadying the patient's head. *(B)* The infra-orbital ridges are lightly palpated using the index, middle, and ring fingers to determine symmetry or fractures. *(C)* The zygomatic arch is palpated on each side to determine continuity and the possible presence of displaced fractures. *(D)* The infra-orbital rims, zygomatic bodies, and maxilla are palpated and examined from the top of the head to determine depressions and fracture displacements. *(E)* The nasal bone and maxilla are examined for stability and possible fracture displacement. *(F)* The nose is examined intra-nasally to determine placement of the nasal septum and possible displacement of nasal bones or disruption of nasal mucosa. *(G)* The occlusion is observed to determine any disturbances of normal teeth relations. *(H)* The mandible is palpated, then distracted to determine sites of discomfort and possible mandibular fractures.

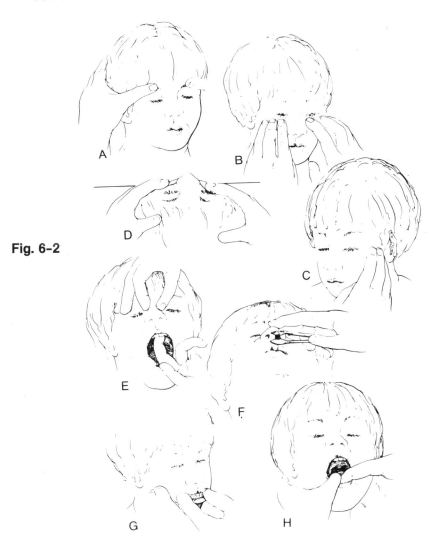

Fig. 6-2

Reference:
    1. Fleisher G, Ludwig S. Textbook of Pediatric Emergency Medicine. Baltimore: Williams & Wilkins, 1983:937. (Figure and text reproduced with permission.)

MANAGEMENT OF EPISTAXIS

A patient presenting to the emergency department with epistaxis may be a frustrating problem. Most cases of epistaxis result in minimal blood loss and are self-limited. However, there is an occasional case of significant hemorrhage. All of these patients are extremely anxious and very difficult to examine. Successful management hinges on a good examination that identifies the hemorrhage site.

The most frequent cause of epistaxis in children is some type of rhinitis (50–75%) associated with dry air or self-inflicted nasal trauma (nose picking or blowing). In adults, epistaxis may be a complication of an unknown or a known medical problem, such as hypertension, a coagulation abnormality, and arteriosclerotic vascular disease. Approximately 90 per cent of epistaxis in those under 20 years of age and 70 per cent in those more than 20 years of age are from the anterior nasal septum (Little's area or Kiesselbach's area). Most cases result from mucosal irritation. Bleeding from the superior or posterior regions of the nose occurs less often, is more difficult to treat, and has a potential for much greater blood loss. Bleeding from these areas more often results from an underlying disorder and occurs more often in older patients.

Anterior Bleeding

Most anterior bleeds originate in Little's area, resulting from irritation or self-inflicted trauma so the bleeding site is easily visualized. Active bleeding can be controlled by pinching the nose for four to five minutes, followed by cauterization of the bleeding site.

Chemical cautery (silver nitrate), thermocautery, or electrocautery may be used. With silver nitrate be sure the field is dry, since oozing blood may wash some of the chemical off the stick and down the nasopharynx, causing mucosal burns. The major hazard with thermocautery and electrocautery is cauterizing too deeply and causing damage to the septum that may lead to later perforation. After cautery, a small patch of compressed Gelfoam should be placed on the bleeding site to control any remaining pinpoint bleeding areas.

If control cannot be obtained by pinching the nose and cautery, an anterior pack should be placed. Use prepackaged half-inch by six-foot petroleum gauze strips coated with antibiotic ointment. Begin by placing a few strips in the nose, then loop the others underneath these, pushing the entire pack upwards with each new strip. Put each new strip as far back as possible in the nostril. Be sure the nostril is full, but do not pack too tightly as this may cause septal ulceration and necrosis. Remember to leave both ends of the pack hanging out the front of the nose. This assures ease of removal and prevents prolapse of the pack into the nasopharynx.

Superior Bleeding

Superior bleeding is typically supplied by branches of the anterior and posterior ethmoidal vessels. This type of bleeding is usually well controlled with an anterior pack. Cautery is not possible in most cases because of the inability to visualize the site of bleeding.

Posterior Bleeding

Posterior bleeding is from the sphenopalatine artery and generally requires a posterior pack for adequate control. Most otolaryngologists believe that those patients who continue to bleed after placement of a posterior pack require surgery or embolization.

The purpose of posterior packing is to seal the posterior choana of the nostril so that, in combination with an anterior pack, the entire nasal cavity is sealed under pressure. Posterior packing may be done with specially made balloon devices (such as a Reuter balloon), a Foley catheter, or a conventional gauze pack. Before using any of these methods, it is important to administer topical anesthetics and a systemic sedative in sufficient amounts to allow a smooth procedure. Useful topical anesthetics include four per cent lidocaine and two per cent cocaine. Cocaine has the advantage of also inducing vasoconstriction.

If packing is performed with one of the balloon devices, simply follow the enclosed instructions. Generally, the balloon is placed in the nose, and the posterior balloon is inflated and pulled anteriorly to seal the posterior choana. You then inflate the anterior balloon. If a Foley catheter is used, a no. 16 French with a 5 cc balloon is adequate. Cut a one-inch piece of surgical tubing and slide it over the balloon end of the catheter all the way up to the valve end. Lubricate the catheter and press it into the nostril until the tip is seen in the nasopharynx. Place 10 to 12 cc of air in the balloon and pull it anteriorly to seal the posterior choana. With constant traction on the catheter, pack the anterior nose around the catheter, being careful to keep the catheter in the middle of the nostril. This procedure prevents pressure-induced damage to the nasal rim or columnella. Next, slide the surgical tubing down against the anterior pack and place an umbilical or other clamp distal to the surgical tubing to hold it in place. To remove it, simply remove the clamp or cut the catheter between the clamp and the surgical tubing.

To place a conventional gauze pack, fold a 4 × 4 inch gauze into a cone-shaped pack, secure it with umbilical tape or 1–0 nonabsorbable suture and lubricate it with antibiotic ointment. Next, pass a small rubber catheter through the anesthetized nostril into the posterior oropharynx and grasp it with a forceps, drawing the end out through the mouth. Tie the pack to the catheter and pull the catheter through the nose, drawing the pack through the mouth into the nasopharynx and against the posterior choana (Fig. 6–3). Place an anterior pack around the ties and firmly tie them around a gauze bolster held firmly against the anterior pack.

POSTERIOR PACKING WITH CONVENTIONAL GAUZE

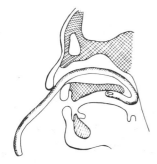
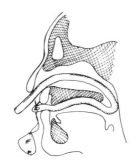
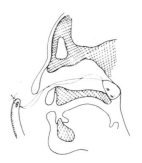

Passing the catheter   Posterior pack tied to end of catheter   Placement of posterior pack

Fig. 6–3

All patients with a posterior pack should be admitted. Those with anterior or posterior packs require prophylactic antibiotics, such as ampicillin, amoxicillin, cefaclor, or erythromycin to prevent possible sepsis.

References:
1. Aghamohamadi A, Marlowe FI. Nasal emergencies and sinusitis. *In:*Tintinalli J (ed.). A Study Guide in Emergency Medicine. Dallas: American College of Emergency Physicians, 1978: *3:*14–23—14–24.
2. Giordano AM, Gaskins RE. Correct, cautious management of epistaxis. Emergency Med Reports 1983;*4,*(1):1–6. (Figure reproduced with permission of American Medical Reports.)

TINNITUS

Tinnitus can be an annoying and frustrating problem both for the patient and for the physician trying to solve it. The accompanying table summarizes the significant features of the various causes of tinnitus. The emergency department physician can immediately treat foreign bodies in the ear canal, middle-ear infections, intoxications, and Meniere's disease. Tinnitus associated with an acute, sudden unilateral hearing loss, however, requires an urgent referral to an otolaryngologist.

Significant Features of Tinnitus

TYPE OF TINNITUS	PROBABLE CAUSE	NOTES
Objective sounds	Vascular origin likely	May be audible to examiner
Subjective sounds	Varies	Most common type by far; may be unilateral or bilateral
Low-frequency (500-1000 c/s)	Wax in ear canal	With history of infection, don't use lavage
	Traumatic perforation of tympanic membrane	If vertigo present, refer for surgery
	Otitis media	
	Acute	Signifies infection
	Chronic	Usually indicates perforated membrane; may require surgery
	Serous	Most common in children
		Concomitant allergy likely
		If unilateral in an adult, look for nasopharyngeal carcinoma
	Otosclerosis	Gradually progressive
		Occurs mostly in Caucasians between 20 and 40 years old
		Female to male ratio is 2:1

Significant Features of Tinnitus (Continued)

TYPE OF TINNITUS	PROBABLE CAUSE	NOTES
High-frequency (2000-6000 c/s)		
Unilateral	Sensorineural hearing loss	
	Acoustic trauma	From firearms or other loud noise; head injury
	Sudden hearing loss	Viral infection
		Vascular problem (thrombosis of internal auditory artery)
		Sudden atmospheric-pressure change
	Acoustic neuroma	Refer for CT scan and microneurosurgery
	Meniere's disease	Medical management (helpful for 70% of patients) with diuretics, vasodilators, histamine; surgery if needed
		Eliminate caffeine, nicotine; prescribe low-sodium diet
Bilateral	Acoustic trauma	Noise-induced
	Presbycusis	Loss of hearing varies with individual; with subjective and objective circumstances, as well as with age
	Intoxication	Lithium Salicylates

References:
1. Liebman EP. Tinnitus: multiple causes, varying significance. Consultant 1984 April;47–59. (Table reproduced with permission.)
2. Tinnitus (editorial). Lancet 1984;*1*:543–545.

FOOD OBSTRUCTION OF THE ESOPHAGUS

Obstruction of the esophagus by a bolus of food is one of the occasional emergencies in the emergency department. Removal of the obstructing bolus by esophagoscopy is the final court of appeal. Dissolution of the food bolus by the use of papain, a trypsin-like enzyme, which is a powerful digestive agent, has been used for more than thirty years, but occasional cases of damage to the esophageal wall have been described with this treatment. Therefore, the use of a muscle relaxant to allow the obstructing bolus to pass through the esophagus by the natural passageway is an important addition to therapy.

Two drugs that are well known in the emergency department have been reported in recent years as being effective muscle relaxants in esophageal obstruction. Nitroglycerin, given in the usual dose of 0.4 mg sublingually, may be effective in minutes but may cause hypotension.

The other drug that has been effective is glucagon, which is given intravenously as a 1 mg dose over one minute with the patient sitting in the upright position to encourage passage of the food bolus. Relief with glucagon is achieved in about two and one-half minutes. Glucagon may cause hypotension and vomiting. We consider glucagon more toxic than nitroglycerin and therefore use nitroglycerin first.

References:

    1. Gibson MS. Nitroglycerin use in esophageal disorders. Ann Emerg Med 1980;*9*:280.

    2. Handal KA, Riordan W, Siese J. The lower esophagus and glucagon. Ann Emerg Med 1980;*9*:577–579.

MISSING TEETH DEPARTMENT

When anterior teeth are avulsed during trauma, the decision to reimplant the tooth depends on the interval between the injury and presentation, and the type of tooth involved. Primary teeth are not reimplanted. Permanent teeth should be replaced as soon as possible after the injury; after four to six hours, the success rate for reimplantation is very low. Patients will often call the emergency department first, asking what to do. They should rinse the tooth in cold tap water, and try to replace the tooth before coming in. If unsuccessful, the tooth should be kept moist, preferably in the mouth under the tongue or inside the cheek, with care not to swallow the tooth.

On arrival in the emergency department, the tooth should be rinsed with saline. Scraping and scrubbing can damage the root and should not be done. Any clotted blood in the socket should be removed with suction and the tooth then replaced. The tooth is held between the thumb and index finger of one hand, while the thumb and index finger of the other hand are placed on the lingual and buccal plates of the alveolar bone. If necessary, alveolar nerve block may be used. Finally, the tooth should be stabilized with a periodontal splint until the patient can be seen by a dentist. Such a splint may be fashioned with Coe-Pak (Coe Laboratories, Inc., Chicago). The splint material is mixed together and formed into a rope. It is applied for a distance of three teeth to both sides of the injured area and molded over the gum line and in between the teeth.

References:

    1. Medford HM. Acute care of avulsed teeth. Ann Emerg Med 1982;*11*:559–61.

    2. Medford HM. Temporary stabilization of avulsed or luxated teeth. Ann Emerg Med 1982;*11*:490–92.

ACUTE EPIGLOTTITIS IN ADULTS

Acute epiglottitis is a disease characterized by sore throat, dysphagia, and respiratory distress. While common in children, it is considered rare in adults, although its incidence in adults appears to be rising, either from increased awareness of the disease or from an absolute increase in incidence. In children, the disease is caused by infection with *Haemophilus influenzae.* In adults, streptococcal and staphylococcal infections have also been documented.

In adults, sore throat and dysphagia are the most common symptoms. In addition, the voice is often muffled. Hoarseness, however, is usually absent, since the vocal cords are usually not involved. While the condition may progress rapidly as in children, the symptoms usually progress over a longer period in adults, typically in 24 to 48 hours. Respiratory distress is less common in adults but carries with it the same risk as with children, so careful attention to the airway is mandatory. On physical examination, patients appear ill. Fever typically is present but may be absent. Oropharyngeal injection and cervical lymphadenopathy findings are variable. A lateral neck x-ray exposed for soft tissue densities may be of some help in diagnosing acute epiglottitis, but false-positive results such as the omega-shaped epiglottis do occur, and any delay in diagnosis of the patient with an unstable airway must be avoided. The diagnosis is made by indirect laryngoscopic examination of the epiglottis, which appears edematous and hyperemic. In the presence of airway compromise, however, this procedure carries the same risk of acute obstruction as it does in children.

Treatment consists of mist tent, intravenous antibiotics, and intubation when necessary. As in children, intubation should be performed in the operating room by skilled personnel with tracheostomy immediately available should intubation be impossible. Tracheostomy will not be necessary in most cases. Steroids have also been helpful and are recommended. The antibiotics of choice are ampicillin and chloramphenicol.

In summary, acute epiglottitis should be considered in any adult who presents with acute sore throat and painful dysphagia, regardless of the presence or absence of respiratory distress or pharyngeal injection. Visualization of the epiglottis by indirect laryngoscopy should allow correct diagnosis and proper treatment of this emergency.

References:
1. Hawkins DB, Miller AH, Sachs GB, Benz RT. Acute epiglottitis in adults. Laryngoscope 1973;*83:*1211–1220.
2. Sarant G. Acute epiglottitis in adults. Ann Emerg Med 1981;*10:*58–61.

THE RED EYE

The causes of a red eye range from those that are not a threat to sight to those that are an immediate threat to sight. Thus, it is of vital importance to recognize those conditions that may be treated by the emergency physician and those that may require immediate referral to a specialist. The table lists the distinguishing characteristics of these conditions.

	ACUTE CONJUNCTIVITIS	UVEITIS, IRITIS, IRIDOCYCLITIS	ACUTE GLAUCOMA	CORNEAL TRAUMA AND ULCER	ORBITAL CELLULITIS
Incidence	Common	Common	Uncommon	Common	Uncommon
Pain	None	+ +	+ + to + + + +	+ to + + + +	0 to + + + +
Vision	Normal	Normal or slightly blurred	Blurred	Blurred	Normal or blurred
Photophobia	0 to + +	+ to + + + +	+ + to + + + +	0 to + + + +	None
Discharge	+ + to + + + +	None	None	+ + (watery or purulent)	None
Injection	Diffuse (lid and eye)	Circumcorneal	Diffuse	Diffuse	Diffuse
Cornea	Clear	Clear	Cloudy	Abrasion, (ulcer or foreign body)	Clear
Pupil size	Normal	Small	Large	Normal	Normal
Pupil response	Normal	Poor or normal	Poor	Normal	Normal
Intraocular pressure	Normal	Normal	Elevated	Normal	Normal

CHEMICAL INJURY TO THE EYE

Chemical injury to the eye is an emergency that requires immediate treatment. Whereas acids and alkali are probably the most harmful, any substance is a threat. Treatment should begin immediately with irrigation of the affected eye with water or saline solution and continue, in transit, to the emergency department. There, normal saline flowing by gravity through intravenous tubing should be directed to all portions of the eye. Topical anesthetic will be helpful in relieving blepharospasm, allowing lid retraction and complete irrigation. Lid retraction can be improved by using specially designed retractors. If these are not available, a suitable retractor may be fashioned from a paper clip as demonstrated in Figure 6–4.

Alkali in the eye is the most serious eye injury problem. The alkali binds with the tissues in the eye and is slowly released so that damage may continue long after the initial insult. In addition, alkali may penetrate to deeper structures, leading, for example, to cataract formation. In this case, irrigation may be required for hours, and a general rule is that irrigation should continue until the consulting

Fig. 6-4. A homemade eyelid retractor. *A.* Open the paper clip to a right angle. *B.* Bend each end down 90 degrees. *C.* The completed lid retractor.

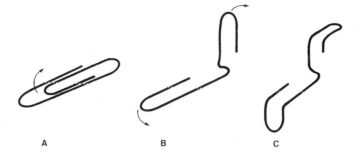

A   B   C

ophthalmologist orders it stopped. Ophthalmologic consultation is mandatory in such cases. No attempt at neutralization of the alkali should be made, as this will result in the release of heat that can cause thermal damage to the eye.

Strong acid in the eye is also a very serious emergency, but generally not as bad as alkali in the eye. Acids do not bind to the tissues and are not as prone to penetrate. Copious irrigation is still necessary and should be continued until a pH test, by touching the globe with pH paper, shows a pH of 7. Again, neutralization is not indicated and may increase ocular damage.

Following adequate irrigation, a thorough ocular examination, including visual acuity testing, funduscopic examination, and fluorescein examination of the cornea, should be performed. Treatment of chemical burns to the eye includes topical antibiotics and patching. Patching should provide sufficient pressure to prevent lid movement.

FLASH BURNS TO THE EYE

Ultraviolet light is absorbed by the corneal epithelium, resulting in cell loosening and faulty cell maturation. The epithelial cells slough, leading to pain, foreign body sensation, and photophobia. This condition may follow any exposure to ultraviolet light, but the typical case is that of the welder who fails to use protective glasses. These patients usually present in the early hours of the morning, for it takes some time for the epithelium to slough; minor irritation while awake and active gives way to considerable discomfort while trying to sleep. The patient has severe pain and photophobia, and examination is often impossible until anesthetic drops are used. Tearing is also prominent. On physical examination, the eyes are red. Visual acuity is usually normal, and the only notable finding is patchy loss of corneal epithelium detected by fluorescein examination. Particular care should be exercised to look for concomitant corneal foreign body. Treatment consists of topical antibiotics and tight patching of both eyes. Often cycloplegics such as homatropine, 5 per cent eye drops, are used to provide pain relief. In addition, analgesics or sedatives may be required in order to provide comfort. Luckily for the patient, corneal healing is rapid and usually uneventful.

TONOMETRY

The Schiotz tonometer is found in many emergency rooms, being relatively inexpensive and easy to use. The instrument is named after its designer, Professor Hjalmar Schiotz, although it has been modified in many ways (Fig. 6–5).

Diagrammatic Drawing of Sklar's Jewel Model Schiotz Tonometer

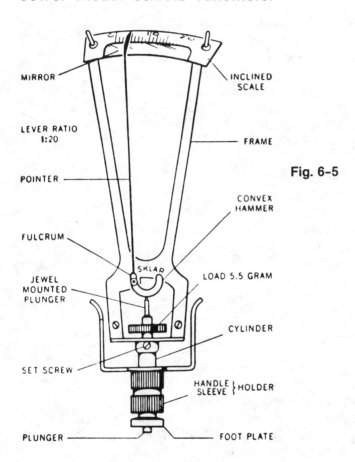

MIRROR

INCLINED SCALE

LEVER RATIO 1:20

FRAME

Fig. 6–5

POINTER

CONVEX HAMMER

FULCRUM

SKLAR

JEWEL MOUNTED PLUNGER

LOAD 5.5 GRAM

CYLINDER

SET SCREW

HANDLE } HOLDER
SLEEVE }

PLUNGER

FOOT PLATE

Concept

The tonometer measures the amount of pressure required for a plunger to indent the cornea: a soft cornea allows deep indentation, a firm cornea allows little indentation. These depths are magnified 20 times through a lever, to give a reading in millimeters. High scale readings (large indentation) reflect low orbital pressures; low scale readings (small indentation) reflect high orbital pressures.

Use

1. Place the plunger on the test block supplied with the instrument. The pointer should be at zero. If not, adjust it by loosening the set screw and turning the frame.

2. Have the patient supine, with clothing loosened around the neck.

3. Anesthetize the eyes with a topical solution.

4. Have the patient fix his gaze on a spot on the ceiling or on his own finger held at arm's length. Caution him against holding his breath.

5. Start with the 5.5 g weight. Hold the tonometer vertically. Retract the lids without pressing on the eyeball. Resting your hand on the patient's forehead or cheek, place the tonometer on the center of the cornea. Lower the handle until it's free. Line up the pointer with its mirror image and take a reading.

6. Other weights may be added to give scale readings of 4 to 10. (Adding the weight labeled 7.5 g to the weight labeled 5.5 g gives a total load of 7.5 g.)

7. Use the chart supplied with the tonometer to calculate intraocular pressures from scale readings. Normal pressures are 10 to 20 mmHg (Fig. 6–6).

8. Clean the instrument after each use according to manufacturer's instructions.

6

CALIBRATION SCALE FOR SCHIOTZ TONOMETERS

Adopted by the Committee on Standardization of Tonometers—JANUARY, 1955.

Table of Intra-Ocular Pressures in mm of Hg for the Four Weights Supplied with Sklar-Schiotz Tonometer

Fig. 6–6

Scale Reading	Plunger Load			
	5.5 GM.	7.5 GM.	10.0 GM.	15.0 GM.
0.0	41.4	59.1	81.7	127.5
0.5	37.8	54.2	75.1	117.9
1.0	34.5	49.8	69.3	109.3
1.5	31.6	45.8	64.0	101.4
2.0	29.0	42.1	59.1	94.3
2.5	26.6	38.9	54.7	88.0
3.0	24.4	35.8	50.6	81.8
3.5	22.4	33.0	46.9	76.2
4.0	20.6	30.4	43.4	71.0
4.5	18.9	28.0	40.2	66.2
5.0	17.3	25.8	37.2	61.8
5.5	15.9	23.8	34.4	57.6
6.0	14.6	21.9	31.8	53.6
6.5	13.4	20.1	29.4	50.0
7.0	12.2	18.5	27.2	46.5
7.5	11.2	17.0	25.1	43.2
8.0	10.2	15.6	23.1	40.2
8.5	9.4	14.3	21.3	38.1
9.0	8.5	13.1	19.6	34.6
9.5	7.8	12.0	18.0	32.0
10.0	7.1	10.9	16.5	29.6
10.5	6.5	10.0	15.1	27.4
11.0	5.9	9.1	13.8	25.3
11.5	5.3	8.3	12.6	23.3
12.0	4.9	7.5	11.5	21.4
12.5	4.4	6.8	10.5	19.7
13.0	4.0	6.2	9.5	18.1
13.5		5.6	8.6	16.5
14.0		5.0	7.8	15.1
14.5		4.5	7.1	13.7
15.0		4.1	6.4	12.6

J. SKLAR MANUFACTURING CO.
Long Island City, N. Y.

Contraindications to Tonometry

1. Eye infection including facial herpes and outbreaks of eye infection in the community.

2. Perforation, abrasion, and chemical burns.

3. Corneal edema, distortion, and scarring.

4. Nystagmus.

5. Uncontrolled coughing.

6. Lack of patient cooperation.

Causes of False Readings

1. Diurnal variation (usual variation is 2–4 mmHg, but may be up to 15–20 mmHg in open angle glaucoma; pressures are highest from 4 to 7 A.M.).

2. Myopia (greater than −8 diopters).

3. Cyclitis.

4. Detachment of choroidal or ciliary body.

5. Systemic dehydration.

6. Hyperglycemia.

7. Impairment of the ipsilateral carotid artery.

8. Myotonic dystrophy.

References:

1. Product information for Sklar's "Jewel" model Schiotz tonometer, J. Sklar Manufacturing Co, Long Island City, NY. (Figure and table reproduced from Sklar catalog with permission.)

2. Keeney AH. Ocular Examination. Basis and Technique. St. Louis: C.V. Mosby Co. 1976:133–152.

3. Spaeth GL, Purcell J. Examination of the eye and its adnexa. *In:*Schwartz GR, (ed.). Principles and Practice of Emergency Medicine. Philadelphia: WB Saunders, 1978:403–404.

7

MEDICINE

SYNCOPE AND PSEUDOSYNCOPE 238

DRUGS AND POSTURAL HYPOTENSION 239

HEADACHE 239

ADMISSION CRITERIA FOR ACUTE ASTHMA ATTACKS 242

AMINOPHYLLINE DOSING 244

PULMONARY EMBOLISM 246

MI OR MSG 247

RIGHT VENTRICULAR INFARCTION 248

LES TORSADES DES POINTES 250

VENTRICULAR ECTOPY OR ABERRATION 251

ANTIARRHYTHMIC DRUGS 254

PREVENTION OF BACTERIAL ENDOCARDITIS 256

TREATMENT OF ACUTE PULMONARY EDEMA 257

PULMONARY EDEMA IN THE ANURIC PATIENT 258

NOMOGRAM FOR DIGOXIN DOSAGE 258

PROPHYLAXIS IN HEPATITIS 260

MANAGEMENT OF NEEDLE-STICK INJURIES 262

PROPHYLAXIS FOR MENINGOCOCCUS 263

BOTULISM 264

TOXIC SHOCK SYNDROME 266

AVAILABLE FROM THE CDC—IMMUNOBIOLOGIC AGENTS
AND ANTIPARASITIC DRUGS 268

SINGLE-DOSE TREATMENT OF UTI'S 270

THE MINDLESS WORKUP OF HEMATURIA 271

HYPONATREMIA 272

ANTACID UPDATE 274

MANAGEMENT OF TONIC–CLONIC STATUS EPILEPTICUS 276

SHINGLES 277

SYNCOPE AND PSEUDOSYNCOPE

When a patient reports a fainting spell, many causes come to mind, some of which require immediate admission and treatment. We like to point out to our residents that the only difference between syncope and death is that in one of them the patient wakes up. Of course, not all syncope is alike, and many "episodes" are not syncope at all. Proper diagnosis depends on such factors as the patient's age, the circumstances preceding the incident, the physical examination, and so forth. The next table lists some of the causes of syncope and some of the problems that may mimic it, with distinguishing characteristics concerning onset and resolution, and brief comments about treatment.

Syncope and Pseudosyncope

CAUSES	ONSET	RESOLUTION	TREATMENT
Decreased Cardiac Output			
Stokes-Adams attacks	Abrupt	Abrupt	Permanent pacemaker
Arrhythmias	Abrupt	Abrupt	Anti-arrhythmia therapy
Tachyarrhythmias			and/or pacemaker
Bradyarrhythmias			
Heart blocks			
Aortic stenosis	Abrupt	Abrupt	Refer for surgery
Congenital heart disease	Abrupt	Abrupt	Refer for surgery
with right-left shunt			
Hypertrophic cardiomyopathy	Abrupt	Abrupt	Beta blocker
Atrial myxoma	Abrupt	Abrupt	Refer for surgery
Myocardial infarction	Abrupt	Gradual or Abrupt	Admit
Pulmonary hypertension	Abrupt	Gradual or Abrupt	Treat cause
Pulmonary embolism			
Decreased Vascular Tone or Volume			
Vasodepressor syndrome (vasovagal episode)	Abrupt	Abrupt	Treat cause
Postural hypotension	Abrupt	Abrupt	
Primary			Primary: Consider mineralocorticoids
Secondary			
Blood, sodium, or fluid loss			Replace blood, sodium, or fluids
Drugs (see next Table)			Stop drugs
Neurogenic			
Cerebral ischemia			
Subclavian steal	Abrupt	Abrupt	Consider surgery
TIA	Abrupt	Abrupt	Medical or surgical treatment
Carotid sinus hypersensitivity	Abrupt	Abrupt	Pacemaker
Other			
Alcohol intoxication	Gradual	Gradual	Hydrate; withdraw alcohol
Hyperventilation	Gradual	Gradual	Reassurance; rebreathing
Seizure	Abrupt	Abrupt	Anticonvulsant medication
Cough	Abrupt	Abrupt	Treat cause
Micturition	Abrupt	Abrupt	Treat cause
Hypoglycemia	Gradual	Gradual	Glucose

DRUGS AND POSTURAL HYPOTENSION

"As yet no drug has been found with a single action and no human body with a single reaction."

Matz

Vasodilators

Prazosin
Hydralazine
Nitrates
Clonidine
Nitroprusside
Diazoxide

Ganglionic blockers

Guanethidine
Methyldopa
Reserpine

Phenothiazines

Diuretics

Calcium blockers

Verapamil
Diltiazem
Nifedipine

Antiarrhythmics

Bretylium
Procainamide
Quinidine

7

HEADACHE

"You won't cure many of them; you won't even know what's wrong with some of them; but you can always be kind to them."

Matz

Headache is one of the common afflictions of man and, thus, a frequent reason for a visit to the emergency department. Determining the significance of a headache can be difficult because of the variability in pain tolerance from person to person. The accompanying table contains valuable information that can be obtained from the history and physical examination, as well as key associated symptoms that assist the emergency physician in finding the correct diagnosis of the cause of a patient's headache.

Synopsis of Headaches

	HISTORY	PHYSICAL EXAMINATION	ASSOCIATED SYMPTOMS	PRECIPITATING FACTORS	OTHER
Common migraine	Builds over several hours, lasts hours to days. Severe pain, unilateral, and usually a daytime headache.	Photophobia, tender scalp, headache behind the eyes and/or over the forehead.	Nausea, vomiting, polyuria, chills, nasal congestion, and tearing.	Life stress, menses, and certain foods.	Decreases during pregnancy, middle age, and menopause. Positive family history is common.
Classic migraine	One hour to reach peak, lasts hours to days, severe throbbing pain, usually unilateral preceded by aura, and may switch sides.	Photophobia, tender scalp, and may have neurologic deficits (hemiplegia, hemiparesis, aphasia).	Nausea and vomiting.	Life stress, pregnancy, menses, and certain foods.	Decreases during middle age.
Cluster headache	Sudden onset, severe headache, usually unilateral, throbbing or constant pain. No aura, lasts 20 minutes to 1 hour, recurrent during the day for weeks to months, and involves the eye.	Hyperemia of one eye, tearing and Horner's syndrome.	No nausea or vomiting; autonomic symptoms, such as red face, stuffy nose, lacrimation on same side as headache.	Alcohol use, nitroglycerin (NTG), and certain foods.	Cutaneous telangiectasias common.
Tension headache	Moderate bilateral band of constriction or tightness, often occipital, and variable in duration.	Contraction of neck or scalp muscles, and greater pain with palpation over area of pain.	Agitation, depression, and sleep disturbance.	Life stress, fixed position, and depression.	

Temporal arteritis	Usually patient over 50 years of age, severe acute headache, one temple only. A headache that is "different from any other."	Tenderness over region of pain or temporal artery.	Transient ischemic attack, syncope, malaise, fever, and fatigue.		Requires immediate treatment to prevent complications, such as blindness and strokes. Elevated ESR characteristic. Arterial biopsy for diagnosis.
Nonmigraine, vascular headache	Throbbing, severe headache, increases with movement and exertion, may be occipital, usually bilateral or generalized.	Hypertension or evidence of infection.	Those related to associated cause.	Sepsis, alcohol use, caffeine withdrawal, carbon-monoxide poisoning, hypercarbia, hypoglycemia, oral contraceptive use, altitude sickness, hypoxia, drugs (NTG), monosodium glutamate, etc.	
Headache secondary to serious intracranial disease	Headache does not fit any of the previous descriptions: recent in onset, patient's age greater than 40 years, always unilateral, never switches sides, and progressive in severity over weeks or months.	Cerebral bruits, weakness, any focal signs; check for otitis media, papilledema, nuchal rigidity, and positive Kernig and Brudzinski signs.	Personality changes, nausea and vomiting, visual disturbances, seizures, and fever.	Trauma, hypertension, ruptured aneurysm, meningitis, tumor, abscess, and subdural hematoma.	Sudden onset with syncope suggests subarachnoid bleed.

7

References:

1. Gallagher EJ. Headache. *In:* Kravis TC, Warner CG (eds.). Emergency Medicine, A Comprehensive Review. Rockville, Maryland: Aspens System Corporation. 1983:627–638.

2. Gottlieb AJ, Zamkoff KW, Jastremski MS, et al. The Whole Internist Catalog. Philadelphia: WB Saunders, 1980:96–97.

3. Tintinalli J. Headache. *In:* Tintinalli J (ed.). A Study Guide in Emergency Medicine. Dallas: American College of Emergency Physicians 1978:1–121 to 1–128.

4. Wolf JK (ed.). Migraine and other headaches. Practical Clinical Neurology. Garden City, New York: Medical Examination Publishing Company. 1980: 298–321.

ADMISSION CRITERIA FOR ACUTE ASTHMA ATTACKS

The initial management of a patient with an acute asthma attack is usually straightforward. Beta-agonist therapy is initiated first, followed by a theophylline-type bronchodilator if the patient has not improved sufficiently. Treatment in the emergency department may continue for 6 to 12 hours before a decision to admit or discharge the patient is made. Decisions relating to the end of emergency treatment—when to discharge a patient, when to admit a patient—are complicated by the fact that many asthmatic patients experience clinical signs of improvement, such as amelioration of wheezes and dyspnea, before significant improvement in airway obstruction occurs. Such patients may be discharged too early, only to soon return in worse condition than at initial presentation. In addition, while most asthmatic patients will respond to prolonged treatment in the emergency department, many will still need to be admitted for care. If those who will need admission can be identified early, they can be admitted sooner, thus allowing emergency department resources to be utilized more effectively. Several approaches to these problems have been reported and are summarized here.

Pre-treatment Admission Criteria

1. Inability to perform spirometry.[7]
2. Patients assume an upright posture and are diaphoretic on admission to the emergency department.[2]
3. $P_{CO_2} > 45$ mmHg.[4]
4. Patient demonstrates four or more of the following:[3]
   a. Pulse 100 beats/min or greater.
   b. Respirations 30/min or greater.
   c. Pulsus paradoxus 18 mmHg or greater.
   d. PEFR = 120 L/min or less.
   e. Moderate to severe dyspnea.

f.   Moderate to severe accessory muscle use.

g.   Moderate to severe wheezing.

Early Post-treatment Admission Criteria (15–20 min after initial beta-agonist therapy)

1. Initial PEFR < 16 per cent of predicted and improvement in PEFR < 16 per cent.[1]

2. Initial PEFR < 100 L/min and increase in PEFR < 60 L/min.[8]

Later Post-treatment Admission Criteria (e.g., at 6 hr)

1. Increase in FEV_1 < 400 cc after treatment.[5]

2. PEFR < 300 L/min or FEV_1 < 2.1 L after treatment.[8]

3. Initial FEV_1 < 600 cc and FEV_1 < 1.6 L after treatment.[7]

4. Deterioration of PEFR > 15 per cent after initial good response to bronchodilators.[6]

PEFR = Peak expiratory flow rate (measured by a Wright peak flow meter in L/min).

FEV_1 = Forced expiratory volume at one second, measured in cc or L.

References:

1. Banner AS, Shah RS, Addington WW. Rapid prediction of need for hospitalization in acute asthma. JAMA 1976;*235*:1337–1338.

2. Brenner BE. Bronchial asthma in adults: presentation to the emergency department. Am J Emerg Med 1983;*1*:50–70.

3. Fischl MA, Pitchenik A, Gardner LB. An index predicting relapse and need for hospitalization in patients with acute bronchial asthma. N Engl J Med 1981;*305*:783–789.

4. Hart GR, Anderson RJ. Emergency management of acute asthma. Emerg Med Annual 1982;*1*:61–93.

5. Kelsen SG, Kelsen DP, Fleegler BF, et al. Emergency room assessment and treatment of patients with acute asthma. Am J Med 1978;*64*:622–628.

6. Lulla S, Newcomb RW. Emergency management of asthma in children. J. Pediatrics 1980; *97*:346–350.

7. Nowak RM, Gordon KR, Wroblewski DA, et al. Spirometric evaluation of acute bronchial asthma. JACEP 1979;*8*:9–12.

8. Nowak RM, Pensler MI, Sarkar DD, et al. Comparison of peak expiratory flow and FEV_1 admission criteria for acute bronchial asthma. Ann Emerg Med 1982;*11*:64–69.

7

AMINOPHYLLINE DOSING

Aminophylline and other xanthines are useful agents in the treatment of bronchospasm. Ideal emergency treatment with this drug involves an initial loading dose to achieve a therapeutic level and a continuous infusion to maintain that level. A number of factors may increase or decrease the clearance of aminophylline and thus affect the maintenance dose. The following tables serve as guides to appropriate aminophylline therapy. The loading dose need not be modified except

Serum Theophylline Levels and Toxicity

SERUM LEVEL (μg/ml)	TOXICITY
0–5	No toxicity. Little or no therapeutic effect.
5–10	No toxicity. Slight improvement in FEV_1.
10–20	Therapeutic range.
15–25	GI Toxic Effects: Nausea, vomiting, abdominal cramps, occasionally hematemesis.
25–35	CNS Toxic Effects: Headache, restlessness, agitation, tremulousness, delirium, hallucinations.
35–50	Cardiovascular Toxic Effects: Sinus tachycardia, hypertension, arrhythmias including supraventricular tachycardia, VPCs.
50 +	Serious to Fatal Toxic Effects: Seizures, coma, cerebral edema, hypotension and shock, hyperthermia, severe cardiac arrhythmias including ventricular tachycardia, fibrillation and asystole, apnea and cardiopulmonary arrest.

Factors Altering Theophylline Plasma Clearance / Serum Half-life

↓ CLEARANCE/ ↑ $T\frac{1}{2}$ (↓ MAINTENANCE DOSE REQUIRED)	↑ CLEARANCE/ ↓ $T\frac{1}{2}$ (↑ MAINTENANCE DOSE REQUIRED)
Prematurity in neonates	Childhood
Hepatic disease	Smoking (tobacco, marijuana)
Heart failure	High protein–low carbohydrate diets
Pulmonary disease	Charcoal-broiled foods
Macrolide antibiotics (erythromycin, clindamycin)	
Obesity	
Dietary methylxanthines (coffee, tea)	
? Thiabendazole	
Cimetidine	

for the patient who is already taking an oral preparation. In these patients it is best to obtain a serum theophylline level, and adjust the dosage accordingly. Remember that these values serve only as a guide to initial dosage. Later adjustments must be based on serum theophylline level determinations.

Aminophylline Dosage Recommendations

	LOADING (mg/kg)	MAINTENANCE (mg/kg/hr)
Children (Age 1-18)	5.6	1.0
Adults		
Nonsmokers	5.6	0.5
Smokers < 40 years old	5.6	0.9
> 40 years old	5.6	0.4
Liver disease—cirrhosis		
Normal bilirubin	5.6	0.25-0.45
Bilirubin > 1.5	5.6	0.20
CHF + liver disease	5.6	0.1-0.3
Heart disease		
CHF	5.6	0.2-0.4
Pulmonary disease		
COPD without cor pulmonale	5.6	0.4
Pneumonia	5.6	0.6
Obesity		
TBW = Total Body Weight	5.6 (Use TBW)	0.6 (Use IBW)
IBW = Ideal Body Weight		
Men = 110 lb + /- 5 lb/in above/below 5 ft		
Women = 100 lb + /- 5 lb/in above/below 5 ft		
Patients Taking Oral Theophylline		
Serum level NOT known, but patient probably *is not* taking adequate doses regularly	2.8	0.5
Serum level NOT known, but patient probably *is* taking adequate doses regularly	None	0.5
No theophylline for 24 hr	5.6	0.5
Serum level known	1.0 for every 2 μg/ml increase in serum level desired (valid up to 10 μg/ml	0.5

7

Note that these dosage modifications will not necessarily result in therapeutic serum levels or prevent toxicity in every patient. Dose adjustments based on indices of liver function (bilirubin, enzymes, serum albumin) are particularly inaccurate. This table should serve as a guide for initial doses only—subsequent adjustments should be based on measured theophylline serum levels.

Reference:
1. Eisenberg MS, Copass MK. Emergency Medical Therapy. Philadelphia: WB Saunders, 1982:236–237. (Tables reproduced with permission.)

PULMONARY EMBOLISM

The diagnosis of pulmonary embolism is one of the more difficult problems for the emergency physician. Many factors account for this. The symptoms and signs of pulmonary embolism are nonspecific for the condition. While most emboli originate in the lower extremities, physical signs of deep vein thrombosis are present in only one half of the patients with pulmonary embolism. In addition, routine diagnostic tests do not add significantly useful information. While normal ventilation-perfusion lung scans are useful in ruling out pulmonary embolism, the false-positive rate is high. Pulmonary angiography, therefore, remains the gold standard for the definitive diagnosis of this disease.

A useful approach to the diagnosis is to consider the patterns of presentation of patients with pulmonary embolism. The data shown here were derived from a national cooperative study of the use of thrombolytic agents in the treatment of angiographically proven pulmonary embolism. Stein and coworkers[1] evaluated 215 adults without pre-existing cardiac or pulmonary disease from among 327 patients included in the trials. They identified three syndromes of the disease. These syndromes, their frequency in the study population, and the frequency of various signs and symptoms of pulmonary embolism in each syndrome are presented in the accompanying tables. While these signs and symptoms may suggest the presence of pulmonary embolism, only more definitive studies, including ventilation-perfusion lung scanning and pulmonary angiography, will give some degree of certainty to the diagnosis. A rational approach to the diagnosis of pulmonary embolism is presented in the accompanying tables.

Initial Syndromes of Acute Pulmonary Embolism in
215 Patients with No Pre-existing Cardiac or
Pulmonary Disease

	PATIENTS	
	Number	*Per cent*
Circulatory collapse syndrome		
Shock	21	10
Syncope	19	9
Pulmonary infarction syndrome		
Hemoptysis ± pleuritic pain	54	25
Pleuritic pain without hemoptysis	88	41
Uncomplicated embolism syndrome		
Dyspnea	26	12
Nonpleuritic pain	6	3
Deep venous thrombosis with tachypnea	1	0.5

Most Frequent Signs and Symptoms in Various
Syndromes of Acute Pulmonary Embolism

	Circulatory Collapse Syndrome		Pulmonary Infarction Syndrome		Uncomplicated Embolism Syndrome	
	Shock	*Syncope*	*Hemoptysis*	*Pleuritic Pain*	*Dyspnea*	*Nonpleuritic Pain or DVT ± Tachypnea*
Dyspnea	71	89	91	82	100*	0*
Pleuritic pain	38	63	91	100*	0*	0*
Apprehension	71	74	63	65	58	0
Cough	33	42	81	39	42	33
Hemoptysis	10	5	100*	0*	0*	0*
Tachypnea > 20/min	81	89	81	84	88	72
Tachycardia > 100/min	86	58	56	49	81	29
Accentuated P₂	62	79	52	53	62	14
Rales	48	47	60	55	42	29
Fever (> 37.5°C)	43	21	58	52	42	29
Deep venous thrombosis	19	42	31	35	38	57

*The presence or absence of this manifestation helped define the syndrome
P_2 = Pulmonary component of second heart sound
DVT = Deep venous thrombosis

Reference:
    1. Stein PD, Willis PW, DeMets DL. History and physical examination in acute pulmonary embolism in patients without pre-existing cardiac or pulmonary disease. Am J Cardiol 1981;*47:* 218–23 (Tables reproduced with permission.)

MI OR MSG?

A patient arrives at your emergency room with substernal chest pain and a pressure sensation radiating to the neck and forearms. He is diaphoretic and complains of numbness around and about his neck, face, and upper chest area. You rapidly begin a standard cardiac injury investigation. Just as you are putting on the chest ECG leads, however, the patient asks, "Could it be something I ate?" He may be correct, providing he just had dinner at a Chinese restaurant. There have been many anecdotal reports in the medical literature describing what has become known as the "Chinese Restaurant Syndrome." Clinical studies have linked its symptoms to monosodium glutamate, a widely used food additive in many Oriental dishes (especially won ton soup). Some individuals are exquisitely sensitive to this product, and specifically order Chinese food without MSG. The common symptoms of Chinese Restaurant Syndrome as described include:

1. A burning sensation in the chest radiating to the neck, shoulders, forearms, and abdomen.

2. Tightness and pressure over the malar areas radiating to the zygomatic and retro-orbital regions.

3. Precordial pressure.

4. Severe headache and dizziness.

5. Palpitations.

6. Nausea and vomiting.

Affected patients experience symptoms within 15 to 45 minutes after eating, with the illness lasting up to several hours with spontaneous resolution. There is even one case reported in an infant. Keep this "syndrome" in mind for your next patient with chest complaints; he may have had won ton too many.

> *"Nor bring, to see me cease to live,*
> *Some doctor full of praise and fame,*
> *To shake his sapient head and give*
> *The ill he cannot cure a name."*
>
> Matthew Arnold

References:
1. Apres RS. Chinese restaurant syndrome in an infant. Clin Pediatr 1980;*13*:705.
2. Schaumberg H. Monosodium glutamate: its pharmacology and role in the Chinese restaurant syndrome. Science 1969;*163*:826–828.

RIGHT VENTRICULAR INFARCTION

Ischemia in the distribution of the right coronary artery may often involve the right ventricle in addition to the inferior wall of the left ventricle. It is important to recognize right ventricular infarction, because the therapy for low cardiac output due to right ventricular failure is somewhat different from the usual therapy for left ventricular failure. The output of the right ventricle will usually respond well to volume loading, but will often become worse with vasodilator therapy.

The diagnosis of right ventricular myocardial infarction can be confirmed by obtaining an ECG tracing of the right chest leads. Right chest leads are obtained by starting the recording in the fourth left intercostal space at the sternal border as V_1R. V_2R is obtained in the fourth right intercostal space at the sternal border. V_3R to V_6R are obtained by placing the ECG electrode in a location that is opposite to the standard V_2 to V_6 positions. For example, V_6R would be the right mid-axillary line. Figure 7–1 illustrates the ECG of a normal patient with right chest leads; Figure 7–2 illustrates the ECG with right chest leads of a patient with a right ventricular myocardial infarction.

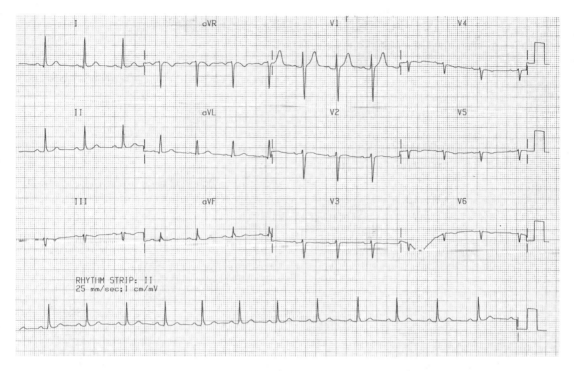

Fig. 7-1. Right precordial leads from a normal subject. Notice that the R wave progression decreases from V_1R to V_6R.

7

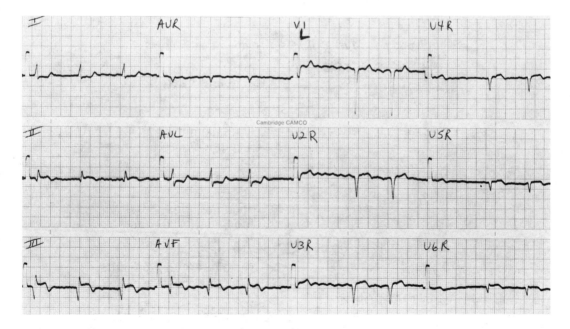

Fig. 7-2. Right precordial leads from a patient with an acute right ventricular infarction. There is ST segment elevation of greater than two boxes and T wave inversion in V_2R through V_6R. The limb leads also show an acute inferior wall myocardial infarction.

LES TORSADES DES POINTES

Les torsades des pointes is an arrhythmia that may resemble either ventricular tachycardia or coarse ventricular fibrillation. It occurs in patients with a prolonged QT interval, probably as a result of a premature ventricular contraction falling on a T-wave. This activity triggers a run of ventricular tachycardia that is remarkable in that the axis of the QRS changes direction during the run (Fig. 7–3). The arrhythmia is usually self-limited but may be prolonged and accompanied by hypotension. Immediate treatment includes cardioversion for prolonged episodes and bretylium or lidocaine to prevent recurrences. Measures that increase the underlying heart rate, such as isoproterenol and overdrive pacing, are also helpful. Treatment should then be geared toward removing the underlying problem causing the prolonged QT interval. A list of predisposing causes of *les torsades des pointes* is presented.

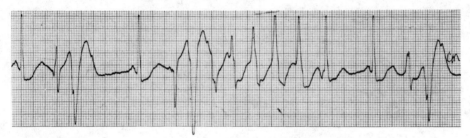

Fig. 7–3. Ventricular tachycardia in which the QRS changes direction.

Predisposing Causes of Les Torsades des Pointes

CARDIAC DISEASES	ASHD
	Complete heart block
	Severe bradycardia
	Myocarditis
METABOLIC DISORDERS	Hypokalemia
	Hypocalcemia
	Hypomagnesemia
DRUGS	Quinidine
	Disopyramide
	Procainamide
	Lidocaine (toxic dose)
	Thioridazine
	Phenothiazine
	Tricyclic antidepressants (overdoses)
CNS DISORDERS	CVA
	Subarachnoid hemorrhage
OTHER	Congenital prolongation of QT

Reference:
1. Parrish C, Wooster WE, Braen GR. Les torsades des pointes. Ann Emerg Med 1982;*11*: 143–146.

VENTRICULAR ECTOPY OR ABERRATION

One of the more difficult problems in arrhythmia identification is deciding if a rapid rhythm with a wide QRS complex is ventricular or supraventricular in origin. Situations in which supraventricular rhythms may have abnormal configurations include pre-existing bundle branch block, rate-dependent bundle branch block, and aberrant conduction of supraventricular beats (Fig. 7–4).

The table lists some useful diagnostic clues to help the physician differentiate between ventricular ectopy and aberrant conduction.

Figure 7–5 demonstrates some morphologic clues one can obtain from V_1 and V_6 that can also be useful in the differential diagnosis.

Ventricular Aberration vs. Ectopy: Diagnostic Clues[1]

FEATURES	VENTRICULAR ECTOPY	SUPRAVENTRICULAR BEATS WITH ABERRANCY
Regularity	Usually regular, but slight variation in cycle length of up to 0.02–0.03 sec may occur	Quite regular unless atrial fibrillation or variable AV block is present
QRS duration	Suggested if $\geq$ 0.14 sec	Suggested if $\leq$ 0.12 sec
QRS axis	High prevalence of left axis in the presence of RBBB or LBBB	Usually normal axis or right axis with RBBB
Relation of P-waves to QRS complexes (if apparent)	AV dissociation in 85%; retrograde P-waves following QRS complex seen in most others	1:1 Relationship unless varying degrees of AV block are present
Capture or fusion beats	Diagnostic if present	Never present
Effect of carotid massage	No response	May convert the arrhythmia or increase the AV block
Direction of initial 0.02 sec of QRS complex*	Almost always different from that of normally conducted beats	Same as that of normally conducted beats
Findings on His bundle ECG	No relationship between "H" deflections and QRS complexes except when retrograde activation is present; in this case, an "H" spike follows each QRS complex	"H" deflection before every QRS complex

*In order to be certain of the direction of the initial QRS forces, more than a single lead, and preferably all 12 standard leads, should be examined.

References:
1. Marriott HJL. Tampa Tracing Tables. (Fig. 7–5 reproduced with permission.)
2. Wellens HJ, Bar FW, Lie KI. The value of the electrocardiogram in the differential diagnosis of tachycardia with a widened QRS complex. Am J Med 1978;*64*:27–33.
3. Wyndham CR. Recognition and management of supraventricular arrhythmias. Res Staff Physician 1980; June: 43S–65S (Fig. 7–4 reproduced with permission).

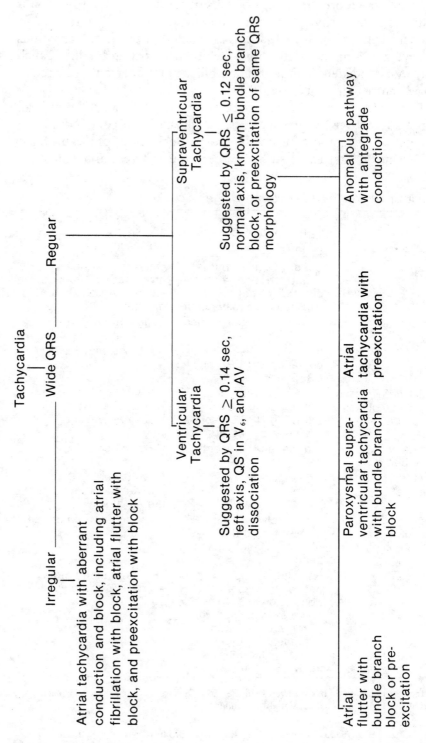

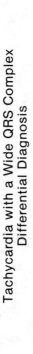

Fig. 7-4. Tachycardia with a wide QRS complex. Differential diagnosis.

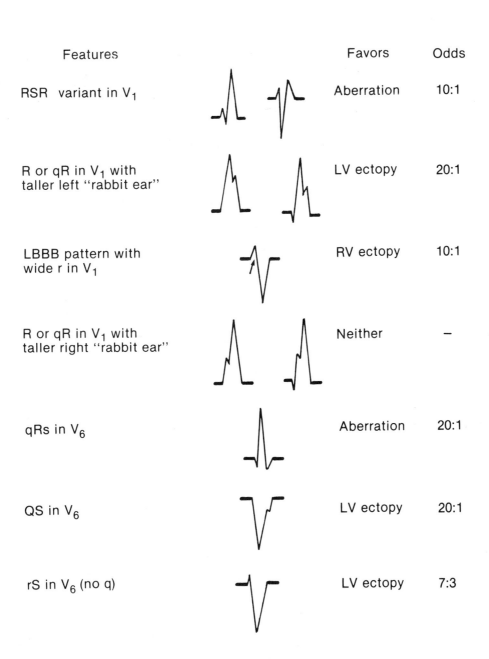

Features		Favors	Odds
RSR variant in V_1		Aberration	10:1
R or qR in V_1 with taller left "rabbit ear"		LV ectopy	20:1
LBBB pattern with wide r in V_1		RV ectopy	10:1
R or qR in V_1 with taller right "rabbit ear"		Neither	–
qRs in V_6		Aberration	20:1
QS in V_6		LV ectopy	20:1
rS in V_6 (no q)		LV ectopy	7:3

Fig. 7-5. Ventricular aberration vs. ectopy: morphologic clues.

ANTIARRHYTHMIC DRUGS *

	QUINIDINE	PROCAINAMIDE	DISOPYRAMIDE	LIDOCAINE	PHENYTOIN	PROPRANOLOL	BRETYLIUM	VERAPAMIL
Dosage								
IV								
Initial	NA†	100 mg IV q5 min to 1000 mg	NA	1-2 mg/kg (50-200 mg)‡	100 mg IV q5 min to 1000 mg	1 mg/min IV q5 min to 5 mg	5 mg/kg with additional doses to 10-20 mg/kg	0.075 to 0.15 mg/kg over 2 min; maximum dose 10 mg
Maintenance	NA	2-4 mg/min	NA	2-4 mg/min	NA	1-3 mg/q4h	5-10 mg/kg q6h	NA
Oral								
Loading	300 mg	0.5-1.0 grams	300 mg	NA	1000 mg in divided doses	None	NA	NA
Daily Total	1.2-3.2 gm	1-4 gm	400-800 mg	NA	300 mg	40-400 and more	NA	80-160 mg
Schedule	q6h	q3-4h	q6h	NA	Daily	q6h	q6h	q6h
Half-life	6h	3-4h	6h	Bolus: 15-30 min; Long-term: 2h	20-26h	IV: 2-3h Oral: 6h	Unknown	IV: 2-5h Oral: 3-7h
Therapeutic plasma levels	2-6 μg/ml	4-8 μg/ml	2-4 μg/ml	1.5-5.0 μg/ml	10-18 ng/ml	Not established§	Not established	Not established
Metabolism	Liver	Liver, plasma hydrolysis	Liver	Liver	Liver	Liver	Unknown	Liver
Renal excretion (unmetabolized)	20-50 %	50-60 %	50 %	< 10 %	< 5 %	< 5 %	Unknown	< 5 %

ECG Effects						
P-R	↑↓	↑↓	↑↓	↑↓	↑↓	↑↓
QRS	→↑	→↑	↑→	↑→	→↑	↑
Q-T	→↑	→↑	↑→	↑↑	↑	↑
Physiologic Effects						
Automaticity	→	→	→	→	→	↓
Conduction velocity	→	→	↑↓	↑	Unknown	↑
Effective refractory period	↑	→	→	→		
					Unknown	↑

*Measure blood level when there is failure to respond at usual dosage level, toxicity at usual dosage level, or suspected altered metabolism. Dosage schedule should not exceed half-life of the drug. A loading dose before starting the maintenance dose is necessary to achieve therapeutic levels rapidly.

†NA—Not applicable.

‡ Pharmacokinetic considerations dictate that a second bolus be given 20 minutes after the first, so that the total loading dose falls within the recommended range.

§ 100–200 ml is the serum level of propranolol required to produce sympathetic blockade.

↑ Increased
↓ Decreased
→ Unchanged

Reference:
1. Treatment of Cardiac Arrhythmias. Med Lett 1983;25:21–28.

"Many clinicians view research in cardiac metabolism the way farmers view studies of the earth's core: It doesn't help much with the plowing."
Anonymous

7

PREVENTION OF BACTERIAL ENDOCARDITIS*

	DOSAGE FOR ADULTS	DOSAGE FOR CHILDREN
Dental and Upper Respiratory Procedures†		
Oral‡		
Penicillin V	2 g 1hr before procedure and 1 g 6 hr later	> 60 lbs: Adult dosage < 60 lbs: Half the adult dose 1 hr before procedure and 6 hr later
Penicillin allergy:		
Erythromycin	1 g 1 hr before procedure and 500 mg 6 hr later	20 mg/kg 1 hr before procedure and 10 mg/kg 6 hr later
Parenteral‡		
Ampicillin	1 g IM or IV 30 min to 1 hr before procedure and repeat once 8 hr later	50 mg/kg IM or IV 30 min to 1 hr before procedure and repeat once 8 hr later
or Aqueous penicillin G	2 million units IM or IV 30 min to 1 hr before procedure and repeat once 8 hr later	50,000 units/kg IM or IV 30 min to 1 hr before procedure and repeat once 8 hr later
plus Gentamicin	1.5 mg/kg IM or IV 30 min to 1 hr before procedure and repeat once 8 hr later	2.0 mg/kg IM or IV 30 min to 1 hr before procedure and repeat once 8 hr later
Penicillin allergy:		
Vancomycin	1 g IV infused *over 1 hr* beginning 1 hr before procedure and repeat once 8 hr later	20 mg/kg IV infused *over 1 hr* beginning 1 hr before procedure and repeat once 8 hr later
Gastrointestinal and Genitourinary Procedures†		
Parenteral		
Ampicillin	2 g IM or IV 30 min to 1 hr before procedure and repeat once 8 hr later	50 mg/kg IM or IV 30 min to 1 hr before procedure and repeat once 8 hr later
plus Gentamicin	1.5 mg/kg IM or IV 30 min to 1 hr before procedure and repeat once 8 hr later	2.0 mg/kg IM or IV 30 min to 1 hr before procedure and repeat once 8 hr later
Penicillin allergy:		
Vancomycin	1 g IV infused *over 1 hr* beginning 1 hr before procedure and repeat once 8 hr later	20 mg/kg IV infused *over 1 hr* beginning 1 hr before procedure and repeat once 8 hr later
plus Gentamicin	1.5 mg/kg IM or IV 30 min to 1 hr before procedure and repeat once 8 hr later	2.0 mg/kg IM or IV 30 min to 1 hr before procedure and repeat once 8 hr later
Oral§		
Amoxicillin	3 g 1 hr before procedure and 1.5 g 6 hr later	> 60 lbs: Adult dosage < 60 lbs: Half the adult dose 1 hr before procedure and 6 hr later

*For patients with valvular heart disease, prosthetic heart valves, most forms of congenital heart disease (but not uncomplicated secundum atrial septal defect), idiopathic hypertrophic subaortic stenosis, and mitral valve prolapse.

†Data are limited on the risk of endocarditis with a particular procedure. For a review of the risk of bacteremia with various procedures, see Everett ED, Hirschmann JV. Medicine 1977;*56*:61.

‡An oral regimen is safer and is preferred for most patients. Parenteral regimens are more likely to be effective; they are recommended especially for patients with prosthetic valves, those who have had endocarditis previously, and those taking continuous oral penicillin for rheumatic fever prophylaxis.

§Parenteral regimens are more likely to be effective.

Reference:
1. Prevention of bacterial endocarditis. Med Lett 1983;*26*:3–4. (With permission.)

TREATMENT OF ACUTE PULMONARY EDEMA

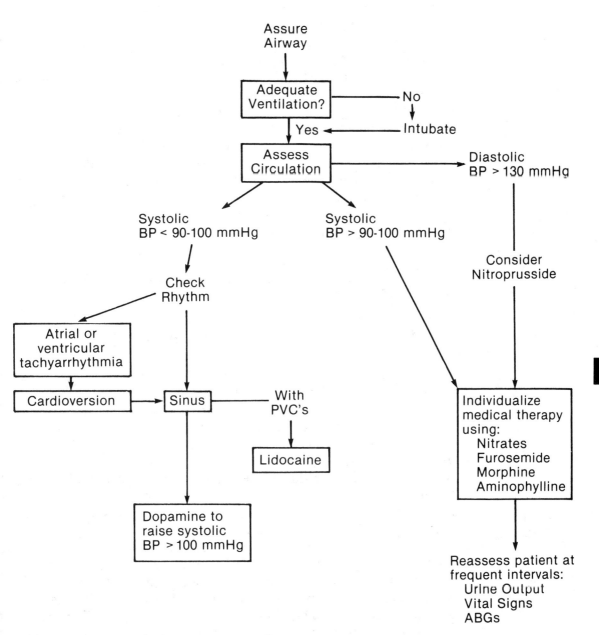

Assure
Airway

Adequate
Ventilation? ————— No

Yes ←———— Intubate

Assess
Circulation ————————→ Diastolic
BP > 130 mmHg

Systolic
BP < 90-100 mmHg

Systolic
BP > 90-100 mmHg

Consider
Nitroprusside

Check
Rhythm

Atrial or
ventricular
tachyarrhythmia

Cardioversion ——→ Sinus ——— With
PVC's

Lidocaine

Individualize
medical therapy
using:
  Nitrates
  Furosemide
  Morphine
  Aminophylline

Dopamine to
raise systolic
BP > 100 mmHg

Reassess patient at
frequent intervals:
  Urine Output
  Vital Signs
  ABGs

7

PULMONARY EDEMA IN THE ANURIC PATIENT

The anuric patient with pulmonary edema is a therapeutic challenge. While vasodilators (morphine, nitrates, nitroprusside), inotropes (digoxin, dobutamine), bronchodilators (aminophylline), and positive pressure ventilation have a role, the dilemma is how to remove body fluid when the traditional route of excretion—the kidney—is not functioning. Phlebotomy, thoracentesis, paracentesis, and dialysis are all possible, although each method has potential complications and may not be readily available. The gastrointestinal tract must then be used as a route for fluid loss. Diarrhea can be induced by the osmotic effects of sorbitol. An oral dose of 50 gm can be given to the patient every half hour if necessary. Patients who have decreased peristalsis (as in hypothermia and opioid use) may need larger doses. Serum electrolyte levels must be monitored carefully. This therapeutic method is simple, available, and effective.

Reference:
1. Anderson CC, Shahvari MBG, Zimmerman JE. The treatment of pulmonary edema in the absence of renal function. JAMA 1979;*241*:1008–1010.

NOMOGRAM FOR DIGOXIN DOSAGE

In Fig. 7–6, the central vertical scale represents the total oral loading dose (mg). The fan-shaped group of lines on the left, leading from the body weight and converging at zero, represents the effect of body weight upon this loading dose, adjusted for oral absorption. The fan of lines thus yields the lower left scale of maximum total body digoxin (maximum total body digoxin [μg/kg]), showing the dilutional relationships that both the 85 per cent effectiveness of oral digoxin (assumed to occur) and the patient's body weight exert upon the oral loading dose. It also provides a computed overall peak total body concentration of digoxin, expressed in μg/kg of digoxin.

To use the nomogram for adult euthyroid patients with reasonably normal hepatic function, normal electrolyte balance, normal gastrointestinal absorption, and no previous digitalis therapy, decide what risks of arrhythmias and of adverse reactions per patient-year you are willing to accept. This depends upon the urgency of the patient's clinical status and your estimate of his possible sensitivity to digoxin. (In general, most patients with normal sinus rhythm have done well with a maximum total body digoxin concentration of 10 μg/kg.) If hypokalemia is present, the selected level should be revised downward somewhat.

The series of arrows shown in the nomogram represents the determination of a dosage regimen for a hypothetical patient weighing 150 lb (68 kg). The patient's creatinine clearance is 100 ml/min, and his selected therapeutic goal corresponds to a maximum total body digoxin concentration of 10 μg/kg, corresponding to a risk of adverse reactions of 0.2 episodes per patient-year, as shown in the lower left scale at the start of the upward vertical series of arrows. Continue to look upward vertically from the chosen maximum total body digoxin concentration, as shown by the sample vertical arrow, until the line corresponding to the patient's body weight is encountered. Once that point is found, proceed horizontally to the right to obtain the suggested total oral loading dose. Here, as shown by the arrow, a loading dose of 0.8 mg is found. Divide this total dose into two or three parts to be given six hours apart, checking carefully for toxicity before giving each new increment.

Once the increments of loading dose have been administered and the patient has tolerated them, the maintenance dose may be determined. Continue horizontally to the right from the point of the loading dose to the line corresponding to the patient's measured or estimated creatinine clearance, or to the patient's serum creatinine level, on the nomogram. In this example, creatinine clearance was assumed to the 100 ml/min. From this point, continue vertically downward to find the appropriate single oral daily maintenance dose, which in this case is 0.27 mg. If the amount shown is difficult to achieve with tablets, continue downward to the appropriate corresponding dose of digoxin pediatric elixir (0.05 mg/ml).

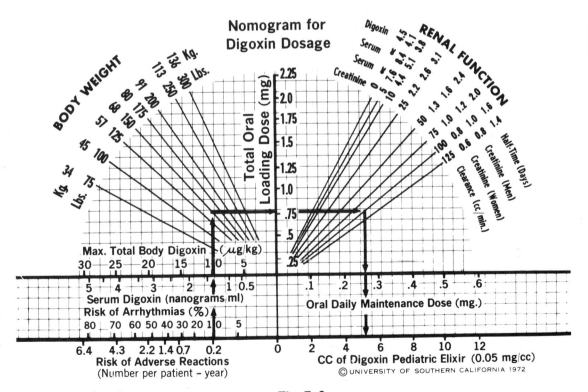

Fig. 7-6.

Reference:
   1. Jelliffe RW, Brooker G. A nomogram for digoxin therapy. Am J Med 1974;57:64. (With permission.)

PROPHYLAXIS IN HEPATITIS

The diagnosis of acute viral hepatitis can usually be established in the emergency department based on the patient's clinical presentation

Serologic Findings in Acute and Convalescent Viral Hepatitis

HEPATITIS A
    Acute: IgM-specific anti-HA
    Convalescent: IgG-specific anti-HA
HEPATITIS B *
    Acute: HBsAg, anti-HBc positive
    Convalescent: anti-HBs, anti-HBc positive
        anti-HBs positive†
NON-A, NON-B HEPATITIS
    Acute: Clinical acute hepatitis in absence of serologic
        markers of acute hepatitis A or B
    Convalescent: No tests available

---

    * For ease in presentation, this has been somewhat simplified. There are 8 possible combinations of the 3 serologic markers (HBsAg, anti-HBc, anti-HBs). The presence of HBsAg with or without either antibody should be taken as evidence of active hepatitis B infection. Anti-HBc in the absence of HBsAG or anti-HBs may be seen at a time during acute disease when HBsAg is no longer demonstrable and also late in convalescence if anti-HBs disappears first.
    †Anti-HBs will also be seen in individuals successfully vaccinated against hepatitis B.

Use of HBIG (Hepatitis B Immune Globulin) in Hepatitis B

CLINICAL SITUATION	DOSE OF HBIG IM
Post-exposure	
Acute hepatitis B	
Spouse (sexual contact)	0.06 ml/kg (immediately and 4 wk later)
Other family contacts	None
Work, school contacts	None
Neonate, exposed during third trimester	0.5 ml (immediately and 4 wk later)
Chronic HBsAg carrier	
Spouse	None (possibly vaccine)
Nonrecurring sexual contact (if susceptible)	0.06 ml/kg (immediately and 4 wk later)
Other family contacts	None
Work, school contacts	None
Neonate—HBeAg positive mother	0.5 ml (at birth, 3 mo, and 6 mo)
Other	
Parenteral and mucosal exposure: HBsAg positive material	0.06 ml/kg (immediately and 4 wk later)
Parenteral and mucosal exposure: unknown source	None (use SIG [serum immune globulin] at 0.06 ml/kg immediately and 4 wk later)
Large dose HBsAg	0.2 ml/kg (times 4 over 1 wk)
Pre-exposure	None (vaccine as indicated)

and liver function test results. Once the diagnosis is made, the patient should be advised about the risks to family members and other contacts of contracting the disease. This advice is best given on the basis of serologic tests that help determine the type of viral hepatitis involved. The appropriate tables given here allow interpretation of the test results and provide recommendations regarding immunoprophylaxis.

Use of SIG in Hepatitis A

CLINICAL SITUATION	DOSE OF SIG IM
Post-exposure	
Household contacts	0.02 ml/kg (once)*
School contacts	None (unless epidemic)
Work contacts	None
Sexual contacts	0.02 ml/kg (once)*
Accidental inoculation	0.02 ml/kg (once)*
Pre-exposure	
Foreign travel (endemic area)	0.02 ml/kg (every 3-4 mo)
Prolonged travel	0.06 ml/kg (every 5 mo)
Primate handlers	0.04 ml/kg (every 4 mo)
Institutional workers	0.04-0.1 ml/kg (every 6 mo)
Health care workers	None

*Should be given within 14 days (ideally within 7 days) of exposure.

Use of SIG in Non-A, Non-B Hepatitis

CLINICAL SITUATION	DOSE OF SIG IM
Post-exposure	
Acute Hepatitis	
Spouse (sexual contact)	0.06 ml/kg (once)
Household contact	0.02 ml/kg (once)
School contact	None
Work contact	None
Neonate, exposed during third trimester	0.5 ml (immediately and 4 wk later)
Presumptive Chronic Carrier	
Nonrecurring sexual contact	0.06 ml/kg (once)
Household contact	None
School contact	None
Work contact	None
Neonate	None
Other	
Parenteral and mucosal exposure	0.06 ml/kg (immediately and 4 wk later)
Pre-exposure	None

Reference:
1. Koretz RL. New developments in the control of viral hepatitis. ER Reports 1982;*3*:65–72. (Tables reproduced with permission.)

MANAGEMENT OF NEEDLE-STICK INJURIES

Accidental needle puncture is one of the commonest work-related injuries in health care personnel. Although usually only a minor annoyance, occasional serious complications may occur. Viral hepatitis is the commonest, but other infections and serious trauma may result from these injuries. (I have treated an ICU nurse who received a right tension pneumothorax resulting from a needle puncture. She required tube thoracostomy and hospitalization.) The following outline provides an approach to the management of this problem.

A. Prevention
1. Educate hospital personnel on epidemiology of and safeguards against needle puncture.
2. Provide easily accessible needle-disposal units (ideally, needle cutter units).
3. Avoid recapping needles.
4. Dispose of all needles in proper receptacles only.
5. Take extreme care in cleaning up after procedures involving needles.
6. Insist on mandatory reporting of all needle punctures.

B. Management
1. For injury caused by clean, unused needle.
   a. Cleanse wound.
   b. Update tetanus immunization if necessary (current recommendation is tetanus toxoid 0.5 ml q 10 years).

2. For injury caused by dirty, used needle.
   a. Cleanse wound.
   b. Update tetanus immunization if necessary (see current recommendation).
   c. Identify the patient in whom the needle was first used.
   d. Determine HBsAg (hepatitis B surface antigen) status of patient (see c) and injured person and anti-HBsAg of injured person (useful only if results are available within seven days).
   e. Give hepatitis B immune globulin (HBIG) (0.06 ml/kg) within seven days and again in 28 to 30 days if:
      1. Patient (see c) is known to have hepatitis.
      2. Patient (see c) is found to be HBsAg-positive and injured person anti-HBsAg–negative.
   f. Give conventional serum immune globulin (0.06 ml/kg) to person who was stuck if the dirty needle was from one of the following:

1. Patient who is HBsAG-negative, but a high risk for non-A, non-B hepatitis (i.e., has active hepatitis, history of previous viral hepatitis, or history of multiple transfusions; drug abuser, homosexual, or on hemodialysis).

2. Patient who is a high risk, and HBsAg status cannot be determined within seven days.

g. Clinical follow-up for hepatitis in personnel punctured by a dirty needle from HBsAg-positive or high-risk patient.

1. Advise them of the symptoms of hepatitis.

2. Obtain a baseline SGOT value.

3. Obtain follow-up SGOT, HBsAg, anti-HBsAg at one, three, and six months post-injury.

h. Clinical follow-up for personnel punctured by a dirty needle from a patient with another infection or unusual trauma.

1. Handle on individual basis.

2. Consultation with an infectious disease specialist may be useful.

i. Both HBIG and gamma globulin can be given safely to pregnant personnel.

An alternative approach to prophylaxis following needle-stick, ocular, or mucous membrane exposure to blood known to contain HBsAg or for human bites from HBsAg carriers has just been suggested by the Immunization Practices Advisory Committee.[3] Instead of the two-dose HBIG regimen recommended previously, a single 0.06 ml/kg dose of HBIG and a 1.0 ml of hepatitis B vaccine should be given intramuscularly at separate sites as soon as possible after exposure (ideally within 24 hours). Hepatitis B vaccine must be repeated one month and six months later.

References:
1. McCormick RD, Maki DG. Epidemiology of needle-stick injuries in hospital personnel. Am J Med 1981;70:928–932.
2. Seeff LB, Hoofnagle JH. Immunoprophylaxis of viral hepatitis. Gastroenterology 1979;77:161–182.
3. ACIP. Postexposure prophylaxis of hepatitis B. Morbid Mortal Wkly Rep 1984;33:285–290.

PROPHYLAXIS FOR MENINGOCOCCUS

Once the diagnosis of meningococcal meningitis has been made, the question of stopping the spread of the disease should be raised. Those at high risk include the patient's immediate family, day-care center contacts, and any others who may have had contact with the patient's oral secretions prior to institution of therapy. This latter group includes medical personnel who were involved in resuscitation, intubation, or suctioning of the patient. The disease may also be spread through kissing and sharing food or drinks.

The best prophylactic drug is sulfadiazine, but unfortunately, only 85 per cent of isolates are sensitive to it. When sulfadiazine sensitivity is known, two days of treatment are adequate to eliminate nasopharyngeal carriage and to prevent meningococcal disease. Doses are listed in the accompanying table.

When sulfadiazine sensitivity is unknown, or when the organism is resistant to sulfadiazine, rifampin is the treatment of choice. Rifampin is also given for two days, and doses are also listed in the table. Unfortunately, it is available only in capsule form, since it is unstable in solution. The capsules may be opened and sprinkled on applesauce or jelly for children. In addition, since rifampin in high doses has been shown to be teratogenic in laboratory rodents, its use in pregnant women is contraindicated. Careful monitoring of pregnant women is recommended, with intravenous penicillin initiated at the first sign of meningococcal disease. Finally, don't forget to tell your patients that rifampin turns the urine orange.

Meningococcal Prophylaxis

SENSITIVE TO SULFADIAZINE		RESISTANT TO SULFADIAZINE OR UNKNOWN SENSITIVITY	
Age	*Dose of Sulfadiazine*	*Age*	*Dose of Rifampin (twice daily)*
<1 mo	500 mg daily	<1 mo	5 mg/kg
1 mo to 12 yr	500 mg twice daily	1 mo to 12 yr	10 mg/kg
12 yr to adult	1 gm twice daily	12 yr to adult	600 mg

Reference:
   1. Preventing spread of meningococcal disease. Med Lett 1981;*23*(8):37–38.

BOTULISM

Botulism is a type of food poisoning caused by ingestion of the endotoxin of *Clostridium botulinum*. It is a rare disease, the mortality is high, and most patients are not diagnosed or are misdiagnosed at initial presentation. This problem is particularly true of incidents involving one person. Outbreaks must be reported to the Centers for Disease Control in Atlanta.

The endotoxin acts by preventing release of acetylcholine from the neuromuscular junction and other cholinergic sites. The toxin is a protein, and seven immunologic types have been identified. Almost all cases in humans are caused by Type A, B, or E. Initial symptoms are nonspecific and include malaise, headache, weakness, dizziness, blurred vision, and dry mouth. An initial diagnosis of flu, viral syndrome, or stroke is common. Dry mouth and blurred vision are important symptoms—all patients in a large outbreak of Type B botulism in Michigan in 1977 had dry mouth, and 86 per cent had either trouble in focusing or diplopia. Onset of symptoms is usually within 24 hours of ingestion of the toxin but may be delayed up to three days.

Symptoms progress to increasing motor weakness and may be manifest by worsening visual problems, slurred speech, trouble in swallowing, and difficulty in walking. Nausea and vomiting occur in less than 50 per cent of patients. Constipation or urinary retention may ensue. Motor findings are usually bilateral and symmetrical, with normal sensorium and memory. The sensory examination findings are normal.

Diagnosis is made based on clinical data. Confirmation depends on the injection of specimens suspected of containing the toxin into mice; they are adversely affected by as little as 900 molecules of the toxin. Specimens from the patient's serum, feces, and vomitus, or food samples and containers, may be sent to the Centers for Disease Control for analysis. For more information, you may contact the Centers for Disease Control during the day at 404-329-3753 and during the night at 404-329-3644.

In the presence of increasing motor weakness, ventilatory insufficiency may develop; therefore, any treatment plan must include frequent assessment of ventilatory status, including serial arterial blood gas values and pulmonary function determinations (forced vital capacity [FVC] and negative inspiratory force). In addition, trivalent antitoxin (antisera to Types A, B, and E), available from the Centers for Disease Control, should be administered to all patients with suspected botulism. This antitoxin is derived from horse serum; therefore, hypersensitivity reactions or serum sickness may be a problem. Hydrocortisone, 100 mg, and diphenhydramine, 50 mg, may be given to patients with known sensitivity to horse serum before the trivalent antitoxin. In addition, although the disease is caused by the endotoxin and not by the infection with *C. botulinum*, penicillin, 1 million units qid, is recommended for five to seven days.

Besides the usual mechanism of endotoxin ingestion, two other types of botulism have been reported: wound botulism and infantile botulism. Wound botulism results from deep contamination of a wound with *C. botulinum*. The wound itself usually appears quite innocuous, without the usual signs of infection. The disease, however, appears in a fashion identical to food-borne botulism. In infants, generally less than 1 year of age, ingestion of spores of *C. botulinum* is followed by absorption of sufficient toxin to cause symptoms which are usually insidious and chronic. The infant may be lethargic and have problems eating; constipation is the most common symptom. Loss of head control may be present, and muscle weakness may progress to respiratory paralysis.

Reference:
   1. Schwartz GR. Food Poisoning: Botulism. *In:*Haddard LM, Winchester JF, (eds.). Clinical Management of Poisoning and Drug Overdose. Philadelphia: WB Saunders, 1983:335–342.

TOXIC SHOCK SYNDROME

"Just because your doctor has a name for your condition doesn't mean he knows what it is."

Murphy

Toxic shock syndrome (TSS) is a disease of acute onset, marked by fever, multiple organ system involvement, rash, and severe hypotension. There has been a plethora of reports and studies since the syndrome was first described in 1978, and to date more than 1600 cases have been reported to the Centers for Disease Control. A primary infection with *Staphylococcus aureus* has been implicated in most cases; however, the production of toxins from this organism appears to be primarily responsible for most of the clinical manifestations. A total of 92 per cent of reported cases of TSS are associated with menstruation and tampon use. It is important to remember, however, that nonmenstrual TSS occurs (in both adults and children) and may occur in patients with burns, postoperative wound infections, post-partum infections, and complications following abortions. Localized *S. aureus* infections in lung, bone, skin, and nasal mucosa have also been implicated. The criteria for the diagnosis of TSS are listed here; preferably, all of those signs listed must be present to assure diagnosis.

Criteria for the Diagnosis of Toxic Shock Syndrome

1. Fever (Temperature $\geq$ 38.9°C [102°F]).
2. Rash: Erythematous macular rash (occasionally petechial).
3. Hypotension: Systolic blood pressure $\leq$ 90 mmHg for adults, $\leq$ 5th percentile for children under 16 years of age, orthostatic drop in diastolic blood pressure $\geq$ 15 mmHg from lying to sitting, or orthostatic syncope.
4. Multisystem involvement (3 or more):
   a. Gastrointestinal: vomiting, diarrhea at onset of illness.
   b. Mucous membrane: vaginal, oropharyngeal, or conjunctival hyperemia.
   c. Muscular: severe myalgia, or creatine phosphokinase level $\geq$ 2× upper limit of normal, or both.
   d. Renal: BUN or creatinine levels $\geq$ 2× the upper limit of normal; urinary sediment with pyuria ($\geq$ 5 WBC/high powered field); or oliguria ($\leq$ 1 ml/kg/hr urine production for 24 hours).
   e. Hepatic: SGOT or SGPT levels $\geq$ 2× the upper limit of normal.
   f. Hematologic: thrombocytopenia (platelets < 100,000/mm³).
   g. Central nervous system: disorientation or alterations in conscious-

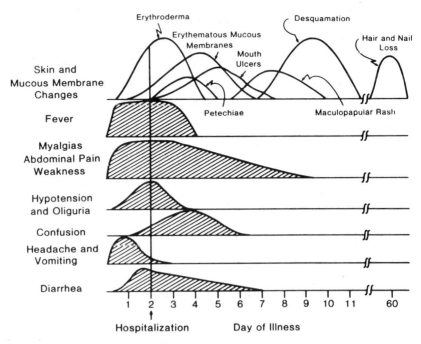

Fig. 7-7. Typical pattern of TSS.

ness without focal findings and in the absence of hypotension and hyperpyrexia.

h. Cardiopulmonary: hypoxemia, myocardial depression.

i. Metabolic: serum calcium level $\leq$ 7.0 mg/100 ml, phosphate level $\leq$ 2.5 mg/100 ml, total serum protein level $\leq$ 5.0 mg/100 ml.

5. Desquamation of palms and soles during recovery phase.

6. Reasonable evidence for the absence of rickettsial disease, leptospirosis, meningococcemia, and rubeola (measles).

The typical clinical pattern is demonstrated in Figure 7-7.

One third of TSS patients will have at least one further episode of TSS. Most of these recurrences are less severe than the original episode. The risk of recurrence is reduced if antistaphylococcal antibiotics are utilized during the primary illness. The criteria for recurrence of TSS are as follows:

A. *Major Criteria*

1. Fever $\geq$ 38.9°C (102°F).

2. Rash.

3. Vomiting or diarrhea.

4. Mucous membrane hyperemia or myalgia.

5. Hypotension.

B. *Definite Recurrence*

1. Desquamation and at least three major criteria.

C. *Probable Recurrence*

    1. Desquamation and two major criteria.

    2. Three major criteria associated with menstruation.

The following diseases would be included in the differential diagnosis of TSS:

1. Scarlet fever.
2. Leptospirosis.
3. Rocky Mountain spotted fever.
4. Septic shock and meningococcemia.
5. Hemolytic uremic syndrome.
6. Mucocutaneous lymph node syndrome (Kawasaki disease).

Steps to be taken in patients suspected of having TSS include:

1. Appropriate cultures from all suspected sites of *S. aureus* infection.
2. Removal of tampons or other foreign objects (wound packs, dressings, nasal packs).
3. Insertion of large-bore venous catheters.
4. Intensive monitoring while in the emergency department.
5. After cultures are obtained, intravenous antibiotics effective against coagulase-positive *S. aureus* should be administered.
6. If shock is present, intravascular volume replacement with crystalloid solutions should be instituted.

References:

    1. Chesney PJ, Crass BA, Polyak MB, et al. Toxic shock syndrome: management and long-term sequelae. Ann Intern Med 1982;*96*(2):847–.

    2. Chesney PJ, Davis JP, Purdy WK, et al. Clinical manifestations of toxic shock syndrome. JAMA 1981;*246*:741–748. (Figure reproduced with permission. Copyright 1981, American Medical Association.)

AVAILABLE FROM THE CDC – IMMUNOBIOLOGIC AGENTS AND ANTIPARASITIC DRUGS

The Centers for Disease Control (CDC) in Atlanta currently distribute four special immunobiologic agents through the Immunobiologics Services, Biologic Products Division, Center for Infectious Diseases (CID), and 13 drugs for parasitic diseases through the Parasitic Diseases Division, CID, and the Quarantine Division, Center for Prevention Services.

The CDC dispenses the agent or drug to the requesting physician for administration to a patient whose situation or condition calls for its use, but only if and when that use is approved by the CDC for that particular patient. Included in the package insert is appropriate information regarding indications and contraindications, dosages, routes, frequency of administration, adverse reactions, toxicity, and other data.

Emergency supplies of four of these products are available at CDC quarantine stations located at airports in Boston, Chicago, Honolulu, Los Angeles, Miami, New Orleans, New York, San Francisco, San Juan, Seattle, and Washington, D.C. To obtain these products, call the CDC.

Products Available for Emergency Use

PRODUCT	TELEPHONE NUMBERS	
	Monday-Friday 8 A.M. to 4:30 P.M.	*After working hours, holidays, and weekends*
Botulinal equine antitoxin (ABE)	404-329-3753	404-329-3311
Diphtheria equine antitoxin	404-329-3687	404-329-3311
Vaccinia immune globulin (VIG)	404-329-2562	404-329-3311
Varicella-zoster immune globulin (VZIG)*		
Pentamidine isethionate and other parasitic drugs	404-329-3670	404-329-3311

*As of February 1, 1981, VZIG is distributed in the United States by the American Red Cross Blood Services-Northeast Region through 13 regional Blood Centers. All requests for VZIG should be directed to the nearest regional distribution center, although physicians experienced with VZIG will continue to be available for consultation at the Immunization Division.

7

Drugs Available for Treating Parasitic Diseases

DRUGS	INDICATIONS
Pentamidine isethionate (Lomidine)	Pneumocystosis, African trypanosomiasis
Sodium stibogluconate (Pentostam)	Leishmaniasis
Suramin (Bayer-205)	African trypanosomiasis, onchocerciasis
Melarsoprol (Mel B)	African trypanosomiasis
Bayer-2502 (Lampit)	American trypanosomiasis
Diloxanide furoate (Furamide)	Amebiasis
Dehydroemetine	Amebiasis
Bithionol, N.F.	Paragonimiasis
Sodium antimony dimercaptosuccinate (Astiban)	Schistosomiasis
Metrifonate (Bilarcil)	Schistosomiasis
Quinine dihydrochloride (parenteral)	Pernicious malaria
Chloroquine hydrochloride (parenteral)	Pernicious malaria

Nonemergency requests for immunobiologics such as anthrax vaccine, botulinal toxoid, eastern equine encephalitis vaccine, tularemia vaccine, and Venezuelan equine encephalitis vaccine may be made by writing or calling the Immunobiologics Services, Biological Products Division, Monday through Friday, 8 A.M. to 4:30 P.M. (Eastern time) at 404-329-3356. For drugs for parasitic diseases, write or call the Parasitic Disease Drug Service, Parasitic Diseases Division, Monday through Friday, 8 A.M. to 4:30 P.M. (Eastern time) at 404-329-3670.

Reference:
1. Available from the CDC. Consultant 1984; Feb: 205. (With permission.)

SINGLE-DOSE TREATMENT OF UTI'S

Recent studies have indicated that single-dose antimicrobial therapy is effective in eradicating uncomplicated urinary tract infections for selected patients. Obvious advantages of single-dose therapy are simplicity, elimination of the need for compliance, low incidence of drug reactions, cost effectiveness, and less chance for the development of resistant organisms.

The following is a list of indications, contraindications, and antibiotics known to be effective for single dose treatment of UTI'S.

I.   Indications
1. Acute uncomplicated cystitis.
2. Asymptomatic bacteriuria in nonpregnant women.
3. Asymptomatic bacteriuria of pregnancy.
4. Asymptomatic pyelonephritis.

II. Contraindications
1. Recurrent urinary tract infections.
2. Acute urethral syndromes.
3. Acute pyelonephritis.
4. Acute and chronic prostatitis.
5. Catheter-associated bacteriuria.
6. Compromised host with acute cystitis.

III. Antibiotics and Doses
1. Most effective.
   a. Amoxicillin, 3 gm orally.
   b. Trimethoprim-sulfamethoxazole, 3 double-strength tablets or 6 regular tablets (total dose 2.4 gm SMX, 480 mg TMP).

2. Others.
   a. Sulfisoxazole, 2 gm orally.
   b. Kanamycin, 500 mg IM, 1 dose.

Patients usually have a bacteriologic cure in 24 to 48 hours; however, symptoms may persist. Follow-up cultures are indicated in all initially asymptomatic patients and in those with persistent or recurrent symptoms 1 week after therapy.

References:
1. Treatment of UTI'S. Med Lett 1981;*24*(23):69.
2. Abraham E, Brenner BE, Simon RR. Cystitis and pyelonephritis. Ann Emerg Med 1983; *12*(4):228–234.
3. Cunha BA. Single dose therapy of urinary tract infections. Hosp Phys 1983;*19*:35–37.

MINDLESS WORKUP OF HEMATURIA

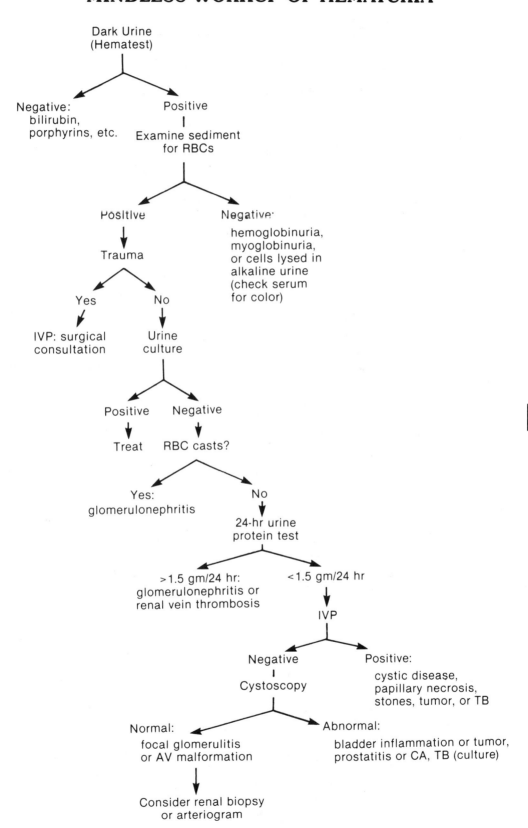

Dark Urine
(Hematest)

Negative:
bilirubin,
porphyrins, etc.

Positive

Examine sediment
for RBCs

Positive

Negative:
hemoglobinuria,
myoglobinuria,
or cells lysed in
alkaline urine
(check serum
for color)

Trauma

Yes

No

IVP: surgical
consultation

Urine
culture

Positive

Negative

Treat

RBC casts?

Yes:
glomerulonephritis

No

24-hr urine
protein test

>1.5 gm/24 hr:
glomerulonephritis or
renal vein thrombosis

<1.5 gm/24 hr

IVP

Negative

Cystoscopy

Positive:
cystic disease,
papillary necrosis,
stones, tumor, or TB

Normal:
focal glomerulitis
or AV malformation

Abnormal:
bladder inflammation or tumor,
prostatitis or CA, TB (culture)

Consider renal biopsy
or arteriogram

7

HYPONATREMIA

The first step in evaluating a low serum sodium level is to satisfy yourself that true hyponatremia exists. This involves eliminating the possibility of the following four factors:

1. *Spurious hyponatremia* occurs with *hyperlipidemia* (when a lipid layer increases blood volume), although sodium concentration in the water compartment is normal. This can also be seen with severe *hyperproteinemia* (serum protein level > 12–15 gm/100 ml) in which there is an increase in plasma volume without an increase in the water compartment. In spurious hyponatremia, the plasma osmolarity is normal.

2. A shift of water out of cells caused by extracellular solutes, such as glucose and mannitol. For every 100 mg/100 ml elevation in serum glucose level, the serum sodium level will drop by 1.6 mEq/L.

3. Laboratory error.

4. Sampling error: Blood is drawn above an intravenous site or through a central line without adequate aspiration.

True hyponatremia represents a disproportion between body water and sodium. This can occur in a patient who is dehydrated or in a patient who is volume expanded. It is essential to determine at the outset whether the patient is hypovolemic, euvolemic, or hypervolemic.

Hypervolemia

If the patient has *edema* and appears to have excess extracellular fluid, he has increased body salt but excessively increased water. Such a patient most likely has (1) cirrhosis, (2) congestive heart failure, or (3) nephrotic syndrome.

In all three conditions, the urinary sodium concentration on a spot sample should be less than 10 mEq/L, and the urinary osmolarity should be high.

If the urinary sodium concentration is greater than 20 mEq/L, suspect that the patient has underlying renal disease and has ingested more water than he can excrete given his glomerular filtration rate (GFR).

Euvolemia

If a patient appears *normally hydrated,* he probably has the syndrome of inappropriate ADH secretion (SIADH). (Excess ADH actually results in a modest, clinically inapparent volume expansion.) The urinary sodium concentration will be high (unless dehydration coexists), and the urinary osmolarity will exceed serum osmolarity. Additional clues are low BUN and uric acid levels. The diagnosis can be confirmed by the water-loading test when the patient is stable.

There are many causes of SIADH. They include solid tumors, lymphomas, and leukemias; all sorts of lung diseases; nearly any intracranial disease; many drugs; and "stress."

Hypothyroidism and glucocorticoid deficiency also impair water excretion and resemble SIADH.

Hypovolemia

If the patient is *clinically dehydrated,* he has lost more salt than water from either a renal or an extrarenal source, distinguishable by the urinary sodium concentration.

Renal salt loss (with high U_{Na}) occurs with (1) diuretic use, (2) interstitial disease, and (3) mineralocorticoid deficiency.

Nonrenal salt loss can occur from (1) the GI tract (diarrhea, vomiting), (2) the skin (severe burns), and (3) "third spacing" of fluid as in pancreatitis, peritonitis, traumatized muscle, and so forth.

The normal kidney has the ability to excrete 15 to 20 ml/minute of excess water. Therefore, water intoxication will occur only if the patient is limited in his ability to excrete free water (decreased GFR, diuretics, SIADH, and so forth), or if the patient is able to maintain a water intake exceeding 2 liters every hour.

7

Thanks to Steve Scheinman, M.D. for this contribution.
References:

1. DeFronzo RA, Thier SO. Pathophysiologic approach to hyponatremia. Arch Intern Med 1980;*140*:897–916.

2. Gottlieb AJ, Zamkoff K, Jastremski MS, et al. The Whole Internist Catalog. Philadelphia; WB Saunders, 1980:360–362.

ANTACID UPDATE

The next two tables compare the acid neutralizing capacity, sodium content, and monthly cost of therapy for the commonly used liquid and tablet antacids. The monthly cost of therapy is based on a standard therapy for duodenal ulcer using antacid at a dosage sufficient to neutralize 140 mEq of acid one and three hours after meals and at bed time for 30 days. Since there is little difference in the cost of the various antacids when calculated per bottle or per tablet,

Neutralizing Capacity, Sodium Content, and Cost Effectiveness of Liquid Antacids

ANTACID	ACID NEUTRALIZING CAPACITY mEq/mL	VOLUME CONTAINING 140 mEq mL	SODIUM CONTENT mg/5 mL	MONTHLY COST OF THERAPY $	COMPOSITION	MANUFACTURER
Maalox TC	4.2	33	1.2	44	Aluminum hydroxide, magnesium hydroxide	W.H. Rorer, Inc., Fort Washington, Pennsylvania
Titralac	4.2	33	11.0	35	Calcium carbonate, glycine	Riker Laboratories, Inc., Northridge, California
Delcid	4.1	34	1.5	57	Aluminum hydroxide, magnesium hydroxide	Merrell-National Laboratories, Cincinnati, Ohio
Mylanta II	3.6	39	1.1	63	Aluminum hydroxide, magnesium hydroxide, simethicone	Stuart Pharmaceuticals, Wilmington, Delaware
Camalox	3.2	44	2.5	55	Aluminum hydroxide, magnesium hydroxide, calcium carbonate	W.H. Rorer, Inc. Fort Washington, Pennsylvania
Gelusil II	3.0	47	1.3	74	Aluminum hydroxide, magnesium hydroxide, simethicone	Parke-Davis, Morris Plains, New Jersey
Basaljel ES	2.9	48	23.0	101	Aluminum carbonate	Wyeth Laboratories Philadelphia, Pennsylvania
Maalox Plus	2.3	61	2.5	68	Aluminum hydroxide, magnesium hydroxide, simethicone	W.H. Rorer, Inc., Fort Washington, Pennsylvania
Gelusil	2.2	64	0.7	80	Aluminum hydroxide, magnesium hydroxide, simethicone	Parke-Davis, Morris Plains, New Jersey
Riopan Plus	1.8	78	0.7	78	Aluminum hydroxide, magnesium hydroxide, simethicone	Ayerst Laboratories, New York, New York
Amphojel	1.4	100	7.0	114	Aluminum hydroxide	Wyeth Laboratories Philadelphia, Pennsylvania
Phosphaljel	0.3	466	12.5	498	Aluminum phosphate	Wyeth Laboratories, Philadelphia, Pennsylvania

the differences in the monthly cost of therapy are caused by wide differences in the neutralizing capacities of the various antacids.

The considerations in advising your patients to use an antacid regimen are cost effectiveness, convenience, taste, and in some patients, sodium content or phosphate binding. The liquid forms are generally more cost effective, because they are better neutralizers. However, one of the high potency tablet preparations may be more convenient for use during the day.

Neutralizing Capacity, Sodium Content, and Cost Effectiveness of Tablet Antacids

ANTACID	ACID NEUTRALIZING CAPACITY mEq/tablet	VOLUME CONTAINING 140 mEq tablets	SODIUM CONTENT mg/5 tablet	MONTHLY COST OF THERAPY $	COMPOSITION	MANUFACTURER
Camalox	16.7	8	1.5	54	Aluminum hydroxide, magnesium hydroxide	W.H. Rorer, Inc., Fort Washington, Pennsylvania
Basaljel	15.4	9	2.0	68	Aluminum carbonate	Wyeth Laboratories, Philadelphia, Pennsylvania
Mylanta II	11.0	13	1.3	85	Aluminum hydroxide, magnesium hydroxide, simethicone	Stuart Pharmaceuticals, Wilmington, Delaware
Tums	10.5	13	2.7	56	Calcium carbonate	Norcliff Thayer, Inc., Tuckahoe, New York
Alka 2	10.5	13	2.0	58	Calcium carbonate	Miles Laboratories, Inc., Elkhart, Indiana
Riopan Plus	10.0	14	0.3	76	Aluminum hydroxide, magnesium hydroxide, simethicone	Ayerst Laboratories, New York, New York
Titralac	9.5	15	0.3	57	Calcium carbonate, glycine	Riker Laboratories, Inc., Northridge, California
Gelusil II	8.2	17	2.1	107	Aluminum hydroxide, magnesium hydroxide, simethicone	Parke-Davis, Morris Plains, New Jersey
Rolaids	6.9	20	53.0	86	Aluminum carbonate	Warner Lambert Company, Morris Plains, New Jersey
Maalox Plus	5.7	25	1.4	106	Aluminum hydroxide, magnesium hydroxide, simethicone	W.H. Rorer, Inc., Fort Washington, Pennsylvania
Digel	4.7	30	10.6	101	Aluminum hydroxide, magnesium hydroxide, simethicone, magnesium carbonate	Plough, Inc., Memphis, Tennessee
Amphojel	2.0	70	7.0	360	Aluminum hydroxide	Wyeth Laboratories, Philadelphia, Pennsylvania

Reference:
1. Drake D, Hollander D. Neutralizing capacity and cost effectiveness of antacids. Ann Intern Med 1981;*94*:215–217. (Tables reproduced with permission.)

MANAGEMENT OF TONIC-CLONIC STATUS EPILEPTICUS *

1. Establish an oral or nasopharyngeal airway. Give oxygen. Draw venous blood for CBC and serum electrolytes, calcium, magnesium, glucose, and BUN levels; and levels of any anticonvulsant drugs prescribed for the patient. Draw arterial blood for gas determinations. Monitor the ECG.

2. Start an intravenous line of normal saline. Give thiamine 50 to 100 mg IM or IV, and glucose (D50W), 50 ml IV.

3. Give diazepam, 2 mg/min IV, until seizures stop or to a total of 20 mg. Also give phenytoin, 50 mg/min, to a total of 18 mg/kg. (If a patient's level of consciousness must be monitored, as in head trauma, use phenytoin alone.)

4. If seizures persist, intubate and ventilate the patient. Give phenobarbital, 100 mg/min IV, until seizures stop or to a total of 20 mg/kg, *or* give diazepam, 8 mg/hr, as a continuous IV drip (e.g., 100 mg diazepam in D5W, 500 ml at 40 ml/hr).

5. If seizures persist, give lidocaine, 50 to 100 mg IV, bolus. If seizures stop, begin a continuous drip of 1 to 2 mg/min lidocaine, *or* give paraldehyde 4 per cent, 5 to 10 ml orally or rectally. (Dilute rectal paraldehyde with 2 volumes olive oil.)

6. If seizures persist, arrange for general anesthesia with halothane and neuromuscular blockade. This should be done only with EEG monitoring.

---

*Adapted from Delgado-Escueta (Table 1, 1339).

References:

1. Delgado-Escueta AV, Wasterlain C, Treiman DM, Porter RJ. Management of status epilepticus. New Engl J Med 1982;*306*:1337–1340.

2. Goodman LS, Gilman A. The Pharmacological Basis of Therapeutics, 5th ed. New York: Macmillan Publishing Co., Inc., 1975:132.

3. Poulton TJ. Management of status epilepticus (Letter). New Engl J Med 1982;*307*:1146.

SHINGLES

Shingles is an excruciatingly painful skin condition caused by activation of latent varicella-zoster (chickenpox and shingles virus). The patient's complaint is that of a sensation described as burning, itchy, prickly, tingling, sharp and knife-like, or various combinations of these sensations associated with a rash that involves one or two adjacent dermatomes. The rash will begin as vesicles that become pustules and then scabs over one to two weeks. Most patients are seen after the rash has developed, making the diagnosis simple. Some patients, however, will experience the pain before the rash develops, which can lead to some diagnostic difficulties. Hyperesthesia in the area of pain sensation is sometimes a clinical clue that the cause is shingles.

The following list contains four considerations for the emergency physician in the management of a patient with shingles.

1. *Relief of acute symptoms:* A cocktail of an analgesic and an antihistamine is often quite effective. We use acetaminophen with codeine and diphenhydramine. Calamine lotion may also be helpful for the itching. One sufferer reported that pressure applied to the rash with an elastic binder provided dramatic pain relief.

2. *Prevention of postherpetic neuralgia.* Postherpetic neuralgia is a dreaded complication of varicella-zoster in older patients. Prednisone 50 to 100 mg daily for 5 days, and then tapered off for another 5 days, definitely reduces the incidence of postherpetic neuralgia and should be given to any immunocompetent patient more than 50 years of age. Prednisone should not be given to any immunosuppressed individual because of the possibility of potentiating systemic dissemination.

3. *Recognition of optic involvement.* Herpes zoster of the ophthalmic branch of the trigeminal nerve may cause permanent visual damage. Clues to ophthalmic involvement are vesicles along the nose and a dendrite pattern of corneal ulceration revealed by fluorescein staining. Ophthalmic herpes requires immediate treatment by an ophthalmologist.

4. *Prevention of systemic spread.* Patients who are immunosuppressed because of other reasons, particularly lymphatic malignancies and drug therapy, are at risk of a generalized herpes infection with CNS involvement or pneumonia that is often fatal. These patients should be admitted and given intravenous vidarabine if it can be started within 72 hours of the onset of the rash.

Reference:
1. Challenge of a painful pox. Acute Care Medicine 1984; March:13–28.

8

PEDIATRICS

THE APPROACH TO THE CHILD IN THE EMERGENCY
DEPARTMENT 280

PEDIATRIC NORMS 282

THE AIRWAY IN PEDIATRICS 284

WORTH ITS WEIGHT 285

MAINTENANCE FLUIDS IN PEDIATRICS 285

BURN ESTIMATES IN CHILDREN 286

DIABETIC KETOACIDOSIS (DKA) IN CHILDHOOD 287

REYES SYNDROME 288

NEWBORN STABILIZATION 289

THE IRRITABLE INFANT 292

OTALGIA IN CHILDREN 293

SINUSITIS IN CHILDHOOD 294

THE SWOLLEN EYE 295

THE UVULA: THE FINAL FRONTIER? .296

HEART FAILURE IN INFANTS AND CHILDREN 297

SICKLE CELL ANEMIA: INFECTION OR INFARCTION? 298

THE CHILD WITH STRIDOR 299

EN FACE OR ON EDGE? 300

FOREIGN OBJECTS IN THE AIRWAY .300

ALL THAT WHEEZES 301

THE ASTHMATIC FLOW SHEET 302

DRIVE–THRU PULMONARY TESTING .304

THEOPHYLLINE TO GO 306

CHLAMYDIAL INFECTIONS IN INFANCY 307

THE RETURN OF THE WHOOP 309

ACUTE PEDIATRIC PNEUMONIA 310

CHEST PAIN IN CHILDREN 312

THE "ACUTE ABDOMEN" IN PEDIATRICS 313

RECTAL BLEEDING IN INFANCY AND CHILDHOOD 314

INFECTIOUS GASTROENTERITIS 317

ORAL REHYDRATION SOLUTIONS 317

THE DYNAMICS OF SEXUAL ABUSE IN CHILDHOOD 318

THE SUPRAPUBIC URINE SPECIMEN 319

STIFF NECK IN CHILDREN 321

NURSEMAID'S ELBOW 321

IF THE CRUTCH FITS 322

CLOSING CUTS IN CHILDREN 322

INCREASED INTRACRANIAL PRESSURE IN INFANCY
AND CHILDHOOD 323

THE COMATOSE CHILD 324

STATUS EPILEPTICUS IN CHILDHOOD 328

KAWASAKI SYNDROME
(MUCOCUTANEOUS LYMPH NODE SYNDROME) 329

SCABIES 331

THE DIFFERENTIAL DIAGNOSIS OF CHILD ABUSE 332

THE AUTOPSY REQUEST IN PEDIATRICS 334

THE APPROACH TO THE CHILD
IN THE EMERGENCY DEPARTMENT

Infants and children often respond poorly to new and threatening environments and people. It is part of our job, therefore, to minimize the trauma for a child being treated in the emergency department. In so doing, we lessen the anxiety of both the child and the parents, a factor that can help maximize the reliability of the physical examination and medical evaluation. Several general principles that should be utilized are as follows:

A. The Emergency Department Environment

    1. Infants and children, if possible, should not share the same waiting area with adult patients.

    2. A patient (of any age) who is loud or abusive should be isolated from all children who are waiting for treatment.

    3. The sound of another child's cry is contagious; examination rooms should be as private as possible to isolate a child's cry.

    4. Equip the examination room with distractions and use them, e.g., posters, paintings, mobiles, toys, books, and hand puppets.

    5. Small infants are sensitive to temperature variations; keep the room warm.

B. The Role of the Parent

    1. A calm interaction between physician and parent will often relax an anxious child.

    2. If a child is resting calmly in the parent's arms when you enter the room, utilize this quiet time to interview the child or parent. Facets of the physical examination that can be performed with the child in this position include the child's color and tone, respiratory rate and effort, fontanelle status, appearance of the pupils, and general state of alertness.

    3. Possible reasons for parental absence during the physical examination include:

       a. Honoring the privacy of an adolescent.

       b. Evaluating potential physical or sexual abuse.

       c. A child who is critically ill.

       d. Parents who are emotionally unable to witness possibly painful procedures.

C. The Role of the Physician

    1. Never isolate yourself from the child emotionally; attempts at communication should be made with patients of all age groups, using eye contact, smiles (with infants), or direct conversation.

2. Tell the truth. If you are going to perform a painful procedure, let the child in on it. There is no quicker way to break a bond of trust than by saying "this won't hurt" when it will hurt.

3. Assume that the school-age child, five to ten years old, (and older) is modest until proved otherwise. A stepwise examination will not heighten this anxiety.

Finally, every age group has characteristics that bear directly on the type of approach the clinician should utilize. The table provides some developmental characteristics to aid in your approach to each group's emergency care.

Approach to Emergency Care of Pediatric Patients

AGE (Years)	IMPORTANT DEVELOPMENTAL CHARACTERISTICS	FEARS	USEFUL TECHNIQUES
Infants 0–1	Minimal language skills Feels like an extension of parents Sensitive to physical environment	Strangers	Keep parents in sight Prevent infants from getting hungry Use warm hands Keep room warm
Toddlers 1–3	Receptive language skills more advanced than expressive language skills See themselves as individuals Assertive	Brief separations Pain	Maintain verbal communication Examine while toddlers are in parent's lap Allow some choices when possible
Preschoolers 3–5	Excellent expressive language skills for thoughts and feelings Rich fantasy life Magical thinking Strong concept of self	Long separations Pain Disfigurement	Allow expression Encourage fantasy, play, and participation in care
School-age children 5–10	Fully developed language Understands some body structure and function Able to reason and compromise Experience with self-control Incomplete understanding of death	Disfigurement Loss of function Death	Explain procedures Explain pathophysiology and treatment Project positive outcome Stress children's ability to master situation Respect physical modesty
Adolescents 10–19	Self-determination Decision making ability Peer group important Realistic view of death	Loss of autonomy Loss of peer acceptance	Respect autonomy Stress acceptance by peers Allow choices and control

Reference:
1. Fleisher G, Ludwig S. Textbook of Pediatric Emergency Medicine. Baltimore: Williams & Wilkins, Company, 1982: XXXI. (Reprinted with permission of Williams & Wilkins Company, Baltimore.)

8

PEDIATRIC NORMS

Normal values for blood pressure, heart rate, and respiratory rate vary according to the age of each infant or child. Use the graphs and tables here to properly assess your pediatric patient's vital signs.

Age-Specific Heart Rates

AGE	HEART RATE (Beats min)	
	MEAN	RANGE
0–24 hr	119	94–145
1–7 days	133	100–175
8–30 days	163	115–190
1–3 mo	154	124–190
3–6 mo	140	111–179
6–12 mo	140	112–177
1–3 yr	126	98–163
3–5 yr	98	65–132
5–8 yr	96	70–115
8–12 yr	79	55–107
12–16 yr	75	55–102

Normal Resting Respiratory Rate Per Minute

AGE (YEARS)	BOYS MEAN ± SD	GIRLS MEAN ± SD
0–1	31 ± 8	30 ± 6
1–2	26 ± 4	27 ± 4
2–3	25 ± 4	25 ± 3
3–4	24 ± 3	24 ± 3
4–5	23 ± 2	22 ± 2
5–6	22 ± 2	21 ± 2
6–7	21 ± 3	21 ± 3
7–8	20 ± 3	20 ± 2
8–9	20 ± 2	20 ± 2
9–10	19 ± 2	19 ± 2
10–11	19 ± 2	19 ± 2
11–12	19 ± 3	19 ± 3
12–13	19 ± 3	19 ± 2
13–14	19 ± 2	18 ± 2
14–15	18 ± 2	18 ± 3
15–16	17 ± 3	18 ± 3
16–17	17 ± 2	17 ± 3
17–18	16 ± 3	17 ± 3

Normal Ranges for the Blood Pressures of Children

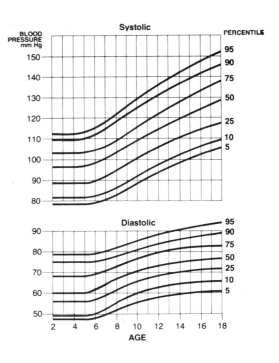

Fig. 8-1. Percentile for normal blood pressure measurement in boys (right arm, seated).

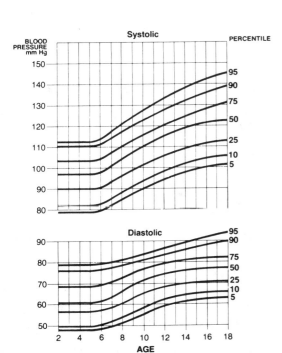

Fig. 8-2. Percentile for normal blood pressure measurement in girls (right arm, seated).

8

THE AIRWAY IN PEDIATRICS

The initial priority in pediatric CPR is the same as that in adult CPR, namely the establishment of an adequate airway. Some basic facts concerning ventilation of the pediatric patient are listed here.

1. The trachea of infants and children lacks the firm cartilaginous support of the adolescent and adult. Marked hyperextension of the neck will therefore collapse the trachea. Place the patient in a "sniffing" position by simply lifting the occiput of the head by the hand or by placing a rolled towel underneath the head.

2. The sole gauge of adequate ventilation is either the visible movement of the chest wall or the auscultation of satisfactory breath sounds.

3. Basic rate differences in the CPR of infants and children, as compared with adults, are outlined.

	HEART BEAT (Beats/min)	RESPIRATORY RATE (Breaths/min)
Infant	120–140	24–30
Young child	100–120	20–24
Older child and adolescent	80–100	12–18
Adult	60–80	8–12

4. The concentration of oxygen delivered to the hypoxic pediatric patient should be the highest possible. There is no need for concern in an emergency situation for the risks of oxygen toxicity.

5. A rough estimate of the correct size endotracheal tube to use is provided by the formula:

$$\frac{\text{Patient's age in years } + 16}{4} = \text{internal diameter of tube (mm)}$$

OR

Width of the patient's small digit = diameter of trachea

6. A more precise list is provided in the table.

Guidelines for Selection of Endotracheal Tubes and Suction Catheters*

AGE†	ENDOTRACHEAL TUBE (mm)	SUCTION CATHETER
Newborn	3.0	6F
6 mo	3.5	8F
18 mo	4.0	8F
3 yr	4.5	8F
5 yr	5.0	10F
6 yr	5.5	10F
8 yr	6.0	10F
12 yr	6.5	10F
16 yr	7.0	10F
Adult (F)	7.5–8.0	12F
Adult (M)	8.0–8.5	14F

*One size larger and one size smaller (0.5 mm) should be allowed for individual variations.
†Uncuffed tubes are utilized in patients less than 7 to 8 years of age.

WORTH ITS WEIGHT

All drugs administered to infants and children are given based on the patient's weight (kg). For some children with cardiac arrest, you may be lucky enough to receive a warning through ambulance radio of their impending ER arrival. One of the most valuable pieces of information you should obtain at this time is the age of the child. The following table allows you to estimate the child's weight from the age. While you await the arrival of the patient, you can prepare the appropriate medications and have them ready to promptly administer when the child arrives. This time-saving maneuver may prove lifesaving.

Average Weight (kg)

AGE	BOYS	GIRLS
1 mo	4	4
3 mo	6	5
6 mo	8	7
9 mo	9	8.5
12 mo	10	9.5
15 mo	11	10
18 mo	11.5	11
2 yr	12.5	12
2½ yr	13.5	13
3 yr	15	14
3½ yr	16	15
4 yr	17	16
4½ yr	18	17
5 yr	20	18
6 yr	21	20
7 yr	23	22
8 yr	25	25
9 yr	28	28
10 yr	32	33
11 yr	35	37
12 yr	40	41
13 yr	45	45
14 yr	50	50
15 yr	57	54
16 yr	63	57

8

MAINTENANCE FLUIDS IN PEDIATRICS

Occasionally, you may be called upon to order maintenance intravenous fluids for pediatric patients in your emergency department. Use the table as a guideline for calculating the appropriate rate of fluid administration. These rates are based on 50th percentile weights for age. It is important to emphasize that these are only *maintenance* rates. Be sure to modify your orders in cases of fluid imbalance, such as shock, dehydration, heart failure, or syndrome of inappropriate antidiuretic hormone secretion (common in infants and children with meningitis, Reyes syndrome, and head trauma).

Pediatric Maintenance Fluid Rates (ml/hr)

AGE	RATE	AGE	RATE
1 mo	15	7 yr	65
3 mo	25	8 yr	70
6 mo	30	9 yr	70
9 mo	35	10 yr	75
12 mo	40	11 yr	80
18 mo	45	12 yr	85
2 yr	45	13 yr	90
3 yr	50	14 yr	90
4 yr	55	15 yr	100
5 yr	60	16 yr	100
6 yr	65		

BURN ESTIMATES IN CHILDREN

We are all familiar with the "rule of nines," a convenient method for estimating the percentage of burned body surface in the adult patient. This rule is not accurate for children less than 14 years of age because of anatomic differences at various stages of growth. Use the table to correctly calculate the extent of burn injury in the pediatric patient.

Percentage of Burn Injury in Relation to Body Part

AREA	0–1 yr.	1–4 yr.	4–9 yr.	10–15 yr.	ADULT
Head	19	17	13	10	7
Neck	2	2	2	2	2
Anterior trunk	13	17	13	13	13
Posterior trunk	13	13	13	13	13
Right buttock	2½	2½	2½	2½	2½
Left buttock	2½	2½	2½	2½	2½
Genitalia	1	1	1	1	1
Right upper arm	4	4	4	4	4
Left upper arm	4	4	4	4	4
Right lower arm	3	3	3	3	3
Left lower arm	3	3	3	3	3
Right hand	2½	2½	2½	2½	2½
Left hand	2½	2½	2½	2½	2½
Right thigh	5½	6½	8½	8½	9½
Left thigh	5½	6½	8½	8½	9½
Right leg	5	5	5	6	7
Left leg	5	5	5	6	7
Right foot	3½	3½	3½	3½	3½
Left foot	3½	3½	3½	3½	3½

Reference:
1. The Harriet Lane Handbook. Chicago: Year Book Medical Publishers, 1981:226 (Reproduced with permission).

DIABETIC KETOACIDOSIS (DKA) IN CHILDHOOD

The infant or child with diabetes is always at risk of developing ketoacidosis. The multitude of infectious diseases that are encountered during childhood are often associated with fluid deficit incurred through emesis and an increase in the patient's insulin requirement. Mortality from DKA in children is estimated at less than 3 per cent. The mainstay of medical therapy for DKA in children is the provision of a constant level of circulating insulin. This is accomplished by the intravenous infusion of continuous low-dose insulin. An outline for management of diabetic ketoacidosis in children is provided.

Protocol for Management of Ketoacidosis

A. First Priority. Reverse or prevent hypovolemic shock or life-threatening acidosis or both.
   1. Begin initial IV fluid therapy of normal saline at 20 ml/kg/hr for 1 hr or until patient is normotensive.
   2. Institute $NaHCO_3$, 0.3 mEq/kg IV push, only if venous pH is $\leq$ 7.10. Continue slow drip of 150 mEq/L of $NaHCO_3$ only until pH reaches 7.10, *THEN STOP!* (Rapid bolus may suddenly increase osmolality, may produce systemic alkalosis with hypokalemia or paradoxical CSF acidosis with obtundation.)
B. Second Priority. Reverse metabolic sequelae of insulin deficiency.
   1. Give crystalline zinc insulin (CZI), 0.1 units/kg IV push.
   2. Administer CZI, 0.1 units/kg/hr constant infusion IV via Harvard pump through tubing preflushed with infusate (to prevent insulin binding to glass and plastic).
   3. Monitor blood glucose levels, venous pH, and potassium levels as indicated.
C. Third Priority. Prevent complications of re-insulinization.
   1. Add IV dextrose when blood glucose level reaches 300 mg/100 ml.
   2. Do not reduce hyperosmolality rapidly because of the increased risk of acute cerebral edema. Keep blood glucose levels between 200 and 300 mg/100 ml for the first 24 hours of therapy.
   3. Replenish fluid and electrolyte losses.
      a. Assume 10 per cent dehydration plus double maintenance fluids in the polyuric, hyperpneic child.
      b. For potassium and phosphate replacement, begin potassium replacement when the urinary output is established and the serum potassium level is $\leq$ 5.0 mEq/L. Replace at 3 to 6 mEq/kg/24 hr. Monitor patient who is receiving any infusate $\geq$ 40 mEq/L or $\geq$ 4 mEq/kg/24 hr with ECG (T waves). Give 50 per cent of the potassium as phosphate, the remainder as chloride.

8

Reference:
   1. Spack NP. Recent advances in the care of patients with juvenile diabetes mellitus. Pediatr Rev 1980; *1*:259–264.

REYES SYNDROME

Reyes syndrome primarily attacks children between the ages of 4 and 17 years. The illness has two major manifestations, hepatic dysfunction and encephalopathy. Morbidity and mortality from this disorder have greatly decreased in proportion to earlier diagnosis and institution of therapy.

Symptoms

Common symptoms include (1) recent URI, flu-like illness, or varicella; (2) protracted vomiting, beginning two to three days later; and (3) behavioral changes, such as lethargy, confusion, combativeness, delirium, and coma.

Very young infants with Reyes syndrome may *not* show the classic symptoms. They more commonly present with irritability, coma, or convulsions.

Stages of Neurologic Dysfunction

Stage 1	Patient is quiet, lethargic, and will not eat but will walk.
Stage 2	Patient is stuporous, has thick speech, is unable to follow commands, will not walk, and is clumsy.
Stage 3	Patient is delirious and combative. Clonus is present, Babinski sign may be positive or negative, pupils are dilated but responsive, and oculocephalic reflex is present.
Stage 4	Coma, decerebration, seizures, brainstem hyperventilation, tachycardia, blurred discs, dilated pupils, and oculocephalic reflexes are present.
Stage 5	Coma, flaccid paralysis, spinal reflexes, fixed dilated pupils, and papilledema are present; respirations and oculocephalic reflexes are absent.

Confirmatory Laboratory Studies

1. SGOT, SGPT levels are elevated.
2. Serum ammonia level is elevated.
3. Bilirubin level is normal.
4. Clotting dysfunction indicated by increased PT and PTT.
5. CPK markedly increased in some patients.

6. CSF may have greater opening pressure than normal, but white blood cell count, glucose level, and protein value are normal.

7. Profound hypoglycemia may be demonstrated.

Management

Once the diagnosis of Reyes syndrome has been made, the child should be transferred to a pediatric intensive care facility, where personnel are experienced in dealing with this disorder. Important management considerations prior to and during transport are as follows:

1. Establish phone contact with the intensive care unit staff to alert them to the patient's impending transport. Clinical advice is also best obtained in this manner.

2. Establish an intravenous line with 10% dextrose in half-normal saline and administer at two-thirds maintenance.

3. Administer Aquamephyton (vitamin K) 2 to 5 mg IM or IV.

4. Combativeness and undue stimulation increase the patient's intracranial pressure. If necessary, diazepam 0.1 to 0.4 mg/kg IV push can be used cautiously for transient sedation.

Reference:
1. Volk D. Reyes syndrome. Clin Pediatr 1981; *20*:505–511.

NEWBORN STABILIZATION

8

The birth of a child is a wonderful event. There is always the possibility, however, that a mother will give birth to an infant who is premature or in neonatal distress. Stabilization of these infants by the emergency department staff, while awaiting the arrival of a transport team from a neonatal special care unit, is a vital step in their management. The following clinical problems are most commonly encountered in these newborns.

Hypothermia

Hypothermia is defined as a rectal temperature below 36°C. It can result in an increased oxygen requirement owing to increased metabolic rate. Hypothermia causes metabolic acidosis, hypoglycemia, hypotension, and apnea.

Treatment

1. Thoroughly dry the newborn with warm, dry towels, and keep replacing them.

2. If oxygen is administered, it should be warmed and humidified.

3. Use an Isolette or overhead warmer if available. Rewarm the infant at 0.5° every half hour. Set the heat source $1^{\circ}C$ above the infant's rectal or axillary temperature.

4. Stabilize the infant at an axillary or rectal temperature of 36.5 to $37^{\circ}C$.

Hypotension

Hypotension is seen in asphyxiated infants and in those with septicemia, congestive heart failure, and respiratory distress. It can also be secondary to blood loss from abruptio placentae, placenta previa, maternal bleeding prior to delivery, or twin-to-twin transfusion.

Signs of hypotension include blanched skin, weak pulse, and cool, mottled extremities. The systolic blood pressure should always exceed 40 mmHg regardless of birth weight.

Treatment

The following are infused over 5 to 10 minutes:
1. Fresh frozen plasma at 10 ml/kg
2. Whole blood at 10 to 20 ml/kg
3. Lactated Ringer's solution at 10 to 20 ml/kg

Repeated infusions may be necessary.

Hypoglycemia

Hypoglycemia is very common in distressed newborns; glycogen stores in this group are easily depleted. Hypoglycemia is also seen in infants of diabetic mothers. Signs of hypoglycemia include apnea, tremors, irritability, lethargy, hypotonia, or seizures. Immediate bedside glucose level determinations using Dextrostix or Chemstrip methods should be made, if available, from blood sampled at the heel. Serum can be sent to the laboratory for confirmation. Hypoglycemia is defined as a blood glucose level of < 30 mg/100 ml in the full-term infant and < 20 mg/100 ml in the infant < 2500 gm.

Treatment

1. Administer an IV bolus of 1 ml/kg of 50 per cent dextrose.
2. Follow initial bolus with a continuous infusion of 10 per cent dextrose at 4 ml/kg/hr.

Altered Acid-Base Status

Newborns with respiratory distress commonly develop hypoxemia, hypercarbia, and acidosis. Infants generally do not become clinically cyanotic until the arterial oxygen concentration is less than 50 mmHg; therefore, arterial blood sampling is the preferred method for the detection of true hypoxemia.

There are toxicities in newborns related to overuse of supplemental oxygen. Arterial blood specimens should be taken for reliable monitoring of the response to therapy. Optimal arterial blood oxygen concentration is 60 to 80 mmHg. The treatment for respiratory acidosis is respiratory support; metabolic acidosis is best corrected *not* by bicarbonate infusion but by assuring adequate oxygenation, by correcting hypotension and hypothermia, and by maintaining normoglycemia.

Indications for positive pressure ventilation include the following:

1. Apnea or gasping

2. Severe shock

3. Hypercarbia with $Pa_{CO_2} > 60$ mmHg with pH < 7.20

4. Hypoxia with $Pa_{O_2} < 50$ mmHg with $F_{IO_2} > 90$ per cent

5. Persistent metabolic or respiratory acidosis

Frequent phone consultations with the staff of the referral center are recommended while you are waiting for the transport team to arrive. Emergency drug doses for newborns are listed next.

DRUG	DOSE
Epinephrine	0.1 ml/kg (1:10,000) IV or ET (endotracheal tube)
Sodium bicarbonate	1–2 mEq/kg IV (dilute 1:1 with sterile water)
Calcium gluconate (10 per cent)	1 ml/kg IV
Dextrose (50 per cent)	1 ml/kg IV (dilute 1:1 with sterile water)
Atropine	0.01 mg/kg IV
Naloxone	0.01 mg/kg IV

Reference:
Contributed by David Clark, M.D.

THE IRRITABLE INFANT

One of the most disturbing sounds is that of an infant who is crying uncontrollably. Parents are not immune to this stress and will frequently bring a baby in for a checkup, especially if the crying is of abrupt onset (often at night). The following is a list of possible causes to aid in evaluation of uncontrollable crying.

I.   Crying with Physical Findings
   A. Infections
       1. Meningitis
       2. Otitis media
       3. Gastroenteritis
       4. Urinary tract infection
       5. Osteomyelitis or septic arthritis

   B. Surgical Problems
       1. Intussusception
       2. Incarcerated hernia
       3. Testicular torsion

   C. Accidents
       1. Long-bone fracture
       2. Skull fracture
       3. Corneal foreign body or abrasion (think eyelash)
       4. Burn
       5. Open diaper pin
       6. Hair tourniquet on finger, toe, or penis

   D. Manifestations of Child Abuse
       1. Subdural hematoma
       2. Unexplained fracture
       3. Retinal hemorrhage

II. Crying without Physical Findings
   A. Hunger
   B. Teething
   C. Cow's milk allergy
   D. Colic
   E. Child abuse

Most infants will have no evidence of physical malady. The most important task of the emergency physician is then to reassure the parents that nothing is seriously wrong and that a clinical follow-up should be obtained if the problem persists. The competency of the parents must be assessed as well, for this stressful event mandates a calm approach within the home environment.

Reference:
   1. Brazelton T. Crying in infancy. Pediatrics 1962; *29*:579–588.

OTALGIA IN CHILDREN

Children who complain of ear pain are most often suffering from a problem within the ear itself. However, many instances occur in which anything but the ear is the culprit. Pain may be referred to the ear along various neurogenic pathways, including the trigeminal, facial, glossopharyngeal, and vagal nerves. Many of the causes of ear pain in children are outlined next.

I. Pain from the Ear Itself
   A. External Ear
      1. External otitis
      2. Foreign body or insect
      3. Trauma
   B. Middle Ear Structures
      1. Acute otitis media
      2. Serous otitis media
      3. Mastoiditis

II. Referred Pain
   A. Trigeminal Nerve
      1. Dental problems (caries, teething, abscess)
      2. Temporomandibular arthritis
      3. Paranasal sinusitis
   B. Facial Nerve
      1. Bell's palsy
      2. Herpes zoster oticus (viral neuritis of the facial nerve)
   C. Glossopharyngeal Nerve
      1. Tonsillar disease
      2. Retropharyngeal abscess
   D. Vagus Nerve
      1. Epiglottitis
      2. Thyroiditis
   E. Cervical Nerves
      1. Lymphadenopathy
      2. Lymphadenitis
      3. Cervical spine disease
   F. Miscellaneous
      1. Migraine
      2. Parotitis
      3. Psychogenic causes

8

SINUSITIS IN CHILDHOOD

As the title states, infections of the paranasal sinuses can occur during infancy and childhood. Clinical suspicion must be high, however, to assure early diagnosis in this age group. A clinical summary is therefore provided.

Anatomical Factors

1. Pneumatization occurs at birth for the maxillary and ethmoid sinuses, at 2 to 3 years of age for the sphenoid sinus, and at 4 to 6 years of age for the frontal sinus.

2. The majority of cases of sinusitis in early childhood involve the maxillary sinus. At 10 years of age, the frontal sinus is the most common site.

Clinical Patterns

1. The classic symptom complex of facial pain, headache, and fever is often absent in young children.

2. The most common clinical pattern in children consists of a protracted cold lasting longer than ten days with a daytime cough that worsens at night. Parents often report that the child has a low-grade fever and fetid breath. The nasal discharge may be thin or thick and can be clear or purulent.

3. A less common presentation is that of a child with a severe cold, a high fever (> 39°C), and a purulent nasal discharge. Periorbital swelling and pain may also be present.

4. The physical findings in many cases may be indistinguishable from those in simple rhinitis.

Diagnosis

1. Transillumination is awkward, requires time and cooperation, and is not very sensitive.

2. Classic x-ray findings include the presence of an air-fluid level, complete opacification, or mucosal membrane thickening (> 4 mm in children older than 1 year of age).

Bacteriology

1. *Streptococcus pneumoniae, Branhamella catarrhalis,* and *Hemophilus influenzae* occur most frequently.

2. Cultures from the throat or nasopharynx are of no clinical value.

Therapy

1. The antimicrobials of choice are ampicillin and amoxicillin.

2. In cases of resistant *B. catarrhalis* or *H. influenzae* and in

patients who are allergic to penicillin, cefaclor, trimethoprim-sulfamethoxazole, or erythromycin-sulfisoxazole may be used.

3. The value of decongestants and antihistamines is equivocal in the treatment of sinusitis in children.

Reference:
   1. Wald ER. Acute sinusitis in children. Pediatr Infect Dis 1983; *2*:61–65.

THE SWOLLEN EYE

Unilateral eye swelling is common in pediatric patients and is a difficult diagnosis for any clinician. The most important causes to exclude are those of either periorbital (preseptal) or true orbital cellulitis. Fortunately, there are many benign conditions that may be at work. The following two tables will assist you in solving the mystery.

Differential Diagnosis of "Swollen Eye" (Excluding Paranasal Sinus-Related Problems)

Periorbital laceration or abrasion	Trauma should be obvious. Cellulitis is most often caused by group A streptococci or coagulase-positive staphylococci.
Insect bite	The site of inoculation is usually evident. The surrounding area is nontender but often pruritic.
Allergy	Systemic allergy is usually not strictly unilateral. Contact allergy does not produce local or systemic signs of infection.
Conjunctivitis	The primary site of involvement is the conjunctiva, not the surrounding soft tissue. Slower progression; no systemic toxicity.
Dacryocystitis	Originates in medial lower lid. May progress to moderately severe cellulitis. Radiographic evidence of sinusitis is usually absent.
Dermatitis	Seborrheic or eczematoid skin changes apparent.
Nasal vestibular infection	Cellulitis begins about nasal vestibular area and produces edema of the lower eye lid prior to development of cellulitis in the upper lid or orbit.
Preseptal or periorbital cellulitis	Intense infection in preseptal area usually caused by *H. influenzae* type b. There is often a violaceous or hemorrhagic appearance to the tense, indurated tissue about the eye.

8

Classification of Orbital Cellulitis

STAGE		
I	Inflammatory Edema	Inflammatory edema beginning in medial or lateral upper eyelid; usually non-tender with only minimal skin changes. No induration, visual impairment, or limitation of extraocular movements.
II	Orbital Cellulitis	Edema of orbital contents with varying degrees of proptosis, chemosis, limitation of extraocular movement and/or visual loss.
III	Subperiosteal Abscess	Proptosis down and out with signs of orbital cellulitis (usually severe). Abscess beneath the periosteum of the ethmoid, frontal, or maxillary bone (in that order of frequency).
IV	Orbital Abscess	Abscess within the fat or muscle cone in the posterior orbit. Severe chemosis and proptosis; complete ophthalmoplegia and moderate to severe visual loss present (globe displaced forward or down and out).
V	Cavernous Sinus Thrombosis	Proptosis, globe fixation, severe loss of visual acuity, prostration, signs of meningitis; progresses to proptosis, chemosis, and visual loss in contralateral eye.

Reference:
1. Wald ER, Pang D, Milmoe GJ. Sinusitis and its complications in the pediatric patient. Pediatr Clin North Am 1981; *28*:777–796. (Tables reproduced with permission.)

THE UVULA: THE FINAL FRONTIER?

When was the last time you thought about the uvula? This forgotten piece of anatomy receives little or no attention in most medical literature; yet, uvulitis does occur and can be associated with significant morbidity. Be the first in your emergency department to know these facts about uvulitis in children.

1. The most common form of severe uvulitis is characterized by marked erythematous and hemorrhagic changes. It is usually associated with group A streptococcal pharyngitis and is rarely accompanied by airway obstruction.

2. A less common variety of severe uvulitis is observed in children with epiglottitis and concomitant *H. influenza* type b bacteremia. Patients with uvular erythema, who also have dysphagia or respiratory

distress, should, therefore, be evaluated radiographically to rule out the possibility of epiglottic swelling.

3. Appropriate surface cultures of the uvula should include plating on chocolate agar as well as on standard sheep-blood agar.

4. An unusual noninfectious cause of uvulitis in children is hashish abuse.

References:
1. Kotloff K, Wald E. Uvulitis in children. Pediatr Infect Dis 1983; *2*:392.
2. Tennant FS, Preble M, Prendergast TJ. Medical manifestations associated with hashish. JAMA 1971; *216*:1965.

HEART FAILURE IN INFANTS AND CHILDREN

Congestive heart failure (CHF) is a rare clinical event in children, as contrasted with its all too frequent occurrence in adults. Whereas most adults with this disease have a prior history of cardiac problems, failure itself may be the initial symptom of cardiac disease in infants. The majority of children ($>$ 90 per cent) with CHF present within the first year of life, usually as a manifestation of congenital heart disease. The older child with CHF is more likely to have myocardial or rheumatic diseases.

The presenting signs and symptoms of CHF in infants and children are listed; they are quite different from those in adults.

Signs and Symptoms of Congestive Heart Failure in Infants and Small Children

Fails to thrive and gain weight
Appears irritable
Tachypnea
   Poor, slow feeder
Tachycardia
Wheezes, gallop (auscultation)
Cardiomegaly
Hepatomegaly
Abnormal pulses
Sweating
Edema
   Decreased urination
Cyanosis
   Increased oxygen extraction

8

The mainstay of medical therapy for CHF in children is digitalization. A diuretic may be instituted as ancillary therapy if necessary. The most commonly used cardiac glycoside in pediatrics is digoxin. The graphs provide guidelines for its administration in the patient with acute CHF.

Digoxin Dosage for Infants and Children*

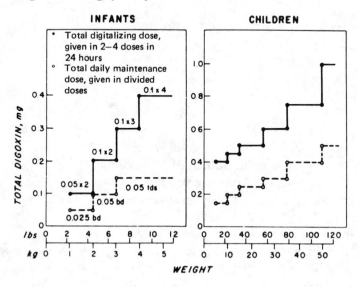

*Courtesy of Dr. Eoin Aberdeen and The Hospital for Sick Children, London, England. (tds = three times daily, bd = twice daily)

References:

1. Fulton D, Grodin M. Pediatric cardiac emergencies. Emerg Med Clin North Am 1983; *1*:45–49.

2. Nadas A, Hauck A. Pediatric aspects of congestive heart failure. Circulation 1960; *21*:424–429.

SICKLE CELL ANEMIA: INFECTION OR INFARCTION?

Infections are the most common cause of death in children with sickle cell anemia. Children with this hemoglobinopathy possess defects in host immunity that involve splenic function, serum factors, and white blood cell mechanics. It is therefore of paramount importance in this group of patients to correctly diagnose and treat any potential infectious process. A diagnostic problem may arise, however, since many vaso-occlusive sickle cell crises episodes mimic localized infections, especially in the lung and bones of children with sickle cell anemia. Use the facts presented in the tables to help distinguish between infarction (a vaso-occlusive crisis) and infection in this high risk population.

Bone

FEATURES INDICATING INFARCTION	FEATURES INDICATING OSTEOMYELITIS	SHARED FEATURES
Multiple sites	Band count	Local pain, tenderness
History of "crisis"	> 1000 cells/mm³	
History of predisposing factors	ESR > 20 mm/hr	Local erythema, swelling
	Culture results positive	Fever
Abnormal marrow scan	Normal marrow scan	Leukocytosis
		Abnormal x-ray findings
Symptoms abate without antibiotics	Antibiotics relieve symptoms	Abnormal bone scan
Culture results negative		

Lung

FEATURES INDICATING PNEUMONIA	FEATURES INDICATING PULMONARY INFARCTION	SHARED FEATURES
Age ≤ 5 yr	Associated, painful bony crisis	Chest pain
Shaking chills		Infiltrate
Upper-lobe disease	Normal x-ray at onset	Fever
Band count > 1000 cells/mm³	Lower-lobe disease	Leukocytosis
ESR > 20 mm/hr		Hypoxia
Gram stain of sputum		Effusion
Cultures		
Cold agglutinins		

Reference:

1. Nathan DG, Oski FA. Hematology of Infancy and Childhood. Philadelphia: WB Saunders, 1981; 702–703.

THE CHILD WITH STRIDOR

Upper airway obstruction is one of the most frightening emergencies in pediatric medicine. Not all stridor is caused by croup or epiglottitis. A careful history and physical examination will often uncover other "less traditional" causes. Use the tables to help make the correct diagnosis.

Clinical Features of Acute Upper Airway Disorders

	SUPRAGLOTTIC DISORDERS	SUBGLOTTIC DISORDERS
Stridor	Quiet and wet	Loud
Voice alteration	Muffled	Hoarse
Dysphagia	+	−
Postural preference*	+	−
Barky cough	−	+ especially with croup
Fever	+	+ usually in croup
Toxicity	+	−
Trismus	+ usually in peritonsillar abscess	−
Facial Edema	−	+ usually with angioedema

Epiglottitis—Patient characteristically sits bolt upright, with neck extended and head held forward. *Retropharyngeal abscess*—Child often adopts opisthotonic posture. *Peritonsillar abscess*—Patient may tilt head toward affected side.

8

Additional Features of Acute Upper Airway Disorders

	AGE GROUP	MODE OF ONSET OF RESPIRATORY DISTRESS
Severe tonsillitis	Late preschool or school age	Gradual
Peritonsillar abscess	Usually > 10 yr	Sudden increase in temperature, toxicity, and distress with unilateral throat pain, following earlier tonsillitis
Retropharyngeal abscess	Infancy to 3 yr	Sudden increase in temperature, toxicity, and distress after preceding URI or pharyngitis
Epiglottitis	2 to 7 yr	Very acute onset of high temperature with rapid progression of dysphagia and distress in previously well child
Croup	3 mo to 3 yr	Sudden onset (usually at night) of loud stridor and barky cough after preceding URI
Foreign body aspiration	Late infancy to 4 yr	Sudden choking episode while eating nuts, carrots, or chewing on small object, followed by onset of distress either immediately or, more typically, following a silent period of a few hours
Angioedema	Usually school age or older	Sudden onset shortly after eating, bee sting, or other environmental exposure

Reference:

1. Davis HW, Gartner JC, Galvis AG, et al. Acute upper airway obstruction: croup and epiglottitis. Pediatr Clin North Am 1981; *28:*859–880. (Tables reproduced with permission.)

EN FACE OR ON EDGE?

The tracheal rings are interrupted posteriorly, giving room for expansion of the tracheal lumen in the anterior-posterior direction. The esophagus is compressed between the trachea and the vertebral bodies, providing for enlargement of the esophageal lumen in the transverse direction.

The orientation of a flat foreign body on x-ray provides clues to its location. For AP and PA views, an object in the trachea will probably be seen on edge; one in the esophagus will probably be seen en face. In fact, one film clearly showed George Washington's profile— and a quarter was retrieved from the patient's esophagus.

FOREIGN OBJECTS IN THE AIRWAY

Aspiration or ingestion of foreign objects kills 2000 children in the United States each year. Those at greatest risk are between 6 months and 5 years of age.

The classic history is an episode of coughing, choking, gagging, or cyanosis after the child has handled food or small objects. Wheezing, stridor, continued coughing, or fever may develop.

The signs of airway obstruction vary with the site of obstruction and the size of the foreign body in relation to the airway. A foreign object in the esophagus can compress the trachea and cause respiratory symptoms.

Mechanisms of obstruction	Inspiration	Expiration	Clinical findings	X-ray findings
Ball valve (airflow blocked on expiration)			Hyperresonance on side of foreign body; wheezing	Unilateral emphysema; mediastinal shift away from foreign body on expiration
Stop valve (no airflow beyond obstruction)		Air reabsorbed slowly	Decreased breath sounds on side of foreign body; asymmetric chest movement	Late atelectasis
Check valve (foreign body impacts on inspiration but dislodges on expiration)		Air reabsorbed rapidly	Wheezing; decreased breath sounds on side of foreign body	Early atelectasis; mediastinal shift to side of foreign body
Bypass valve (airflow impeded on both inspiration and expiration)			Decreased breath sounds on side of foreign body; asymmetric chest movement; wheezing	Diffuse opacity on affected side

Chest x-rays should be taken of the patient during inspiration and expiration. If the patient cannot cooperate, expiration may be forced by epigastric pressure. (Beware of making the patient vomit.) Films taken by horizontal beam with the patient in the lateral decubitus position show expiration simulated in the dependent lung.

The physical examination and the chest x-ray findings may be normal, even though a foreign body is in the airway. The object may be demonstrated by fluoroscopy, lung perfusion scanning, or lung CT scanning.

If the upper airway is completely occluded, manual thrusts and back blows must be done immediately. Bronchoscopy is recommended for removal of objects from large airways. Bronchodilators and postural drainage may dislodge foreign bodies from segmental bronchi. The patient must be observed closely, as the freed object may lodge in the subglottic area, causing complete airway obstruction. (Also see Management of Airway Obstruction, pages 44 and 72.)

References:
1. Blumhagen JD, Wesenberg RL, Brooks JG, Cotton EK. Endotracheal foreign bodies. Clin Pediatr 1980; 19:480–484.
2. Stanford CC. Aspirated foreign bodies in children. Am Fam Physician 1979; 20:104–108. (Figure reprinted with permission.)

ALL THAT WHEEZES

All that wheezes in childhood is not necessarily asthma. In the pediatric patient, involvement of any branch of the respiratory tract may be accompanied by enough obstruction of outflow to induce wheezing as shown in the outline.

Differential Diagnosis of Wheezing in Children

A. Congenital anomalies
   1. Choanal atresia
   2. Laryngeal stridor
     a. Glottic abnormalities
     b. Chondromalacia
     c. Mandibular hypoplasia
     d. Congenital laryngeal web
     e. Subglottic hemangioma
   3. Tracheal abnormalities
     a. Tracheal or bronchial stenosis
     b. Tracheoesophageal fistulae
   4. Anomalies of the great vessels
B. Bronchial asthma
C. Infections
   1. Bronchiolitis
   2. Croup syndromes
   3. Pneumonia
   4. Bronchitis
     a. Infectious
     b. Chemical, including aspiration of gastric contents
     c. Allergic (asthmatic)
   5. Endobronchial disease
   6. Retropharyngeal and peritonsillar abscess
   7. Adenoid and tonsil hypertrophy
D. Foreign bodies
   1. Upper and lower airways
   2. Esophagus
E. Miscellaneous
   1. Cystic fibrosis
   2. Hypersensitivity pneumonitis
   3. Allergic bronchopulmonary aspergillosis
   4. Gastroesophageal reflux
   5. Alpha$_1$-antitrypsin deficiency
   6. Bronchiectasis

Reference:
   1. Howard WA. Differential diagnosis of wheezing in children. Pediatr Rev 1980; *1*:239–244.

THE ASTHMATIC FLOW SHEET

Children with asthma are frequent emergency patients. Although therapy for such patients varies from center to center, clinical evaluation is improved immeasurably if objective findings are recorded and compared in an orderly manner. The following two flow charts have been utilized with great success in our facility. The first provides a synopsis of the most pertinent historical facts; the second provides an ongoing record of the patient's response to medications.

Asthmatic History

Previously Diagnosed	_____	Duration of Respiratory Symptoms	_____
Age at Initial Diagnosis	_____	(cough, wheezing, dyspnea)	
Last Pediatric ED Visit	_____	Fever	_____
Hospitalizations per Year	_____	Vomiting	_____
Family History of Atopic Disease	_____	Emesis (fluids and medications)	_____

Precipitating Event   Yes   No   Oral Intake past 24 hours (specify) _____

    Medications (dose, dose interval, time of last dose)

	Yes	No	
URI	___	___	
Inhalant	___	___	Theophylline _____
Temperature and Humidity	___	___	Inhalant _____
Medications and Foods	___	___	Steroids _____

Additional Comments: _____

_____

_____

Asthmatic Patient's Response to Medication

	Admitting Examination R_x	Interval Examination R_x	Interval Examination R_x	Interval Examination R_x
Time				
Pulse				
BP				
Respirations				
Alert				
Cyanosis				
Retractions				
Air Movement				
Present				
Equal				
Wheezing				
Rales				
I/E Ratio				
Pulsus Paradoxus				
PEFR (peak expiratory flow rate)				

Hydration in ER

    PO _____

    IV _____

O_2 Used _____

Arterial Blood Gas Results

    (1) _____

    (2) _____

Theophylline Level _____

Final Discharge Diagnosis _____

Discharge Plans

    Medications _____

_____

    Fluids _____

    Follow-up MD _____

      when _____

8

DRIVE-THRU PULMONARY TESTING

Lower airway disorders (such as asthma and pneumonitis) are among the most common problems in children brought to pediatric emergency departments. Measurement of a child's peak expiratory flow rate (PEFR) provides a simple and reliable method of assessing obstructive pulmonary disease. The apparatus of choice is the Wright Peak Flow Meter,* a device that records the maximal flow rate during a forced expiration following a maximal inspiration. Here are some directions for its use.

1. The flow meter is available in two model sizes (for different ages) that are calibrated in liters of flow per minute. One reads the results directly from the meter without performing calculations.

---

*Available from Armstrong Industries: Northbrook, Illinois.

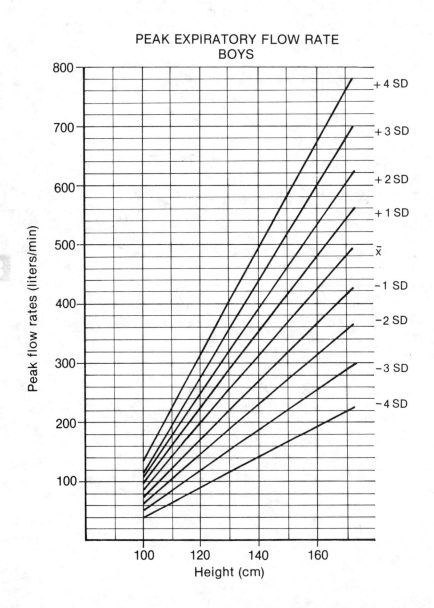

PEAK EXPIRATORY FLOW RATE
BOYS

Fig. 8-3 (A)

Illustration continued on opposite page

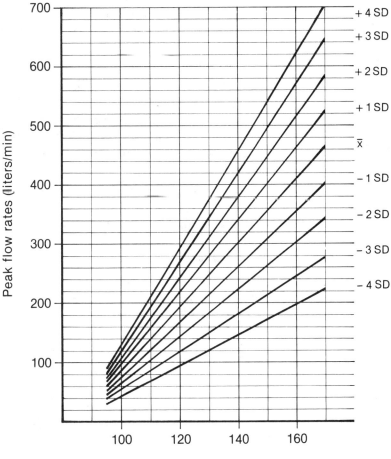

PEAK EXPIRATORY FLOW RATE
GIRLS

Fig. 8-3 (B) *Continued*

2. Instruct the child to take as deep a breath as possible and then to blow through the mouthpiece as fast and as hard as possible.

3. Encourage children to attempt to better their results with each successive measurement (4 to 5 attempts are recommended).

4. Children younger than 4 years of age may be unable to perform this test reliably.

5. The best PEFR obtained is then plotted on a graph that relates flow rate to height (cm) for boys and girls (Fig. 8-3 A & B).

6. A flow rate less than 2 SD below the mean is considered abnormal.

7. Use the PEFR in asthmatic children to determine their clinical status before and after bronchodilator therapy.

8. The older child with pneumonia whose PEFR is abnormal will have a difficult time generating an effective cough; consider admission for such a patient.

THEOPHYLLINE TO GO

You have just informed the parents of a wheezing child that he is most likely an asthmatic. You tell them that the drug of choice for the outpatient management of bronchospasm in children is theophylline. Before sending the family home with the patient's theophylline prescription, be sure to alert them to the following:

1. Asthma itself is a chronic disease with acute exacerbations. The "trigger" events that are reported to induce bronchospasm should be identified, since there are some that can be removed immediately from the child's environment (smoke, dust, mold, aspirin use, or animal hair products).

2. The importance of a follow-up visit (within 3 to 5 days) with the child's regular pediatrician should be stressed. Proper patient education mandates reinforcement, and this is best done in the outpatient setting.

3. Wheezing is often subclinical in character. Advise the parents to continue theophylline therapy for at least two days *after* the wheezing stops.

4. Theophylline therapy is not intermittent; it must be continued at the prescribed dosing intervals to provide maximal benefit.

5. Enumerate the expected side effects of theophylline, e.g., upset stomach, nausea, vomiting, headache, CNS stimulation, and increased urination.

6. Stress the importance of hydration in the asthmatic child. During the acute period, clear liquids are advisable; milk should be avoided.

7. Finally, the effectiveness of any medication is directly related to the compliance of the patient. For this reason, liquid preparations of theophylline are attractive for pediatric use. However, they are not very pleasant in flavor. Fortunately, the advent of bead-filled capsules has made it possible to administer theophylline to even the most reluctant child. The capsule can be opened and its contents can be "hidden" in attractive foods (ice cream, pudding) that the child will accept. Keep the use of these capsules in mind if liquid preparations are rejected by the child.

Both long- and short-acting formulations of theophylline are available for prescription. Recommended theophylline dosages and schedules for children are listed next.

1. Short-acting preparations: 4 to 6 mg/kg/dose, every 6 hours.

2. Long-acting preparations: 16 to 24 mg/kg daily, divided doses every 8 *or* 12 hours (some children are rapid metabolizers of theophylline).

Theophylline therapy should be individualized. Serum theophylline concentrations are the only reliable method for dosage adjustment; these determinations can be made for the child on an outpatient basis.

A table listing the more commonly prescribed theophylline preparations is provided.

Theophylline Preparations

	NAME	THEOPHYLLINE PER TEASPOON, TABLET, OR CAPSULE (MG)
Short-acting liquids	Elixophyllin Elixir	26
	Somophyllin Oral Liquid	90
	Theolair	26
Short-acting tablets or capsules	Elixophyllin Capsules	100, 200
	Somophyllin Capsules	50, 100, 200, 250
	Theolair Tablets	125, 250
Long-acting tablets or capsules	Elixophyllin-SR Capsules	125, 250
	Somophyllin-CRT Capsules	50, 100, 250
	Theo-Dur Tablets	100, 200, 300
	Theo-Dur Sprinkle	50, 75, 125, 200, 300
	Theolair-SR Tablets	250, 500
	Slo-bid Gyrocaps	100, 200, 300
	Slo-phyllin Gyrocaps	60, 125, 250
	Slo-phyllin Tablets	100, 200

CHLAMYDIAL INFECTIONS IN INFANCY

Chlamydia trachomatis is now recognized as one of the most prevalent sexually transmitted diseases in the United States. It is a major cause (40 to 50 per cent of cases) of nongonococcal urethritis in men and is a mainly asymptomatic cervical infection in women. Chlamydial cervical infection is more common in young, married, primiparous black women. If present in the cervix during vaginal delivery, it can be transmitted to the infant during passage through the birth canal. The infant may be inoculated in either the eyes or nasopharynx, or both. The major clinical manifestations of perinatal chlamydial infection are conjunctivitis and pneumonia. Both clinical syndromes are best diagnosed by cultures from conjunctival or nasopharyngeal scrapings of affected patients. The availability of the chlamydial culture technique in your laboratory will greatly aid in diagnosis. The most salient features of both syndromes are summarized in the next two sections.

8

A. Chlamydial Conjunctivitis

   1. Most prevalent infectious cause of neonatal conjunctivitis

   2. Not prevented by the silver nitrate drops administered to the newborn in the delivery room

   3. Incubation period of 5 to 14 days after delivery

   4. Can be unilateral or bilateral

   5. Mild to severe conjunctival reaction

   6. Gram's stain of conjunctival scraping specimens does not demonstrate bacteria or marked white blood cell response

   7. Treatment consists of *oral* erythromycin, 30 to 50 mg/kg daily in 4 divided doses for 10 days (topical therapy is not effective)

B. Chlamydial Pneumonitis

   1. Onset at 4 to 12 weeks of age

   2. Clinical presentation

     a. Afebrile

     b. Subacute onset

     c. Nasal congestion

     d. Staccato cough

     e. Poor weight gain

   3. Physical examination

     a. Tachypnea

     b. Rales

     c. Wheezing uncommon

   4. Hyperinflation and variable alveolar-interstitial infiltrates seen radiographically

   5. Laboratory findings

     a. Eosinophils $\geq$ 300/mm^3

     b. Elevated IgG $\geq$ 500 mg/100 ml

     c. Elevated IgM $\geq$ 110 mg/100 ml

   6. Treatment consists of *oral* erythromycin, 30 to 50 mg/kg daily in 4 divided doses for 10 days

---

References:

   1. Arth C, Von Schmidt B, Grossman M, Schachter J. Chlamydial pneumonitis. J Pediatr 1978; *93:*447–450.

   2. Hammerschlag M. Chlamydial infections. Pediatr Rev 1981; *3:*77–84.

THE RETURN OF THE WHOOP

With the standardization of the pertussis (whooping cough) vaccine in 1951, the incidence of pertussis has been steadily declining. At the present time, however, the United States is witnessing a documented rise in case reports. Would you recognize a case of pertussis? Keep these features in mind when evaluating an infant or child with respiratory complaints.

1. The disease has a triphasic course, beginning with a catarrhal stage (1 to 2 weeks) followed by a paroxysmal cough (2 to 4 weeks) and, finally, a period of convalescence (4 to 12 weeks).

2. The classic cough of pertussis is paroxysmal in nature, often accompanied by a low-grade fever. The cough is violent, abrupt in onset, and easily triggered by even the mildest stimulus.

3. The coughing episodes are often (but not always) followed by a "whoop" or high-pitched inspiratory noise.

4. Post-tussive emesis is frequent.

5. A marked lymphocytosis accompanies the paroxysmal stage.

6. Major complications are apnea, pneumonia, seizures, intracranial bleeding, and subconjunctival hemorrhages.

7. The diagnosis is confirmed by immunofluorescent antibody staining of nasopharyngeal specimens.

8. Erythromycin therapy (7 to 14 days) has been reported to lessen the infectivity of the index case; however, the course of the disease may not be changed.

9. Deaths occur most frequently in children 9 months old and younger. This population is also most often admitted for observation.

10. Previous immunization for pertussis never precludes the possibility of acquiring the disease.

8

Reference:
1. Geller RJ. The pertussis syndrome: a persistent problem. Pediatr Infect Dis 1984; 3:182–186.

ACUTE PEDIATRIC PNEUMONIA

You have just diagnosed pneumonia in your pediatric patient and must decide what treatment course to employ. The majority of cases of pneumonia in children are nonbacterial in origin and require no antibiotic therapy. Bacteria are the major cause of pneumonia in the perinatal period only and, after that age, account for less than 20 per cent of lower respiratory infections. Some features that can help differentiate between the major classes of pneumonia in children are summarized in the next table.

Epidemiologic, Clinical, and Laboratory Findings of Acute Pneumonia in Otherwise Normal Infants and Children According to Causative Agent

	BACTERIA	VIRUS	MYCOPLASMA
Historical Clues			
Age	Any, but especially infants		School age, adolescents
Fever	Majority $\geq$ 39°C	Majority < 39°C	Majority < 39°C
Onset	Abrupt, may follow URI	Gradually worsening URI	Gradually worsening cough
Others in home ill	Infrequent	Frequent, concurrent	Frequent, weeks apart
Associated signs, symptoms	Infrequent; meningitis, otitis, arthritis	Frequent; myalgia, rash, conjunctivitis, pharyngitis, mouth ulcers, diarrhea, cystitis	Frequent; headache, sore throat, myalgia Occasional rash, conjunctivitis myringitis, enanthem
Cough	Productive	Nonproductive	Hacking, paroxysmal, sometimes productive
Pleuritic chest pain	Frequent	Infrequent	Infrequent
Physical Findings			
Auscultatory	Confined rales, no rales. Occasional dullness to percussion, diminished or tubular sounds.	Diffuse, bilateral rales, not anatomically confined. Wheezing in young infant.	Unilateral rales in most patients but frequently in more than one lobe
Toxicity	Degree illness > findings	Degree illness $\leq$ findings	Degree illness < findings
Radiographic Findings			
Initial examination	Hyperaeration ± alveolar infiltrate in patchy or consolidated distribution of lobe or sub-segment	Hyperaeration ± interstitial infiltrate in diffuse or perihilar distribution	Alveolar-interstitial patchy infiltrate in single or contiguous lobes
Progression	Frequent, rapid	Infrequent	May occur; may be migratory
Pleural fluid	May occur; may be large, rapidly progressive	Infrequent; majority small, not progressive	Infrequent; majority small, not progressive
Laboratory Findings			
WBC/mm³	Majority > 15,000 granulocytes predominate	Majority < 15,000 lymphocytes predominate	Majority normal or less than 15,000
C-reactive protein elevated	Majority	Infrequent	Infrequent
ESR $\geq$ 30 mm/hr	Majority	Majority	Majority

If it appears that a bacterial pathogenesis is most likely, the following table will serve as a guide to antibiotic therapy.

Agents	UNCOMPLICATED PNEUMONIA			COMPLICATED PNEUMONIA		HOSPITAL-ASSOCIATED PNEUMONIA
	< 3 mo	3 mo–5 yr	5–19 yr	Pleural Fluid	Lung Abscess	
S. pneumoniae	+ + +	+ + + +	+ + + +	+ +	+	+ +
H. influenzae	+	+ + +	+	+ + +	+	+
Group A streptococci	–	+	+	+ +	–	–
Mouth flora	–	+	+	+ + +	+ + + +	+ + +
S. aureus	+ +	+	+	+ +	+ +	+ +
Groups B and D streptococci	+ + +	–	–	–	–	–
Enteric bacilli	+ + +	–	–	+	+ +	+ +
Tuberculosis	–	+	+	+	+	–
Initial Therapy						
Outpatient		Amoxicillin Consider erythromycin-sulfamethox-azole, TMP-SMX, cefaclor	Penicillin V Consider erythromycin			
Inpatient	Ampicillin + aminoglycoside	Ampicillin	Penicillin G	Ampicillin + nafcillin	Clindamycin	Nafcillin + aminoglycoside
	Consider adding methicillin	Consider adding chloramphenicol, nafcillin	Consider nafcillin, ampicillin	Consider substituting chloramphenicol for ampicillin	Consider penicillin G or cefoxitin alone or adding aminoglycoside	Consider cefoxitin alone or clindamycin for nafcillin

Key to table: + + + + most frequent cause; + + + frequent cause; + + less frequent cause; + occasional cause; – rare cause

The following patients would benefit by admission to the pediatric ward for observation and therapy.

1. Infants less than 3 months of age with pneumonia and rectal temperature greater than 38.5°C.

2. Any infant or child with hypoxia or poor air exchange noted on auscultation.

3. Any infant or child who is dehydrated or is unable to tolerate oral fluid intake. Children with respiratory rates greater than 70 should not be encouraged to drink; aspiration of fluids is quite possible.

4. Any patient in whom good follow-up or competent parental care at home is in doubt.

Reference:
1. Long SS. Treatment of acute pneumonia in infants and children. Pediatr Clin North Am 1983; *30:*297–321. (Tables reproduced with permission.)

CHEST PAIN IN CHILDREN

Children who present with chest pain are rarely the victims of heart disease. Most prospective studies have shown that childhood chest pain is usually idiopathic (up to 50 per cent in one study), directly related to problems with the chest wall itself (costochondritis and muscle strain), or secondary to direct trauma. A careful history and physical examination will usually uncover the cause, although a chest x-ray and an ECG may occasionally also be needed. Whatever the cause, it is important for the clinician to remember that chest pain is viewed as a serious omen and, as far as the parents and child are concerned, a cardiac problem is to blame until proven otherwise. These fears may be chronic, as many of these children will have symptoms that have been present for more than six months; it is this group that contains most of the idiopathic cases. Careful nonemergency follow-up should be arranged for these children. The next table summarizes the most common organic causes of chest pain in children.

CATEGORY	TYPICAL CLINICAL PATTERN
Chest wall complaints	
Muscle strain	Recent history of vigorous new exercise.
Costochondritis	Point tenderness at costochondral junctions.
Herpes zoster infection	Pain and varicelliform rash along a dermatome.
Pulmonary causes	
Pneumonia	Fever, tachypnea, cough, and abnormal x-ray findings.
Pleurodynia	Pleuritic pain worsened by cough and inspiration; a friction rub may be present. Associated with enteroviral infections (usually coxsackie virus).
Pneumothorax	Sudden onset of sharp pain, dyspnea, and orthopnea; pain may radiate to back and shoulders.
Cystic fibrosis	Pneumothorax is a common complication with cystic fibrosis.
Asthma	Chest pain associated with cough, wheezing, and expiratory prolongation.
Pulmonary infarction	A sequela of a vaso-occlusive pulmonary crisis in sickle cell anemia.
Cardiac causes	
Aortic stenosis	Harsh, systolic murmur in second right intercostal space and through carotid arteries; diminished pulse pressure. Left ventricular hypertrophy (LVH)
Idiopathic hypertrophic subaortic stenosis (IHSS)	No murmur or, if present, will increase in systole with standing or Valsalva maneuver. ECG may show LVH or deep Q waves in anteroseptal leads.

costal space and through carotid arteries; diminished pulse pressure. Left ventricular hypertrophy (LVH)

CATEGORY	TYPICAL CLINICAL PATTERN
Mitral valve prolapse	Apical click followed by a late systolic murmur. Chest x-ray normal. ECG may show T-wave inversion in inferior leads. Frequent PVCs and PACs are not uncommon.
Pericarditis	Sharp, sudden chest pain associated with inspiration, relieved by leaning forward. Usual history of a recent URI. An end expiratory friction rub may be present.

References:
1. Bisset GS. Mitral valve prolapse in 119 children. Circulation 1980; *62*:423–429.
2. Driscoll D. Chest pain in children: a prospective study. Pediatrics 1976; *57*:648–651.

THE "ACUTE ABDOMEN" IN PEDIATRICS

The physical examination of the child with acute abdominal pain is quite a challenge for even the most experienced clinician. Children less than 2 years of age are often unable to describe their symptoms or localize their complaints. Since the physical and laboratory findings are often inconclusive in this age group, the key to diagnosis (as any good surgeon will tell you) often lies in the sequential examination of the abdomen over an extended period. The causes of the acute abdomen in the pediatric age group are highlighted in the table.

Etiologic Classification of Acute Abdomen in the Pediatric Age Group

MECHANICAL OBSTRUCTION		INFLAMMATORY DISEASES AND INFECTIONS			
Intraluminal	Extraluminal	Gastrointestinal Disease	Paralytic Ileus	Blunt Trauma	Miscellaneous
Foreign body	Hernia	Appendicitis	Sepsis	Accident	Lead poisoning
Bezoar	Intussusception	Crohn's disease	Pneumonia	Battered-child	Sickle-cell crisis
Fecalith	Volvulus	Ulcerative colitis	Pyelonephritis	syndrome	Familial Mediterranean fever
Gallstone	Duplication	Henoch-Schönlein	Peritonitis		
Ascariasis	Stenosis	purpura and	Pancreatitis		Porphyria
Meconium ileus	Tumor	other causes of	Cholecystitis		Diabetic acidosis
equivalent	Mesenteric	vasculitis	Renal and		Addisonian
Tumor	cyst	Peptic ulcer	gallbladder		crisis
Fecaloma	Superior	Meckel's	stones		Torsion of testis
	mesenteric	diverticulitis	Pelvic inflammatory disease		Torsion of ovarian
	artery syndrome	Acute gastroenteritis	Mittelschmerz		pedicle
		Food poisoning			Hydronephrosis
		Pseudomembranous enterocolitis			Rheumatic fever
					Streptococcal infection
					Nodular lymphoid hyperplasia

Reference:
1. Roy CC, Morin CL, Weber AM. Gastrointestinal emergency problems in pediatric practice. Clin Gastroenterol 1981; *10*:225–254. (Table reproduced with permission.)

RECTAL BLEEDING IN INFANCY AND CHILDHOOD

Rectal bleeding in infancy and childhood is a frightening event for the child, the parents, and the physician. These patients will often be rushed to your emergency room by the parents who have diaper in hand and, it is hoped, a stool specimen for your examination. Most patients will appear clincially well, since the leading cause of rectal bleeding in infants and preschool children is blood from an anal fissure. A complete listing of possible causes is provided in the table that follows.

Clinical Clues to the Causes of Rectal Bleeding

ENTITY	AGE	AMOUNT; APPEARANCE	CLINICAL FEATURES	CAUSE
Acute colitis	Any age	Variable; red	Sickly, "toxic" appearance, diarrhea, abdominal pain	Infection, allergy, isosensitization, chronic ulcerative colitis, chronic active hepatitis, ischemia
Infectious diarrhea	Any age	Small; red	Diarrhea, fever	Bacterial (*Salmonella, Shigella,* pathogenic *Escherichia coli, Campylobacter),* viral, or parasitic infection
Milk (cow's) or protein (soy) intolerance	Neonate and infant	Occult to small; red	Colic, diarrhea, vomiting, edema, rhinitis, asthma, atopic dermatitis	Cow's milk or soy-protein intolerance
Midgut volvulus	Neonate	Variable; red to tarry	Shock, bile-stained vomitus, pain, obstruction	Malrotation with malfixation of mesentery
Anal fissure	Infant	Small; red	Constipation, rectal pain	Constipation; trauma
Cryptitis, proctitis	Any age	Small; red	Colicky episodes, rectal pain, diarrhea	Gastroenteritis, ulcerative colitis, Crohn's disease, venereal disease
Polyps	Any age	Small to moderate; red	Absence of pain, mucus, intermittent diarrhea	Idiopathic, genetic, or familial
Intussusception	Usually < 2 yr	Variable; red, currant-jelly red, tarry	Colicky pain, abdominal distention, vomiting, "knocked-out" look	Idiopathic, polyps, Meckel's diverticulum, lymphonodular hyperplasia, tumors
Intestinal parasites	Any age	Occult to small; red	Diarrhea, cramps, weight loss	Amebiasis, *Trichuris,* hookworm, other
Meckel's diverticulum	Usually < 2 yr	Large; red to tarry	Usually absence of pain; pale, shock-like appearance; anemia	Congenital

Clinical Clues to the Causes of Rectal Bleeding (Continued)

ENTITY	AGE	AMOUNT; APPEARANCE	CLINICAL FEATURES	CAUSE
Duplications	Usually < 2 yr	Variable to large; red to tarry	Mass, intestinal obstruction, rarely pain	Congenital
Nodular lymphoid hyperplasia	Usually < 2 yr	Small; red	Appears well, post-infection diarrhea	Disrupted mucosa, idiopathic, immune deficiency state
Hemangioma and telangiectasia	Any age	Occult to large	Absence of pain, mucocutaneous lesions, hemihypertrophy	Congenital
Peptic ulcer	Any age (most 5 to 15 yr)	Occult to large; tarry	Epigastric pain	Idiopathic; CNS disease, steroid use, burns, sepsis
Henoch-Schönlein purpura	3 to 10 yr	Small to large; red to tarry	Abdominal pain, vomiting, arthritis, purpura, hematuria	Idiopathic
Chronic ulcerative colitis	Any age (most 10 to 19 yr)	Small to occult; red	Abdominal pain, tenesmus, diarrhea	Idiopathic
Crohn's disease	Most 10 to 19 yr	Occult to small, sometimes large; red	Abdominal pain, diarrhea, anorexia, weight loss	Idiopathic
Esophagitis	Any age	Occult to small	Dysphagia, vomiting, heartburn	Hiatal hernia, pyloric outlet obstruction
Esophageal varices	Any age (most 3 to 5 yr)	Large; tarry	Hematemesis, signs of portal hypertension	Cirrhosis or portal vein obstruction
Hemorrhoids	Adolescent	Small; red	Pain on defecation	Constipation, perianal disease, portal hypertension, Crohn's disease
Foreign body	Toddler to school age	Variable; red	Rectal pain	Irritation effect of foreign body
Hemolytic-uremic syndrome	Usually < 5 yr	Small to large; red	Post-infection diarrhea, edema, hematuria	Postgastroenteritis effect (?), platelet thrombi (?)
Antibiotic-associated colitis	Any age	Occult, small to moderate; red	Diarrhea, abdominal distention, cramps, recent antibiotic use	Use of almost any antibiotic, especially ampicillin and cephalosporins in children

Reference:
1. Silverman A, Roy C. Pediatric Clinical Gastroenterology. St. Louis: C.V. Mosby Co., 1983; 23. (Table adapted with permission.)

8

Clinical Features of Acute Infectious Gastroenteritis

CLINICAL FEATURES	ROTAVIRUS	SALMONELLA	CAMPYLOBACTER	YERSINIA	SHIGELLA	ESCHERICHIA COLI Enteropathogenic	Enterotoxigenic	Enteroinvasive
Age	Any age but most < 2 yr	Any age	1–5 yr (most)	Any age	Any age but most < 6 yr	< 1 yr	All ages but most < 1 yr	All ages
Diarrhea in contacts	30 %	Variable	10 %	< 10 %	> 50 %	—	—	—
Fever (> 38.5°C)	Rare	Variable	Rare	About 50 %	Frequent	Rare	Rare	Variable
Concomitant URI	Common	—	—	—	Common	—	—	—
Convulsions	—	Rare	—	—	Common	—	—	—
Vomiting	Invariable	Usual	About 30 %	About 40 %	Absent	Common	Common	Rare
Abdominal pain	Mild	Moderate	Severe	Crampy	Severe	—	—	—
Tenesmus	—	Rare	Frequent	—	Frequent	—	—	Frequent
Diarrhea	Watery	Loose and slimy	Mucoid and watery	Greenish	Mucoid and watery	Watery	Watery	Mucoid and watery
Blood	—	Rare	Usual	25 %	>50 %	—	—	Common
Fecal leukocytes	Unusual	Always	Always	Usual	Always	—	—	Usual

References:
1. Plotkin GR, Kluge RM, Waldman RH. Gastroenteritis: etiology, pathophysiology, and clinical manifestations. Medicine 1979; 58:95–114.
2. Silverman A, Roy C. Pediatric Clinical Gastroenterology. St. Louis: C.V. Mosby Co., 1983; 103. (Table reproduced with permission.)

INFECTIOUS GASTROENTERITIS

In the pediatric patient, infectious gastroenteritis is second only to viral upper respiratory disease as a cause of illness, accounting for 3 to 5 per cent of all hospital admissions. Surveys estimate that less than 15 per cent of all cases are bacterial in origin, while the vast majority (> 50 per cent) are viral in origin. Parasitic infestations (especially *Giardia lamblia* in the Northern Hemisphere) usually result in chronic diarrhea and can occur in epidemic form. A knowledge of the various clinical patterns associated with each particular organism will often aid in an accurate diagnosis. The table describes the clinical features of the more common causes of acute infectious gastroenteritis.

ORAL REHYDRATION SOLUTIONS

The two major objectives in treating an infant or child with acute diarrhea are the replacement of water and electrolyte deficits and the maintenance of ongoing caloric intake. At present, it is well established that it is safe to feed a child who has diarrhea, since there is no physiologic basis for resting the gut during the acute illness. In the United States today, commercially available oral glucose-electrolyte solutions are commonly used as the first step in re-establishing oral intake. The table lists the composition and cost of these solutions.

Some Oral Rehydration Solutions

	INGREDIENTS (mEq/l)							
Solution	Na+	K+	Other Cations	Cl−	Base	Other Anions	Carbo-hydrates	Cost/Quart*
HYDRA-LYTE—Jayco Powder (packet dilutes to one quart)	84	10	—	59	HCO₃ 10 Citrate 20	—	Glucose plus sucrose: 2 %	$ 1.23
INFALYTE—Pennwalt Powder (packet dilutes to one quart)	50	20	—	40	HCO₃ 30	—	Glucose 2 %	1.20
LYTREN—Mead Johnson Liquid (ready to use)	30	25	Ca (4 mEq) Mg (4 mEq)	25	Citrate 36	SO₄ 4 PO₄ 4	Glucose plus corn syrup: 7.7 %	2.73
ORAL ELECTROLYTE-SOLUTION—Wyeth Liquid (ready to use)	30	20	Ca (4 mEq) Mg (4 mEq)	30	Citrate 23	PO₄ 5	Glucose 7.5 %	1.20
PEDIALYTE—Ross Liquid (ready to use)	30	20	Ca (4 mEq) Mg (4 mEq)	30	Citrate 28	—	Glucose 5 %	2.02
PEDIALYTE R.S.—Ross Liquid (ready to use)	60	20	—	50	Citrate 30	—	Glucose 2.5 %	2.02
WHO Oral Rehydration Salts † Powder (packet dilutes to 1 liter)	90	20	—	80	HCO₃ 30	—	Glucose 2 %	.25‡

*Cost to the pharmacist according to *Drug Topics Red Book* 1983 or the manufacturer.

†Oral Rehydration Salts—Jianas Brothers Packaging, 2533 SW Blvd., Kansas City, MO; KBI, Berlin; ALLPACK, Waiblingen, West Germany; Geymont Sud, Anagni, Italy. Also available as *Oralite*—Beecham; *Elotrans*—Fresenius, Bad Homburg; *Oral Rehydration Salts*—Servipharm, Basel; *Salvadora*—LUSA, Lima.

‡Approximate cost per quart in the USA when purchased in lots of 5000 packets.

General recommendations regarding the use of these products include the following:

1. Solutions should contain 50 to 60 mEq/l of sodium. The more concentrated forms (sodium = 90 mEq/l) should be reserved for patients with diarrhea due to cholera, which results in large losses of sodium in the stool.

2. Potassium replacement should approximate 20 mEq/l to adequately compensate for the large stool losses.

3. Products with high concentrations of glucose and other carbohydrates (5 to 7.7 per cent) may worsen diarrhea by osmosis.

Reference:
1. Oral rehydration solutions. Med Lett 1983; *25:*19–20. (Table reproduced with permission.)

THE DYNAMICS OF SEXUAL ABUSE IN CHILDHOOD

The investigation of a case of suspected childhood sexual abuse is a true pediatric psychosocial emergency. In most instances, this is a chronic problem, and physical evidence is often absent at the time of presentation. Skillful history taking will often uncover the extent of the problem and can be of critical importance in legal documentation. Be aware of the dynamics of sexual abuse as described next.

1. Fifty per cent of reported cases involve children less than 13 years of age.

2. The age at which sexual abuse is identified is in no way the same as the age of the child at the onset of the abuse.

3. Concomitant physical abuse must be looked for in all cases of sexual abuse.

4. Most incidents do not involve the use of physical force, and the absence of genital trauma does not exclude the possibility of sexual abuse. Only 7 per cent of girls and 15 to 35 per cent of boys will demonstrate physical indicators of assault.

5. In older children, fear of family disintegration often precludes voluntary reporting. Younger children are often silenced with bribery.

6. Children almost never fabricate or fantasize about sexual abuse.

7. In most cases, male adults are the perpetrators.

8. Eighty per cent of cases involve a person known to the child and family.

9. Most incidents take place within the home environment.

10. Seventy-five per cent of reported cases of incest are between father and daughter. This relationship is often of long standing, and the family, although aware of it, may be forbidden to discuss the relationship.

11. It is not unusual for a child to wait days or even weeks before

reporting an event. It is unusual for a parent to delay in seeking help, once aware of the possibility.

Situations to investigate include the following:

1. A family or child who complains of abuse.

2. A patient less than 12 years of age with venereal disease.

3. Adolescent pregnancy.

4. Patients with genital lesions or injuries that are inconsistent with the history.

5. Any children who demonstrate unusually promiscuous behavior for their age (acting out sexually in school).

6. A parent who expresses excessive concern regarding their child's genital status, perineal itching, dysuria, or pain on defecation.

7. Preschool children with a history of night terrors, clinging behavior, encopresis, or secondary enuresis.

8. School-age children with insomnia, runaway behavior, or school failure.

9. Adolescents who run away, have sleep disturbances, and have begun patterns of drug abuse and prostitution.

From a lecture by Celeste M. Madden, M.D. (Used with permission.)

THE SUPRAPUBIC URINE SPECIMEN

Needle aspiration of urine from the bladder of infants less than 2 years of age has become a standard method for obtaining reliable urine culture material. This procedure is possible because the bladder of children in this age group is predominantly an anterior abdominal organ. The technique is described next.

1. Place the infant in the supine position, immobilized in a frog-leg alignment.

2. Prepare the lower abdominal wall with iodine and wipe off with alcohol.

3. While wearing surgical gloves, locate the aspiration site 1 to 2 cm above the pubic symphysis in the midline.

4. Insert a 22G needle perpendicular to the abdominal wall, advancing to a maximum of 2.5 cm. Begin gentle aspiration immediately after penetrating the skin.

5. If the first attempt is unsuccessful, a second attempt is warranted. This approach should be adjusted so that the needle is at an angle of 10 to 15 degrees toward the pelvis (caudad).

6. After the specimen is obtained, the needle is withdrawn and the site is covered with a Band-Aid.

7. Complications caused by this procedure, although quite rare, include gross hematuria, anterior abdominal wall abscess, and peritonitis.

Differential Diagnosis of Stiff Neck in Children

	ACUTE STIFF NECK					Chronic Stiff Neck
CNS Infection	Non-CNS Infection	Mass Lesion	Inflammation	Toxin or Drug	Trauma	Chronic Stiff Neck
Meningitis	Osteomyelitis of cervical spine	CNS herniation	Juvenile rheumatoid arthritis	Phenothiazines	Spinal injury	Spastic cerebral palsy
Encephalitis	Cervical adenitis	Cervical or paracervical tumor	Kawasaki syndrome	Lead	Subluxation	Myositis ossificans
Abscess	Retropharyngeal abscess	Neuroblastoma		Black-widow spider bite	Post-lumbar puncture	Sternocleidomastoid tumor of infancy
Brain	Discitis	Medulloblastoma		Scorpion bite	Subarachnoid hemorrhage	Congenital vertebral anomaly
Epidural	Otitis media	Hemorrhage		Tick bite		Klippel-Feil syndrome
Poliomyelitis	Pneumonia	Foreign body				Sprengel deformity
Postinfectious encephalomyelitis	Pyelonephritis	Meningeal leukemia				Lead poisoning
	Tonsillitis	Ruptured arteriovenous malformation				Juvenile rheumatoid arthritis
	Tetanus	Intussusception				Arnold-Chiari malformation
	Parotitis					Dystonia musculorum
	Scarlet fever					Wilson's disease
	Other viral infections					Multiple sclerosis
	Influenza					Huntington's disease
	Roseola infantum					
	Infectious mononucleosis					
	Cat-scratch disease					
	Paroxysmal torticollis					
	Malaria					
	Typhoid fever					
	Shigellosis					
	DPT immunization					
	Epidemic cervical myalgia					
	Dental abscess					
	Epiglottitis					
	Herpes zoster					
	Appendicitis					
	Typhus					
	Acute cerebellar ataxia					

Reference:

1. Stein MT, Trauner D. The child with a stiff neck. Clin Pediatr 1982; 21:559–563. (Table reproduced with permission.)

STIFF NECK IN CHILDREN

An infant or child with a stiff neck can be quite a challenge to a diagnostician, since this problem is present in a diverse group of pathologic processes. Any anatomic alteration in the head or neck may produce rigidity. The causes of rigidity include inflammation, a mass effect, a direct irritation or stretching of cervical musculature, and a limitation of cervical vertebral movement. The table on the opposite page enumerates the diagnostic possibilities. When all organic causes have been eliminated, consider a psychogenic cause.

NURSEMAID'S ELBOW

Dislocation of the radial head (nursemaid's elbow) is a common orthopedic problem in toddlers. The injury is usually incurred as a result of abrupt and excessive axial traction across the elbow joint, often seen in "yanking" the child's arm in situations of discipline, abuse, or restraint from danger. The injured child will usually refuse to use the affected arm, preferring to hold the arm at rest on its side in pronation. Reduction of a nursemaid's elbow can be accomplished in the following manner:

1. With the child sitting in the parent's lap, grasp the child's hand as if to shake it.

2. With your other hand, encircle the elbow, placing your thumb over the annular ligament of the radius (lateral).

3. At the same time, and in one continuous motion, supinate the child's hand while flexing the elbow.

4. A "pop" will be felt in the area of the radial head when reduction is accomplished.

5. Most children resume using the arm within 10 to 15 minutes following reduction. More prolonged dislocations will require more time after reduction to return to normal function. The maneuver may be repeated if the clinical response is unsatisfactory.

6. If point tenderness is documented, radiography is recommended.

8

IF THE CRUTCH FITS

Anyone who has had the misfortune of using a set of crutches is aware of the discomfort caused by a poor fit. Use the table to guide you in providing your injured patients with appropriately sized pairs.

"Crutch Sizes"

HEIGHT	CRUTCH SIZE (in)
4' 10"	44
4' 11"	45
5' 0"	45
5' 1"	46
5' 2"	47
5' 3"	48
5' 4"	49
5' 5"	51
5' 6"	51
5' 7"	52
5' 8"	53
5' 9"	54
5' 10"	56
5' 11"	56
6' 0"	58

CLOSING CUTS IN CHILDREN

"The secret of the care of the patient is in caring for the patient."

Francis Peabody

1. Talk to the patient and the parent first. You can create rapport with most children before you touch the wound. Don't display the instruments—never show the child the needle or syringe. Keep talking during the repair, explaining each move.

2. Keep a parent close to the child—separating them may be more traumatic for the child than the laceration. Be sure the parents remain seated, and lessen the chances of their feeling faint by discouraging both parents and child from watching the repair. Have the child lie flat (remove any pillows). Encourage hand contact between the parent and the child and conversation about home events or pets.

3. Adhesive-tape closure of wounds has a lower infection rate and a better healing result than sutures: so whenever tape provides good closure that can be maintained for about one week, use it.

4. Avoid using any solution that hurts. Be patient when you are introducing local anesthetic. Inject through the cut into the subdermis—not through the skin. Don't inject fast; never inject intra-dermally (that really hurts). Watch the child's face—if there is any sign of distress, change the position of the needle, because it may be too near to a nerve. Wait a few minutes for the anesthetic to take effect. Use 1 per cent lidocaine without epinephrine.

5. Some children (mostly toddlers) will need restraining. The papoose splint or a firm body wrap to restrain the arms is best. Talk to the child before applying the splint, and explain what you are doing.

6. A few children will need sedation, especially if the laceration is through the edge of the lip, and you need a non-moving target. A useful cocktail for sedating children is demerol 1–2 mg/kg, phenergan 1 mg/kg, and thorazine 1 mg/kg (DPT IM to maximum doses of 50 mg, 25 mg, and 25 mg, respectively. Morphine is also an effective drug. Give 0.05 mg/kg intramuscularly and repeat in 15 to 20 minutes if needed—you may have to repeat once more for some patients. Respiratory depression is *very* rare in children when this amount of morphine is used. Observe the child until he is wakeful—usually in 60 to 90 minutes.

7. You should be able to complete wound care and suture in about three quarters of the children without any of them crying. Even those who cry are not considered complete failures as long as they have not had a screaming terror.

Don't allow anyone to persuade you to use solutions or techniques that hurt and make children scream (unless you are a card-carrying masochist).

8. If a tetanus shot is needed, delay it until after the wound repair. This shot could be the most painful event of the child's visit.

Thanks to Eoin Aberdeen, M.D. for this contribution.

INCREASED INTRACRANIAL PRESSURE IN INFANCY AND CHILDHOOD

8

The infant or child with increased intracranial pressure is a true emergency; failure to recognize and treat this neurologic problem may result in serious morbidity and, possibly, mortality. Symptoms and signs of elevated intracranial pressure in children are listed next.

Infants	Children	Infants and Children
Full fontanelle	Headache	Altered states of consciousness
Split sutures	Stiff neck	Persistent emesis
Paradoxical irritability	Photophobia	Cranial nerve involvement (VI, III)
Macrocrania	Papilledema	The "setting sun" sign
Papilledema		The triad of hypertension, bradycardia, and hypoventilation
		Decorticate or decerebrate posturing

Once recognized, the following medical techniques may be instituted. The order in which they are utilized varies from one health center to another.

THERAPY	DOSE	MECHANISM OF ACTION
Head elevation (30°)	—	Lowers intracranial venous pressure
Head in midline	—	Prevents jugular vein compression
Hyperventilation	Reduce $PaCO_2$ to 20–25 mmHg	Promptly decreases cerebral blood volume and thus intracranial pressure
Mannitol OR	0.5–1.0 g/kg IV	Both agents effect rapid osmotic diuresis
Glycerol	0.5–2.0 g/kg IV	
Pentobarbital	1–3 mg/kg (loading dose)	Thought to lower cerebral metabolism; may also have some effect on free radical formation Other barbituates (phenobarbital) have also been utilized
Dexamethasone	0.2 mg/kg IV	Slow onset of action May act to reduce CSF production
Hypothermia (27–31°C)	—	Thought to decrease cerebral blood flow and metabolic rate Can cause cardiac arrhythmias

References:

1. Bruce DA. Management of cerebral edema. Pediatr Rev 1983; *4:*217–224.
2. Rosman NP, Oppenheimer EY, O'Connor JF. Emergency management of pediatric head injuries. Emerg Med Clin North Am 1983; *1:*141–174.

THE COMATOSE CHILD

An unconscious infant or child is rushed to your emergency department, and you are called to evaluate the patient. Your mind races through a differential diagnosis of coma in pediatrics, and you draw a blank. Some of the more likely causes are listed here.

Traumatic Causes

The most worrisome sequelae of head injury in children are those that result in intracranial bleeding. The two most important clinical syndromes to recognize are epidural and subdural hematomas, as described in the table.

Clinical Features of Acute Epidural and Subdural Hemorrhages[1]

	EPIDURAL	SUBDURAL
Supratentorial		
Incidence	Less frequent	More frequent
Skull fracture	75 %	30 %
Source of hemorrhage	Usually arterial	Venous
Age	Usually older than 2 yr	Usually younger than 1 yr
Location	Usually unilateral	Usually bilateral
Seizures	< 25 %	75 %
Retinal or preretinal hemorrhages	< 25 %	75 %
Increased intra- cranial pressure	Present	Present
Configuration on CT scanning	Usually lenticular	Usually crescentic
Mortality	25 %	< 25 %
Morbidity	Low	High
Infratentorial		
Frequency	More frequent	Less frequent
Skull fracture	Almost always	Usually
Source of hemorrhage	Venous	Venous

Reference:

1. Rosman NP, Oppenheimer E, O'Connor JF. Emergency management of pediatric head injuries. Emerg Med Clin North Am 1983; *1*:141. (Table reproduced with permission.)

Classic epidural hematomas are thought to follow a pattern of unconsciousness followed by a lucid interval followed by unconsciousness. It is important to realize that this pattern usually does not occur in pediatric patients. The majority of subdural hematomas occur in infancy and, if present, require a careful examination for child abuse as the cause. Finally, severe head trauma of any type can result in generalized cerebral edema, a clinical state without focal neurologic signs.

Intracranial Causes

1. Cerebrovascular accident—although rare in childhood, this entity is seen in children with sickle cell anemia and in children with cyanotic heart disease.

2. Subdural empyema—this can be a sequela of basilar skull fracture or secondary to chronic middle ear infections.

3. Tumors—intracerebral or posterior fossa tumors usually are characterized by a chronic course of neurologic depression. They can cause coma rapidly if hemorrhage within the tumor mass occurs suddenly.

8

Metabolic Causes

This category encompasses most causes of coma in children. A careful history and physical examination will clarify the diagnosis in most cases. Pertinent features are outlined.

CAUSATIVE FACTOR	CLINICAL PATTERNS IN PEDIATRICS
Hypoglycemia	Glycogen stores are quite limited in infants and children and are easily exhausted in any stressful clinical situation (shock, sepsis, meningitis, multiple trauma).
	Unconscious infants and children are considered hypoglycemic until proven otherwise.
Diabetic ketoacidosis	Most patients are known diabetics; frequent inter-current viral illnesses predispose pediatric patients to secondary emesis and resultant ketoacidosis.
Hypernatremia	Common in infants with severe gastroenteritis.
	Also seen in children fed improperly mixed infant formula concentrates, resulting in an underdiluted food source.
	Symptoms can vary, ranging from lethargy and irritability to muscle weakness, convulsions, and coma.
Hyponatremia	Overuse of clear (hypotonic) fluids as oral rehydration therapy in gastroenteritis can rapidly lower serum sodium level.
	The syndrome of inappropriate antidiuretic hormone secretion (SIADH) occurs in children, causing a marked, dilutional hyponatremia.
	Symptoms include muscle cramps, lethargy, agitation, decreased deep tendon reflexes, and seizures.
Meningitis	Classic symptoms (fever, headache, stiff neck, photophobia) may be absent in a child less than 2 years old.
	A child less than 2 years old is more likely to present with fever, paradoxical irritability, lethargy, and poor feeding as historical clues.
Encephalitis	Can accompany any viral disease; more common in mumps, measles, varicella, and any enteroviral infection (coxsackievirus, echovirus).
	Encephalitis with focal deficits and focal seizures can be herpetic in origin.
Reyes syndrome	Look for the classic pattern of a viral prodromal illness (flu or varicella) followed by persistent emesis and progressive neurologic deterioration.
	An elevated serum ammonia level is a classic sign in this disorder.
	See Reyes syndrome, page 288.
Postictal states	Severe seizures can be followed by prolonged periods of unresponsiveness
	Usually a diagnosis of exclusion (if the seizure was unwitnessed).

Exogenous Poisonings

Accidental poisonings are quite common in infants and children and are usually not witnessed. Breakdowns in the "poison-proof" home commonly occur during times of family stress or change (holidays, new home, depression or illness of a family member), and these times must be recognized as risk periods. In addition, surrogate caretakers, such as babysitters and grandparents, are sometimes less vigilant than parents, and there is a greater potential for childhood poisonings to occur at their residences. Ingested drugs that can cause altered states of consciousness are listed next.

DRUG	FINDINGS
Opiates	Pinpoint reactive pupils, hypotension, hypoventilation, bradycardia
Barbiturates	Small reactive pupils, flaccidity, hypothermia
Amphetamines	Dilated pupils, tachycardia, tremors, hypertension
Hallucinogens	Small reactive pupils, hyperventilation, hypertension, abnormal posturing
Atropine agents	Dilated pupils; flushed, dry, warm skin; hyperthermia, tachycardia
Phenothiazines	Dystonia, hypotension
Tricyclic anti-depressants	Hyperthermia, hypotension, tachycardia

A general outline for the sequential management of the comatose infant or child should include

1. Stabilization of the airway (assume cervical spine injury has occurred)
2. Normalization of circulation and body temperature
3. After blood has been drawn for baseline chemistry determinations, administer 50 per cent dextrose, 1 ml/kg *and* naloxone, 0.01 mg/kg intravenously
4. If there is a suspicion of sepsis or meningitis, immediately obtain blood cultures and administer intravenous antibiotics. A lumbar puncture can be performed up to 4 hours after antibiotic administration and still provide reliable bacteriologic results
5. If focal neurologic deficits are present, or there are clinical signs of increased intracranial pressure, you may choose to
   a. Hyperventilate the patient
   b. Administer mannitol, 0.5 to 1.0 g/kg IV
   c. Insert a Foley catheter if mannitol is given
   d. Arrange for a CT scan
6. Investigate the possibility of toxic ingestion by
   a. Performing a urinary ferric chloride test if available
   b. Obtaining (and keeping on ice) serum and urine specimens for toxicologic screens
7. Obtain serum ammonia level and liver function determinations

STATUS EPILEPTICUS IN CHILDHOOD

Status epilepticus is a medical emergency requiring prompt and rational therapy. The various causes of these episodes and corresponding percentage within the pediatric population are listed as follows:

CAUSE	PERCENTAGE (%)
Trauma	2
Tumor	< 1
Vascular	< 1
Infectious (meningitis, encephalitis)	12
Toxic, metabolic	11
Chronic encephalopathy	17
Degenerative	4
Idiopathic with fever	28
Idiopathic without fever	25

Estimates of mortality resulting from tonic-clonic seizures have ranged from 6 to 18 per cent. There is no doubt that prolonged seizure activity can result in systemic hypoxia, local and systemic hypotension, hyperthermia, hypoglycemia, and metabolic acidosis. The guidelines for management can assist in the control of most episodes of status epilepticus, and therein greatly reduce the associated morbidity and mortality.

Guidelines for Management of Convulsive Status Epilepticus[2]

STABILIZATION 0–10 min	Secure airway, blood pressure, nasal O_2, intubate as needed
	Sample blood for complete blood count, electrolytes, BUN, drugs, calcium, magnesium, glucose (serum Dextrostix) levels, and toxic screen
	Start intravenous infusion with 5% dextrose in normal saline (if indicated use 50% dextrose, 1 ml/kg)
	Obtain blood gas values
	Monitor respirations, blood pressure, and ECG
CONTROL SEIZURES 10–25 min	Diazepam, 0.3–0.5 mg/kg (10 mg maximum in 1 dose, to be given no faster than 2 mg/min), may repeat every 10 min for maximum of 3 doses
	Be prepared to intubate patient
	Phenytoin, start after first dose of diazepam; give 18–20 mg/kg, no faster than 50 mg/min; if bradycardia or hypotension occurs, slow infusion rate
25–40 min	If seizures persist, intubate and then continue phenytoin infusion until seizures stop or to a maximum dose of 25 mg/kg
40–60 min	If seizures continue, start infusion of phenobarbital, loading dose of 15–25 mg/kg, no faster than 30 mg/min; monitor respirations and blood pressure
60–90 min	If seizures continue, start infusion of 4–10% solution of paraldehyde diluted in normal saline; administer at rate fast enough to control seizures

Guidelines for Management of Convulsive Status
Epilepticus² (Continued)

CONTROL SEIZURES > 90 min	If paraldehyde has not terminated seizures within 20 min from start of infusion, institute general anesthesia and neuromuscular blockade; EEG monitoring; keep EEG near flat for at least 2 hr, then begin slow withdrawal of anesthesia.
DIAGNOSTIC EVALUATION	Should coincide with control of seizures; detailed history, physical examination, and consideration of further diagnostic work-up with special consideration to treatable conditions (meningitis, encephalitis, metabolic disorders, overdoses, and mass lesions with cerebral edema)

Modified from Treiman and Delgado-Escueta.³

References:
1. Aicardi J, Chevrie JJ. Convulsive status epilepticus in infants and children. Epilepsia 1970; *11*:187–197.
2. Barbosa E, Freeman J. Status epilepticus. Pediatr Rev 1982; *4*:185–189. (Table reproduced with permission.)
3. Treiman DM, Delgado-Escueta AV. Current concepts in neurology: management of status epilepticus. N Engl J Med 1982; *306*:1337–1342.

KAWASAKI SYNDROME (MUCOCUTANEOUS LYMPH NODE SYNDROME)

Kawasaki syndrome was first recognized in Japan in 1967 as an acute, febrile, exanthematous illness of children. Since its first description, many cases have been described in the United States. The diagnosis of Kawasaki syndrome is based upon adherence to clinical criteria together with the exclusion of other clinically similar diseases. The principal findings in this syndrome are outlined as follows:

I. Fever
  1. Abrupt in onset, temperature reaches 40°C
  2. Persists for > 5 days (average 11 days)
  3. Generally unresponsive to standard dosages of antipyretic drugs
II. Conjunctival Injection
  1. Onset within 2 days
  2. May last 3 weeks
  3. Not associated with purulent discharge or corneal damage
III. Oral Signs
  1. Occur within 1 to 3 days of the onset of fever
  2. Erythema and fissuring of the lips
  3. Diffuse erythema of the oropharynx
  4. Hypertrophic papillae of the tongue ("strawberry tongue")
IV. Extremity Signs
  1. Firm indurative edema of hands and feet
  2. Deep erythema of palms and soles
  3. Late (14 to 20 days) desquamation of toe and finger tips
  4. Transverse grooves across fingernails 2 to 3 months after onset
V. Exanthem
  1. Onset with fever

2. Deeply erythematous; can take many forms (scarlatiniform, papular, morbilliform, multiform iris lesions)
3. Frequently pruritic

VI. Lymphadenopathy
1. Usually cervical, involving one node > 1.5 cm in diameter

VII. Variable Associated Features
1. Pyuria (70 per cent of cases)
2. Arthritis and arthralgia involving large joints (30 per cent of cases)
3. CNS irritability (25 per cent of cases have aseptic meningitis)
4. Diarrhea and abdominal pain (25 per cent of cases)
5. Hepatitis (↑ SGOT and ↑ SGPT, 10 per cent of cases)
6. Cardiac abnormalities
    a. Minor ECG abnormalities in 60 per cent of cases; usually seen in second to fifth week of disease, including increase in PR interval, LVH, nonspecific ST changes
    b. Congestive heart failure occurs in 10 per cent of cases
    c. Coronary artery aneurysm and thrombus formation in some cases

The most important sequela of this disease is the development of chronic coronary artery disease in some patients. Individual high-risk factors are as follows:
1. Sex: male
2. Age: < 1 year
3. Initial fever: > 15 days
4. Recrudescent rash and fever
5. WBC: > 30,000/mm^3
6. Cardiomegaly, arrhythmias
7. Prolonged QR interval on ECG
8. Hemoglobin: < 10g/100 ml
9. Elevated ESR for > 5 weeks

Abnormal laboratory test results of patients with Kawasaki syndrome are generally nonspecific and nondiagnostic. One interesting finding, however, is the occurrence of a marked thrombocytosis. This may not develop until after the tenth day of the illness, and will not peak until the fifteenth to twenty-fifth day. This period of hyper-coagulation coincides with the period of highest risk for coronary artery thrombosis.

Treatment for Kawasaki syndrome is supportive and is expected to be more specific as more cases are investigated. Present recommendations include the following:
1. Institute aspirin therapy with "anti-inflammatory" dosages (80 to 100 mg/kg daily in 6 divided doses)
2. Avoid steroid therapy (shown to increase aneurysm formation)
3. Schedule follow-up examinations for monitoring of any cardiac changes

---

References:
1. Fujiwara H, Hamashima Y. Pathology of the heart in Kawasaki disease. Pediatrics 1978; *61:*100–107.
2. Melish M. Kawasaki syndrome. Pediatr Rev 1980; *2:*107–114.

SCABIES

Scabies is an extremely contagious disorder caused by the mite *Sarcoptes scabiei,* which attacks infants and children as well as adults. Infestation is begun by a newly fertilized female mite. It is hoped that we are, at present, near the end of a worldwide pandemic.

I. Clinical Presentation
  A. Primary Lesions
    1. Pruritic papules
    2. Burrows
    3. Pustules
    4. Vesicles
  B. Secondary Changes
    1. Excoriations
    2. Eczematization
    3. Crusts
    4. Secondary infections

II. Distribution of Lesions
  A. Older Children and Adults
    1. Interdigital webs
    2. Flexurae of wrists and arms
    3. Axillae
    4. Belt line
    5. Genitals
    6. Buttocks
  B. Infants
    1. Trunk and extremities
    2. Head and neck
    3. Palms and soles

III. Diagnosis
  A. History of intractable itching (worse at night)
  B. History of exposure
  C. Character and distribution of lesions
  D. Burrows
  E. Microscopic examination of skin scrapings

IV. Treatment
  A. Gamma benzene hexachloride cream or lotion, one application to be left on for 12 hours and then rinsed off. (A second treatment may be required 7 days later.) Gamma benzene hexachloride is absorbed percutaneously and should be avoided in pregnant patients; use crotamiton as an alternative.
  B. Eurax (10 per cent crotamiton) for use in young infants.
  C. Antipruritics (systemic and/or topical).
  D. Antibiotics if secondary infection occurs.
  E. Thorough laundering of bed clothes, bedding, towels.

Reference:
1. Hurwitz, S. Scabies in childhood. Pediatr Rev 1979; *1:*91–94.

8

THE DIFFERENTIAL DIAGNOSIS OF CHILD ABUSE

"Any parent who wants to sign his child out of the ED LWOT [leave without treatment] within ten minutes after signing in is suspect of child abuse or carbon monoxide poisoning until proven otherwise."

Marshall B. Segal, M.D., J.D.

For the emergency department physician, the task of diagnosing child abuse is difficult at best. Initiation of proper management requires an awareness that abuse occurs on a frequent basis and is often associated with classic symptoms and signs. It is also important to examine for and to rule out the presence of any potentially organic cause at the time of presentation for legal, medical testimony at a later time. The next outline lists the major alternative diagnostic possibilities to be considered in all cases of suspected child abuse.

Differential Diagnosis of Child Abuse

CLINICAL FINDINGS	DIFFERENTIAL DIAGNOSIS	DIFFERENTIATING FACTORS
Cutaneous lesions		
Bruising	Trauma	
	Hemophilia	PT, PTT
	Von Willebrand's disease	Bleeding time
	Anaphylactoid purpura	Rule out sepsis
	Ehlers-Danlos disease	Hyperextension
Local erythema or bullae	Burn	
	Staphylococcal impetigo	Culture, Gram's stain
	Bacterial cellulitis	Culture, Gram's stain
	Frostbite	Clinical history and characteristics
	Herpes zoster and/or herpes simplex	Scraping
	Epidermolysis bullosa	Skin biopsy
	Contact dermatitis (allergy or irritant)	Clinical characteristics
Ocular findings		
Retinal hemorrhage	Shaking or other trauma	
	Bleeding disorder	Coagulation studies
	Neoplasm	
Conjunctival hemorrhage	Trauma	
	Bacterial or viral conjunctivitis	Culture, Gram's stain
	Severe coughing	History
Orbital swelling	Trauma	
	Orbital or periorbital cellulitis	CBC, culture, sinus x-rays
	Metastatic disease	X-ray, CT scanning, CNS examination

Differential Diagnosis of Child Abuse (Continued)

CLINICAL FINDINGS	DIFFERENTIAL DIAGNOSIS	DIFFERENTIATING FACTORS
Hematuria	Trauma	Rule out other diseases
	Urinary tract infection	Culture
	Acute or chronic forms of glomerular injury (glomerulonephritis)	Renal function tests, biopsy
Acute abdomen	Trauma	Rule out other diseases
	Intrinsic gastro-intestinal disease (peritonitis, obstruction, inflammatory bowel disease, Meckel's diverticulum)	X-ray, stool tests
	Other (mesenteric adenitis, strangulated hernia, anaphylactoid purpura, pulmonary disease, pancreatitis, lead poisoning, DKA)	Test as appropriate
Osseous lesions		
Fractures (multiple or in various stages of healing)	Trauma	
	Osteogenesis imperfecta	X-ray and blue sclerae
	Rickets	Nutritional history
	Birth trauma	Birth history
	Hypophosphatasia	Low alkaline phosphatase level
	Leukemia	CBC, bone marrow
	Neuroblastoma	Bone marrow, biopsy
	Osteomyelitis or septic arthritis	History
	Neurogenic sensory deficit	Physical examination
Metaphyseal and/or epiphyseal lesions	Trauma	X-ray and history
	Scurvy	Nutritional history
	Menkes' syndrome	Decreased copper and ceruloplasmin levels
	Syphilis	Serology
	Little-league elbow	History
	Birth trauma	History
Subperiosteal ossification	Trauma	
	Osteogenic malignancy	X-ray and biopsy
	Syphilis	Serology
	Infantile cortical hyperostosis	No metaphyseal irregularity
	Osteoid osteoma	Response to aspirin
	Scurvy	Nutritional history
Sudden infant death	Unexplained	Autopsy
	Trauma	Autopsy
	Asphyxia (aspiration, nasal obstruction, laryngospasm, sleep apnea)	"Near-miss" history
	Infection (botulism ?)	Bacterial and viral cultures
	Immunodeficiency (?)	Immunoglobulins
	Cardiac arrhythmia (?)	Autopsy
	Hypoadrenalism (?)	Electrolyte levels

8

Adapted from Bittner S, Newberger EH. Pediatric understanding of child abuse and neglect. Pediatr Rev 1981; 2:197–207.

THE AUTOPSY REQUEST IN PEDIATRICS

Requesting an autopsy from the family of a child who has died in the emergency department is a task viewed with anxiety, ambivalence, and distaste by most physicians. We often consider the request as an unnecessary emotional burden imposed on an already grieving family. These drawbacks are overshadowed, however, by the immense importance of the autopsy in pediatrics, a field wherein every cause of death may have serious psychological, legal, and genetic implications. Many publications exist concerning all facets of the value of the autopsy. Although there is no perfect way to handle the request for an autopsy, the points discussed here may prove helpful.

The Law

The first issue to address is whether or not the child's death is a "medical examiner's case." In some states, for example, any sudden, unexplained childhood death is required by law to have a post-mortem examination under the direction of the medical examiner. In these situations, the physician should contact the medical examiner before approaching the parents; the decision is therefore a legal one. It is the reponsibility of all physicians to be aware of local and state laws concerning these circumstances.

The Autopsy and its Medical Value

1. Establishes the cause of death
2. Enhances the family's adaptation to their loss
3. Uncovers associated conditions
4. Provides epidemiologic data
5. Educates physicians and medical students

The Autopsy and the Family

1. Surprisingly, the autopsy can provide great comfort to both the parents and the physicians because of its precision and finality.
2. The autopsy bears a ritual similarity to the funeral in the grief

process. It may answer the question that all parents ask, namely whether or not they were responsible for or could have prevented the death.

3. Some families actually anticipate the request for an autopsy.

4. In the case of neonatal deaths (first 28 days of life), the autopsy results may help answer questions concerning the roles of maternal medications, genetic defects, and perinatal events.

5. In some cases, however, pursuit of permission to autopsy is not warranted, as in the case of a child who has died after a chronic, identified illness.

What to do at the Time of Death

1. The role of the physician at the time of death should never be primarily one of obtaining autopsy permission. Rather, he should spend some time with the parents and allow them to adequately express their grief, anger, shame, or relief. He should encourage them to verbalize their feelings and ask questions.

2. The regular family pediatrician should be notified immediately in order to provide the family with a familiar medical authority.

3. If applicable, point out that the child did not suffer at the time of death and that the parents had no role in the final outcome.

4. Provide logistic guidance to the family at this time. Explain that the funeral home personnel will make all arrangements with the hospital. Offer to call other family members or friends for additional support for the parents.

5. Clarify what an autopsy entails; point out that it is a surgical procedure designed to examine the internal organs. It does not preclude the option of an open casket at the funeral, and the results, when complete, will immediately be forwarded to the parents.

6. Finally, be sure to offer the family the last opportunity to see their child while in the emergency department.

References:
1. Berger LR. Requesting the autopsy: a pediatric perspective. Clin Pediatr 1978; *17:*445–452.
2. Friedman SB. Psychological aspects of sudden death in infants and children. Pediatr Clin North Am 1974; *21:*103–111.

9
LABORATORY

WHY DO PHYSICIANS ORDER LABORATORY TESTS? 337

DO-IT-YOURSELF LABORATORY WORK 338

DETECTION OF FECAL BLOOD 343

DISORDERS OF POTASSIUM BALANCE 344

SIMPLETON'S APPROACH TO ACID-BASE BALANCE 345

CLINICAL FORMULAS FOR RESPIRATORY MANIPULATION . . . 346

CORRECTIONS 348

FAMOUS GAPS 349

WHY DO PHYSICIANS ORDER
LABORATORY TESTS?

"Once you order a test you are committed to know the results and act accordingly."

Marshall B. Segal M.D., J.D.

The range of answers includes:

Confirmation of clinical opinion
Diagnosis
Monitoring
Screening
Prognosis
Prior result unavailable
Prior result abnormal
Prior result questionable
Patient and family pressure
Peer pressure
Pressure from recent medical
   articles
Personal reassurance
Patient and family reassurance
Public relations
Ease of performance with
   ready availability
Hospital policy
Legal requirement
Medicolegal requirement

CYA (in Munich)
Documentation
Personal profit
Hospital profit
Attempt to defraud
Research
Curiosity
Insecurity
Frustration at having nothing
   else to do
To buy time
Hunting (in Fresno) or
   fishing (in Seattle) expeditions
To establish a baseline
To complete a data base
Personal education
To report to an attending
   physician
Habit
Other

"I was brought up in an older tradition. I was told, before ordering the test decide what you do if it is (1) positive, or (2) negative, and if both answers are the same don't do the test."

Cochrane's Aphorism

9

Which of these reasons have prompted *you* to order laboratory tests?

Reference:
   1. Lundberg GD. Perseveration of laboratory test ordering: a syndrome affecting clinicians. JAMA 1983;*249*:639. (With permission: copyright 1983, American Medical Association.)

DO-IT-YOURSELF LABORATORY WORK

Hematocrit (Packed Cell Volume)

Equipment. (1) Capillary tube (plain if blood has been collected in a tube with EDTA; otherwise, heparinized); (2) clay sealant or Bunsen burner; (3) centrifuge for microhematocrit; and (4) microhematocrit reader.

1. Place the tip of the capillary tube just under the surface of the blood sample, filling it to about 1 cm from its end.

2. Seal the empty end of the tube by filling it with clay or by heating it in a Bunsen burner.

3. Place the capillary tube in one of the slots of the centrifuge, with the sealed end toward the outer rim. Balance it with a tube of the same size on the opposite side of the centrifuge. Secure the head cover and close the centrifuge lid.

4. Run the centrifuge for two to five minutes (or according to manufacturer's instructions). Remove the capillary tube.

5. Read the hematocrit using a hematocrit reader. Align the capillary tube so that the base of the red blood cells (near the sealed end) is at 0 percent on the scale, and the top of the serum (near the open end) is at 100 percent on the scale.

Read the value at the red blood cell–serum interface. That reading is the hematocrit, and it should be expressed as a percentage of whole blood.

Cell Counts

Equipment. A hemocytometer with Neubauer ruling (Fig. 9–1) with volumes of sections labeled for the cytometer (i.e., section 1 = 0.10 mm³ and section 5 A = 0.0040 mm³) is required.

Areas should be scanned in a pattern by moving the slide back and

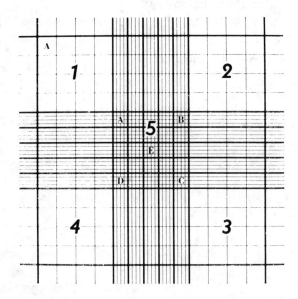

Fig. 9-1. Neubauer ruling of hemocytometer. Note section 1 (0.10 mm³) and section 5A (0.0040 mm³).

forth. Read the first row of a section by moving the slide to the right; next, move down to the second row. Read the second row by moving the slide to the left. Count the cells touching the upper and left-hand lines, but don't count the cells touching the lower and right-hand lines.

Diluting pipettes for red and white blood cells; diluting solutions for red cells (0.85% saline, Hayem's solution, or Gower's solution) and for white cells (glacial acetic acid 1% or Turk's solution) are needed.

Red Blood Cell Count

1. Collect blood in a tube with EDTA. Mix well.

2. Fill the red blood cell diluting pipette with blood to the 0.5 mark. Wipe the pipette clean with dry gauze.

3. Draw up diluting fluid so that the total sample meets the 101 mark. This gives a dilution of 1:200.

4. Shake the pipette for three minutes.

5. Clear the mixture from the stem of the pipette by expelling four to six drops.

6. Place the coverslip over the hemocytometer. Place the tip of the pipette at an open end of the counting chamber and allow the chamber to fill. Let the cells settle for a few minutes.

7. Count the red blood cells in areas A, B, C, D, and E.

8. Calculate the number of red blood cells per mm^3 in whole blood by multiplying the total count in areas A, B, C, D, and E by 10,000. This value is derived:

$$\text{red cells /mm}^3 = \frac{\text{red cells counted} \times \text{dilution factor}}{\text{volume counted}} = \frac{\text{red cells counted} \times 200}{4/1000 \text{ mm}^3/\text{chamber} \times 5 \text{ chambers}}$$

White Blood Cell Count

1. Collect blood in a tube with EDTA. Mix well.

2. Fill the white blood cell diluting pipette with blood to the 0.5 mark. Wipe the pipette clean with dry gauze.

3. Draw up the diluting fluid so that the total sample meets the 11 mark. This gives a dilution of 1:20.

4. Shake the pipette for three minutes.

5. Clear the mixture from the stem of the pipette by expelling four to six drops.

6. Place the coverslip over the hemocytometer. Place the tip of the pipette at an open end of the counting chamber and allow the chamber to fill. Let the cells settle for a few minutes.

7. Count the white blood cells in areas 1, 2, 3, and 4.

8. Calculate the number of white cells per mm^3 in whole blood by multiplying the total count in areas 1, 2, 3, and 4 by 50. This value is derived:

$$\text{white cells /mm}^3 = \frac{\text{white cells counted} \times \text{dilution factor}}{\text{volume counted}} = \frac{\text{white cells counted} \times 20}{1/10 \text{ mm}^3/\text{chamber} \times 4 \text{ chambers}}$$

9

Cerebrospinal Fluid (CSF)

If CSF appears clear, use it undiluted. Use a pipette and cytometer as described for red and white blood cell counts.

1. Fill the counting chamber.

2. Count all the cells in the chamber (areas 1–5 and unnumbered areas between 1 and 2, 2 and 3, 3 and 4, 4 and 1).

3. Calculate the cell count per mm³ by multiplying the total counted by 10/9.

This value is derived:

$$\text{white cells /mm}^3 = \frac{\text{cells counted} \times \text{dilution factor}}{\text{volume counted}} = \frac{\text{cells counted} \times 1}{1/10 \text{ mm}^3/\text{chamber} \times 9 \text{ chambers}}$$

If CSF appears purulent, dilute it, count it, and calculate as for white blood cell count.

Correction for Blood in the CSF (Traumatic Tap)

1. Determine the red and white cell counts for blood and CSF.

2. Use ratios to calculate the CSF white cell count that can be attributed to blood in the CSF.

$$\frac{\text{WBC (CSF)}}{\text{RBC (CSF)}} = \frac{\text{WBC (blood)}}{\text{RBC (blood)}}$$

$$\text{WBC (CSF)}_{calc} = \frac{\text{WBC (blood)} \times \text{RBC (CSF)}}{\text{RBC (blood)}}$$

3. Take the difference between the calculated WBC (CSF) and the measured WBC (CSF) for the true white cell count of CSF.

Red Blood Cell Indices

These indices can be calculated from the red blood cell count (RBC), hemoglobin (HgB) level, and hematocrit (Hct).

$$\text{Mean cell volume (MCV)} = \frac{\text{Hct \% } \times 10}{\text{RBC}}$$

This value is the volume of an average cell and should be expressed in cubic micra, $c\mu$.

$$\text{Mean cell hemoglobin (MCH)} = \frac{\text{HgB} \times 10}{\text{RBC}}$$

This value is the weight of hemoglobin in an average red blood cell and should be expressed in picograms of hemoglobin (pg hemoglobin).

$$\text{Mean cell hemoglobin concentration (MCHC)} = \frac{\text{HgB} \times 100}{\text{Hct}}$$

This value should be expressed as a percentage.

The following chart can be used to help interpret red blood cell indices.

TYPE OF ANEMIA	INDEX (normal range)		
	MCV (80–96 cμ)	*MCH* (27–33 pg)	*MCHC* (32–36%)
Microcytic, hypochromic (iron deficiency, thalassemia trait, lead poisoning)	↓	↓	↓
Macrocytic, normochromic (B$_{12}$ or folate deficiency, reticulocytosis, liver disease, hypothyroidism, Down's syndrome, drugs, "preleukemia")	↑	↑	Normal
Normocytic, normochromic (blood loss, chronic disease, hemolysis, myelosuppression)	Normal	Normal	Normal
Spherocytosis	↓ or Normal	↑	↑

Erythrocyte Sedimentation Rate (ESR)

Equipment. The following equipment is needed: Wintrobe tubes, pipettes, tube rack, and a timing device.

1. Collect blood sample in a tube with EDTA.

2. Fill a Wintrobe tube with whole blood, using a pipette.

3. Place the tube vertically in the rack, in an area away from sunlight and vibrations.

4. After one hour, read the number at the red blood cell–plasma interface. This value is the ESR and should be recorded in mm/hr.

Gram Stain

Equipment. Crystal violet, Gram's iodine, ethyl alcohol (95%) or acetone:alcohol (1:1), safranin O, microscope slide, and a Bunsen burner are needed for Gram staining.

1. Make a thin smear of the material to be stained on a clean glass slide. Allow it to air dry, then fix it by passing it quickly through the top of the Bunsen burner's flame. Allow the slide to cool.

2. Stain the slide with crystal violet for one minute.

3. Rinse the slide with tap water for two seconds.

4. Stain the slide with Gram's iodine for one minute. Rinse with tap water.

5. Decolorize with ethyl alcohol or acetone:alcohol until blue dye has been rinsed off.

6. Rinse in tap water for two seconds.

7. Stain with safranin O for one minute. Rinse with tap water.

8. Blot dry.

9

Acid-Fast Stain

Equipment. Carbolfuchsin, acid alcohol (3% HCl, 97% ethyl alcohol), methylene blue, and a Bunsen burner are needed for acid-fast staining.

1. Make a thin smear of the material to be tested on a clean glass slide.

2. Fix the smear by heating it in a slide warmer for two hours or at room temperature overnight.

3. Flood the slide with carbolfuchsin. Heat to steaming over a low flame, then let stand for five minutes *or* allow to stand with carbolfuchsin for three to five minutes.

4. Rinse in tap water.

5. Rinse with acid-alcohol until no more stain comes off.

6. Cover the slide with methylene blue. Let stand 30 to 60 seconds.

7. Rinse with tap water. Allow to air dry.

Urine Sediment

Equipment. Centrifuge tubes (15 ml), centrifuge, pipette, glass slide, and coverslip are required to prepare a urine sediment sample.

1. Fill the centrifuge tube to about 2 cm from the top. Place it in the centrifuge with a tube filled to the same height, placed opposite for balance.

2. Centrifuge for three minutes at 1800 rpm.

3. Remove the tube. Pour off the supernatant.

4. Hold the top of the tube with one hand and flick the bottom with the other hand to mix the sediment.

5. Use the pipette to place a drop of the sediment on a glass slide. Cover the sample with a coverslip.

Urine Specific Gravity

Equipment. A urinometer or refractometer is required to measure specific gravity of urine.

Urinometer

1. Fill the cylinder with urine about three-quarters full.

2. Float the urinometer in the urine. Spin it so that it doesn't stick to the sides.

3. Read the number on the stem of the urinometer where the bottom of the urine meniscus crosses it. This value is the urine specific gravity.

Correct for temperature. For each 3°C of urine temperature above or below 20°C, add or subtract 0.0001, respectively. For each 1 per cent glucose subtract 0.004 and for each 1 per cent protein subtract 0.003.

Refractometer

1. Clean the urine and scale plates.

2. Place a drop of urine on the urine plate.

3. Turn the scale plate over the urine plate.

4. Look through the viewing lens to read the specific gravity where the urine meniscus crosses the scale.

Correct for temperature. For each 1 per cent glucose subtract 0.004 and for each 1 per cent protein subtract 0.003.

References:

1. Bauer JD. Clinical Laboratory Methods. 9th ed. St. Louis: C.V. Mosby, 1982; 19:145–151, 155–159, 609–610.

2. Faulkner WR, King JW, Manual of Clinical Laboratory Procedures. Cleveland: Chemical Rubber Co, 1970; 157–162, 165–166, 269–272, 349.

3. Gottlieb AJ, Zamkoff KW, Jastremski MS, et al. The Whole Internist Catalog. Philadelphia: WB Saunders, 1980; 375–378.

4. Page LB, Culver PJ. A Syllabus of Laboratory Examination in Clinical Diagnosis. Cambridge, Massachusetts: Harvard University Press, 1960;28. (Figure reprinted with permission.)

5. Paget GE, Thomson R. Standard Operating Procedures in Pathology. Baltimore: University Park Press, 1979; 236–239, 246–248, 255–257.

Sattinger's Laws:
A. If it doesn't work we need a new one.
B. It works better if you plug it in.
C. If at first you don't succeed, try looking in the waste basket for the directions.

9

DETECTION OF FECAL BLOOD

A normal healthy person may lose up to 2 ml of blood in the stool each day. Fecal blood can be quantified radioactively by labeling red blood cells, injecting them intravenously, and measuring fecal radio-activity. A simple method for qualitative detection of fecal blood is the guaiac test. Kits containing a bottle of stabilized peroxide and slides impregnated with guaiac are available from several manufacturers and are widely used.

The guaiac test is based on the following reaction:

$$HgB + 2 H_2O_2 \rightarrow 2 H_2O + O_2$$
$$O_2 + \text{guaiac (colorless)} \rightarrow \text{oxidized guaiac (blue)}$$

After the stool sample is smeared on the guaiac slide, two to three drops of stabilized peroxide are added. The result is positive if a blue color develops within 30 seconds. "Trace" results should be considered negative.

One study used 2 ml fecal blood per day as the limit between positive and negative results. For any single stool tested using guaiac slides (Hemoccult), there was a false-positive rate of 8 per cent and a false-negative rate of 16 per cent. Manufacturers recommend that a series of stool samples be tested in order to lower the rate of false-negative results for any individual.

False-negative results may occur for the following reasons: (1) gastrointestinal lesions bleed intermittently, and some stool samples may not contain any blood; (2) hemoglobin loses its reactivity as it passes through the gastrointestinal tract (< 1/6 hemoglobin from the upper tract is intact in stool); and (3) large amounts of ascorbic acid interfere with the color-change reaction.

The guaiac slide test is not affected by the red meat in a patient's diet, by barium, or by fecal fat. If a patient takes iron preparations or laxatives, the sensitivity of the guaiac slide test is actually improved.

Test kits designed for fecal occult blood should not be used for gastric occult blood, because erroneous results may be obtained. Kits designed specifically to test for gastric occult blood are available.

References:

1. Gottlieb AJ, Zamkoff KW, Jastremski MS, et al. Testing for fecal blood. *In:* The Whole Internist Catalog. Philadelphia: WB Saunders, 1980:257.

2. Iacocca VF. Hemoccult tests not to be used on gastric juices (letter). N Engl J Med 1984; *310*:125.

3. Morris DW, Hansell JR, Ostrow JD, Lee CS. Reliability of chemical tests for fecal occult blood in hospitalized patients. Am J Dig Dis 1976;*21*:845–852.

4. Ostrow JD, Mulvaney CA, Hansell JR, Rhodes RS. Sensitivity and reproducibility of chemical tests for fecal occult blood with an emphasis on false-positive reactions. Am J Dig Dis 1973;*18*:930–940.

5. Stroehlein JR, Fairbanks VF, McGill DB, Go VLW. Hemoccult detection of fecal occult blood quantitated by radioassay. Am J Dig Dis 1976;*21*:841–844.

6. Winawer SJ. Fecal occult blood testing. Am J Dig Dis 1976;*21*:885–888.

DISORDERS OF POTASSIUM BALANCE

The serum potassium determination reflects total body potassium in a complex way. The calculation of total body potassium excess or deficit from the serum potassium value depends on the patient's general nutritional status and serum pH. The following table and nomogram provide the information that is necessary to determine the potassium excess or deficit represented by the serum potassium level and pH.

Total Body Potassium

NUTRITIONAL STATUS	MALE (mEq/kg)	FEMALE (mEq/kg)
Normal	45	35
Moderate Wasting	32	25
Very Marked Wasting	23	20

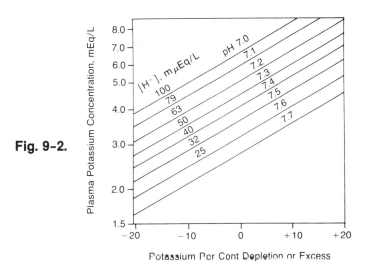

Fig. 9–2.

Example: A 50 kg, moderately wasted male has a plasma potassium concentration of 3.0 mEq/L and a pH of 7.3. Normal total body potassium for a male with moderate wasting (see table) is 32 mEq/kg $\times$ 50 kg = 1600 mEq. Per cent deficit from nomogram is -15%. (Horizontal line from potassium concentration of 3.0 mEq/L intersects diagonal line of pH 7.3 at -15%.) Total deficit calculation is as follows:

$$\% \text{ Deficit} \times \text{Normal Total Body Potassium} = \text{Deficit}$$

$$15\% \times 1600 \text{ mEq} = 240 \text{ mEq}$$

Reference:
1. Chapman WH, Bulger RE, Cutler RE, Striker G. The Urinary System: An Integrated Approach. Philadelphia: WB Saunders, 1973:112–113. (With permission.)

SIMPLETON'S APPROACH TO ACID-BASE BALANCE

GOLDEN RULES

1. $Paco_2$ $\triangle$ 12 mmHg (from normal) = pH $\triangle$ 0.1 in the opposite direction: i.e., $Paco_2$ 52 = pH 7.3

2. pH $\triangle$ 0.1 = base $\triangle$ 6 mEq/L in the opposite direction.

3. mEq $NaHCO_3$ *replacement* = $\dfrac{\text{base } \triangle \times \text{wt (kg)}}{4}$

Arnold's Method

Example: ABGs of $Paco_2$ 52, pH 7.2.

Part A

Problem: What is the measured $Paco_2$? If >40, respiratory acidosis. If <40, respiratory alkalosis.

Solution: 52, therefore respiratory acidosis is present.

Part B

Problem: Calculate the pH expected for Pa_{CO_2} of 52 using Golden Rule no. 1.

Solution: 7.3, Pa_{CO_2} Δ 12 = pH Δ 0.1 in the opposite direction.

Part C

Problem: Are the calculated and measured pH the same?
If yes, there is pure respiratory derangement; if no, a metabolic derangement is also present.

Solution: No, therefore metabolic and respiratory acidosis are present.

Part D

Problem: If a metabolic derangement is present, use Golden Rules nos. 2 and 3 to determine the dose of $NaHCO_3$ to correct fully. *It is usually wise to give only half this dose initially and then reassess.*

Solution: Metabolic pH Δ = 0.1 (7.3 − 7.2 = 0.1) equals a base deficit of 6 mEq/l.

Assume weight equals 70 kg, then

$$\text{mEq } NaHCO_3 = \frac{6 \times 70}{4} = 105$$

Reference:
1. Sladen A. Acid–base balance. *In:* McIntyre KM and Lewis AJ (eds). Textbook of Advanced Cardiac Life Support. Dallas: American Heart Association, 1983.

CLINICAL FORMULAS FOR RESPIRATORY MANIPULATION

I. Oxygenation

    A. Alveolar Air Equation

$$P_{AO_2} = (PB - P_{H_2O})\, F_{IO_2} - \frac{Pa_{CO_2}}{R}$$

P_{AO_2} — alveolar partial pressure of oxygen
PB   — barometric pressure (760 mmHg at sea level)
P_{H_2O} — partial pressure water vapor (usually 47 mmHg)
F_{IO_2} — fractional concentration of inspired oxygen
Pa_{CO_2} — partial pressure of carbon dioxide
R   — respiratory quotient (usually 1.0)

Example: Calculate P_{AO_2} of patient with a Pa_{CO_2} of 25 who is breathing 35 per cent oxygen.

$$P_{AO_2} = (760 - 47)\, 0.35 - \frac{25}{1}$$

$$P_{AO_2} = 224.6 \text{ mmHg}$$

B. a/A Ratio — useful in adjusting F_{IO_2}. (Normal 0.8–0.9).

$$a/A \text{ Ratio} = \frac{\text{Measured } P_{aO_2}}{\text{Calculated } P_{AO_2}}$$

P_{aO_2} — partial pressure of oxygen in arterial blood
P_{AO_2} — calculated from alveolar air equation

Example: Calculate the a/A ratio of a patient with P_{aO_2} 90 and P_{aCO_2} 38 who is breathing 40 per cent oxygen.

$$P_{AO_2} = (760 - 47)\, 0.4 \ - \ \frac{38}{1}$$

$$= 247$$
$$a/A = \frac{90}{247}$$
$$= 0.36$$

What would this patient's P_{AO_2} be on room air (21% oxygen)?

1. Calculate new P_{AO_2}

$$P_{AO_2} = (760 - 47)\, 0.21 \ - \ \frac{38}{1}$$
$$= 112$$

2. a/A $= 0.36$
  a/112 $= 0.36$
  a (on 21%) $= 40$ mmHg

What F_{IO_2} would be required to give a P_{aO_2} of 70 mmHg?

1. a/A $= 0.36$
  70/A $= 0.36$
  A $= 194$ mmHg

2. Substituting into the alveolar air equation

$$194 = (760 - 47)\, F_{IO_2} \ - \ \frac{38}{1}$$
$$F_{IO_2} = 0.32$$

II. Ventilation

$$(P_{aCO_2} \bullet \dot{V}_e) \text{ measured} = (P_{aCO_2} \bullet \dot{V}_e) \text{ desired}$$

P_{aCO_2} = Arterial partial pressure of carbon dioxide
$\dot{V}_e$ = expired minute ventilation = tidal volume $\times$ rate

Example: A patient on a ventilator with a tidal volume of 800 cc and a rate of 10 breaths per minute has a Pa_{CO_2} of 70 mmHg. What new settings would give a Pa_{CO_2} of 40 mmHg?

$$70 \times 800 \text{ cc} \times \text{ten} = 40 \times \dot{V_e} \text{ desired}$$
$$\dot{V_e} \text{ desired} = 14 \text{ liters}$$

New $\dot{V_e}$ of 14 liters can be achieved by increasing tidal volume to 1400 or rate to 17.

Thanks to Kathy Beney, RRT, for this contribution.

CORRECTIONS

Sodium for Hyperglycemia

When the glucose level is very high, water will be drawn into the extracellular fluid and the serum sodium will be diluted. The "true" sodium level can be calculated from the measured sodium and the glucose levels using the following equation:

$$Na_{measured} + \frac{[\,(glucose - 100) \times 1.6]}{100} = \text{true Na}$$

This calculation gives an important clue to the degree of dehydration in hyperglycemic patients; in general, the more dehydrated the patient is, the higher the true sodium level will be.

Remember that the measured, rather than the true, sodium should be used to calculate the anion gap (see Famous Gaps).

Calcium for Albumin and pH

Since 40 per cent of calcium is bound, mainly to albumin, a drop in serum albumin concentration means that the serum has to contain less total calcium to maintain the same ionized calcium. Thus, when the serum albumin concentration drops by 1 mg/dl from the lower limit of the normal range, it is as if the total serum calcium concentration had fallen by 0.8 mg/dl. Similarly, hyperglobulinemia raises the total serum calcium level by 0.16 mg/dl for every 1 gm/dl rise in the globulin.

Serum pH also affects the manifestations of hypocalcemia and hypercalcemia. Acidemia has a minor effect in displacing calcium from albumin and thereby raising the ionized calcium; conversely alkalemia will lower the ionized calcium level. A change in pH by 0.1 will alter the calcium concentration by 0.12 mg/dl. *Alkalemia will enhance neuromuscular irritability, thereby causing tetany.* This is why patients who are hyperventilating may complain of arm and leg cramps and manifest frank tetany.

Osmolarity for Alcohol

If sodium, glucose, and urea do not account for all of the measured osmolarity, the solute most likely to make up the difference is ethanol.

The equation can be used to estimate serum alcohol levels using serum osmols (S_{osm}) and an SMA–6, if direct determination of alcohol concentration is not readily available.

$$S_{osm} = (\, [Na] \times 2) + \frac{[glucose]}{18} + \frac{BUN}{2.8} + \frac{ethanol}{4.6}$$

FAMOUS GAPS

The Anion Gap

The anion gap, which is easily calculated from routine laboratory data, can yield vital information about a patient's acid-base status.

Most laboratories measure serum concentrations of sodium (Na), potassium (K), chloride (Cl), and bicarbonate (HCO_3). Principles of chemical neutrality require that the sum of all serum cations must equal the sum of all serum anions. Thus, the measured cations (MC) Na and K, together with all serum cations that are not immediately measured (UC), must balance the measured anions (MA) Cl and HCO_3, together with all serum anions that are not immediately measured (UA). The sum of MCs is usually greater than the sum of MAs. This difference is called the anion gap.

$$MC + UC = MA + UA$$
$$\text{(by subtraction)} \; MC - MA = UA - UC$$
$$\text{(by substitution)} \; (Na + K) - (Cl + HCO_3) = UA - UC$$

Since the serum concentration of K is a small number that varies little within the physiologic range, its value is often omitted. The formula becomes:

$$\text{anion gap} = Na - (Cl + HCO_3) = UA - UC$$

The value of the anion gap defined in the second equation has been calculated for healthy individuals. Within 2 SDs the normal range is 8 to 16 mEq/L.

By examining the equation, we see that the anion gap will increase if there is an increase in unmeasured anions, a decrease in unmeasured cations, or alterations in the measurement of Na, Cl, and HCO_3.

9

Causes of Increased Anion Gap

DECREASED UNMEASURED CATION	Hypokalemia, hypocalcemia, hypomagnesemia
INCREASED UNMEASURED ACID ANION	Lactic acidosis Ketoacidosis Uremia Hyperosmolar, hyperglycemic-nonketotic coma Salicylate, methanol, ethylene glycol, or paraldehyde intoxication
OTHER UNMEASURED ANIONS	Albumin Penicillin, carbenicillin, nitrate, and citrate
LABORATORY ERROR	Falsely increased serum sodium level Falsely decreased serum chloride or bicarbonate level
DEHYDRATION	

A decrease in the concentration of the unmeasured cations K, Ca, or Mg significant enough to alter the anion gap would rarely occur physiologically.

Unmeasured anions accumulate in several situations. Many disease states involve a combination of factors: acute alcoholism produces both lactic acid and ketoacids; salicylate intoxication causes accumulation of the anion itself and metabolic acids.

Lactic acidosis is the result of inhibition of oxidative metabolism. Lactic acid production may be stimulated by respiratory or metabolic acidosis.

Causes of Lactic Acidosis[1]

INCREASE IN SERUM LACTATE	
Less than 5 mEq/L	*More than 5 mEq/L*
Alkalosis	Shock
Carbohydrate infusion	Severe anemia
Exercise	Hypoxia
Catecholamines	Glycogenoses
Diabetic ketosis	Malignancies
Alcohol	Phenformin
	Idiopathic

Ketoacidosis results from the metabolism of fatty acids to acetoacetic acid and β-hydroxybutyric acid.

Uremic acidosis occurs when renal glomeruli fail to secrete urea, and renal tubules fail to secrete hydrogen ions. Sulfate and phosphate also accumulate in renal failure.

The metabolites of certain medications and toxins are organic acids, e.g., methanol forms formaldehyde and formic acid; ethylene glycol forms glycoaldehyde, oxalic acid, and hippuric acid; and paraldehyde probably forms acetic acid.

Albumin carries a negative charge at physiologic pH levels. Hyper-albuminemia is usually transient.

The anions of therapeutic or preservative salts (penicillin, carbenicillin, salicylate, and nitrate) may accumulate. Some anions, such as citrate (as would be given in blood transfusions), lactate, and acetate, are usually rapidly buffered by HCO_3. If reactions are slowed by hypoxia or hypoperfusion, however, they may also accumulate.

If water loss exceeds salt loss in dehydration, the increase in Na concentration is proportionately greater than the increase in Cl and HCO_3 concentrations. Change is due to the initially higher value of Na.

Another look at the equation shows that a decrease in the anion gap may occur through an increase in the concentrations of unmeasured cations, a decrease in the concentrations of unmeasured anions, and alterations in the measurement of Na, Cl, or HCO_3 as presented in the next table.

Causes of Decreased Anion Gap[3]

INCREASED UNMEASURED CATION	Hyperkalemia, hypercalcemia, hypermagnesemia
RETENTION OF ABNORMAL CATION	IgG globulin, tromethamine (TRIS buffer), lithium
DECREASED UNMEASURED ANION	Hypoalbuminemia
LABORATORY ERROR	*Systematic error:* Hyponatremia because of viscous serum, hyperchloremia in bromide intoxication
	Random error: Falsely decreased serum sodium, falsely increased serum chloride, or bicarbonate
	Hemodilution

Increases in the concentration of K, Mg, Ca, and Li rarely occur physiologically in amounts great enough to alter the anion gap. The alkalinizing agent tromethamine and gamma globulins may accumulate.

Albumin contributes 11 mEq/L of anion; therefore, hypoalbuminemia affects the anion gap significantly.

If an automatic diluter is used with very viscous serum (as in myeloma), an unusually small amount of fluid is delivered for analysis; the amount of sodium estimated in the small sample will be falsely low for standard volumes. Laboratory apparatus tends to produce under-estimated values for very high (>170 mEq/L) values of sodium.

Colorimetric techniques measure halides, which react more strongly with iodide and bromide than with chloride. In iodinism and bromism, a falsely elevated halide reading is obtained. The total halide measurement, however, is attributed to chloride. When the anion gap is calculated, it is low or even negative.

In hemodilution, the concentration of Na is lowered proportionately more than the concentrations of Cl and HCO_3.

9

Anion Gap and Metabolic Acidosis

In those causes of increased anion gap listed in the previous table as "increased unmeasured acid anion," hydrogen ions are buffered by HCO_3. They are lost as water and carbon dioxide, while the unmeasured anion is retained. The level of chloride remains stable, and normochloremic metabolic acidosis develops.

Metabolic acidosis can also occur when the anion gap is normal, if bicarbonate is lost or chloride is added. Again, principles of chemical neutrality require that they balance.

Metabolic Acidosis with Normal Anion Gap (Hyperchloremic Acidosis)[3]

Renal tubular acidosis, including the acidosis of aldosterone deficiency.

Early uremic acidosis.

Acidosis after respiratory alkalosis.

Intestinal loss of bicarbonate and organic acid anions.

Carbonic anhydrase inhibitors: acetazolamide (Diamox), mafenide (Sulfamylon).

Ureterosigmoidostomy.

Dilutional acidosis.

Administration of chloride-containing acid: HCl, NH_4Cl, arginine HCl, lysine HCl.

Administration of non–chloride-containing acid with good renal clearance: sulfuric acid, phosphoric acid, sulfur-containing amino acid.

Use of anion-exchange resin: cholestyramine.

Some ketoacidosis.

Acidosis because of a shift of $H+$ from the cell.

Bicarbonate is lost enterically in diarrhea, pancreatic fistulas, and ureteroenterostomies. It is lost through the kidney with carbonic anhydrase inhibitors (acetazolamide, mafenide), in renal tubular acidosis, and in hypoaldosteronism. If only small degrees of ketosis or uremia are present, the anions instead of accumulating, are excreted. This is also the case with sulfuric acid, phosphoric acid, and sulfur-containing amino acids. The acids are buffered by HCO_3, which is lost. As the acids' anions are excreted, the chloride level rises proportionately.

If a patient is hydrated rapidly with isotonic NaCl, the relative concentration of Cl rises, HCO_3 falls, and Na remains stable. Acids containing Cl are buffered by HCO_3, which is lost as chloride accumulates. Cholestyramine is a chloride salt anion-exchanger, and its use can also produce hyperchloremic acidosis.

The Osmolal Gap

The principal osmotically active particles in serum are sodium salts, urea, and glucose. If their concentrations are known, the serum osmolality can be calculated. All values must be expressed in mOsm/L. The concentrations of molecules reported in mg/dl can be converted by dividing them by their atomic weights and by dividing that value by ten (to convert metric units). BUN is divided by 2.8 (atomic weight of the nitrogen in urea, $N_2H_4CO = 28$); glucose is divided by 18 (atomic weight of $C_6H_{12}O_6 = 180$). The concentration of sodium is given in mEq/L. Since it is a monovalent ion, that is equivalent to mOsm/L. The value of sodium is doubled to include its accompanying anions. The equation for osmolality is then as follows:

$$\text{Osmolality} = 2\,\text{Na} + \frac{\text{BUN}}{2.8} + \frac{\text{glucose}}{18}$$

The calculated value is usually within 10 mEq of the measured value. If the difference is greater, the presence of other osmotically active substances, such as ethylene glycol, methanol, or ethanol, should be suspected. If a mixed overdose including ethanol is suspected, the osmotic effects of ethanol can be included in the calculation. (The concentration of ethanol in mg/dl is divided by 4.6, as the atomic weight of $C_2H_5OH = 46$.)

Isopropyl alcohol is metabolized to acetone and gives a positive reaction to ketone tests. Acetone, however, is not an acid and does not alter the anion gap. Ethylene glycol and methanol are osmotically active; their metabolites produce metabolic acidosis and an increased anion gap. The metabolites of ethylene glycol also produce crystalluria. Identifying these substances, as well as ethanol, can be done on the basis of clinical evidence and simple laboratory tests.

Characteristics of Toxins[1]

TOXIN	ANION GAP	EYE PAPILLITIS/ EDEMA	CHARAC- TERISTIC BREATH ODOR	URINALYSIS CaOx/ HIPPURIC ACID	KETONES	SERUM OSMOLALITY (MEASURED > CALCULATED)
Methanol	+	+	0	0	0	+
Ethylene glycol	+	0	0	+/+	0	+
Ketoacids	+	0	+	0	+	0
Isopropyl (rubbing) alcohol	0	0	+	0	+	?
Ethanol	+	0	+	0	+	+

The Cumberland Gap

The Cumberland Gap is a pass in the Appalachian Mountains near the junctions of Kentucky, Tennessee, and Virginia. The Wilderness Road, which allowed many pioneers access to the American interior, was built through this pass.

References:
1. Emmett M, Narins RG. Clinical use of the anion gap. Medicine 1977;56:38–54. (Tables reprinted with permission of The Williams & Wilkins Co., Baltimore.)
2. Fischman RA, Fairclough GF, Cheigh JS. Iodine and negative anion gap (Letter). New Engl J Med 1978;298:1035–1036.
3. Oh MS, Carroll HJ. The anion gap. New Engl J Med 1977;297:814–817. (Tables reprinted with permission of the New England Journal of Medicine.)

10
PSYCHIATRY

EVALUATION OF THE SUICIDAL PATIENT 355
MANAGEMENT OF THE VIOLENT PATIENT 358
DEPRESSION 360

EVALUATION OF THE SUICIDAL PATIENT

A suicidal patient may be seen at any stage—during suicidal ideation—after an attempted but unsuccessful suicide—or after a completed suicide.

A person with suicidal ideation may not express those thoughts openly. He may complain of those minor problems that are so annoying to a physician but that may be symptoms of depression. Such symptoms include insomnia, hypersomnia, anorexia, weight loss, gastrointestinal problems, diffuse aches and pains, impotence, lack of energy, inability to concentrate or remember, and lack of interest. Rather than being exasperated by such seemingly trivial complaints, the physician should search for organic causes and question the patient further about depression and suicidal inclinations.

Other patients are seen after suicide has been attempted. These attempts may be disguised as dangerous behavior (reckless driving, walking along a busy highway) or poor medical compliance (indiscreet activity by a patient with angina, improper use of insulin by a diabetic).

An attempted suicide should not be considered an unsuccessful suicide: most people who attempt suicide have no real intention of being successful. Most attempts are designed subconsciously to change the behavior of the patient's friends and relatives: to make them pay attention, feel guilty, or forgive the patient for other misdeeds.

For those who have suicidal ideation as well as those who have attempted suicide, the risk of their successfully completing the act should be carefully evaluated. A rating scale as presented in the next two tables can be used. Successful suicides occur most frequently among older males who are socially isolated. They are strongly associated with depression and alcoholism. Those who have a well-developed plan and who have obtained the means to carry it out are at particular risk. The suicide plan itself should be evaluated by the physician for its potential lethality and the patient's chances of being rescued. A rating scale is presented in the Risk-Rescue Rating table. Those whose plans for suicide have no apparent effect on others are at a special risk—they are *not* just attempting to manipulate.

The disposition of the patient who has been cleared medically is often decided with difficulty. A patient may be sent home if the suicide risk is low, if he shows an interest in the future, and if there are caring people to be with him. This action avoids the problems of hospitalization, i.e., loss of self-esteem, economic burden, job compromises, and family friction. Since it carries some risk, however, the decision to allow a patient to go home should be made only with a psychiatrist's assessment and agreement.

The patient may be admitted to a general hospital ward if he is at low risk. This avoids the stigma of psychiatric admission. However, a psychiatric unit is usually the best place for the suicidal patient to be evaluated and treated. The psychiatric unit is attuned to the standard

10

precautions that must be taken to avoid another suicide attempt. If a patient seems to be at high risk for suicide and refuses hospitalization, he may be admitted against his will.

It is rarely the role of the emergency physician to prescribe mood-altering drugs for a suicidal patient. These may provide the means for a subsequent suicide attempt. Medication should be used in conjunction with ongoing therapy, which cannot be provided by the emergency physician. If medication is given in the emergency department, the patient may have less incentive to seek the help of a therapist.

HIGH RISK FACTORS IN ATTEMPTED SUICIDES[5]*

Older than 45 years
Male
White
Separated, divorced, or widowed
Lives alone
Unemployed or retired
Poor physical health in past six months
Mood disorder, alcoholism, or other mental disorder
Medical care in past six months
Firearms, jumping, or drowning used in attempt
Attempt made during warm months
Attempt made during daylight
Attempt made at own or other's home
Reported attempt himself almost immediately
Denies intent to kill self
Suicide note
Previous attempts

*To rate a patient on these factors, score one point for each item that describes the patient and compare the patient's score with the data in the next table to determine the degree of risk. (The general population has a suicide rate of about 11 per 100,000; the low rate for suicide attempts in the table is 63.5 times that of the general population.)

Risk Score and Death Rate per 1000 Population among Attempted Suicides and Degree of Risk[5]

SCORE	SUICIDE RATE	DEGREE OF RISK
0–1	0.00	
		Low
2–5	6.98	
		Medium
6–9	19.61	
		High
10–12	60.61	

Risk-Rescue Rating[5]*

Risk Factors	Rescue Factors
Agent used	*Location*
Ingestion, cutting,	Familiar (3)
stabbing (1)	Nonfamiliar,
Drowning, asphyxiation,	nonremote (2)
strangulation (2)	Remote (1)
Jumping, shooting (3)	*Person initiating rescue*
Impaired consciousness	Key person (3)
None in evidence (1)	Professional (2)
Confusion, semicoma (2)	Passerby (1)
Coma, deep coma (3)	*Probability of discovery*
Lesions, toxicity	*by rescuer*
Mild (1)	High, almost certain (3)
Moderate (2)	Uncertain discovery (2)
Severe (3)	Accidental discovery (1)
Reversibility	*Accessibility to rescue*
Good, complete recovery	Asks for help (3)
expected (1)	Drops clues (2)
Fair, recovery expected	Does not ask for help (1)
with time (2)	*Delay until discovery*
Poor, residuals expected	Immediate, within
if recovery occurs (3)	one hour (3)
Treatment required	Less than four hours (2)
First aid, emergency	Greater than four hours (1)
department care (1)	
Hospital admission, routine	
treatment (2)	
Intensive care, special	
treatment (3)	
Degree of risk by risk	*Degree of risk by rescue*
score (points)	*score (points)*†
High risk: 13–15	Least rescuable: 5–7
High moderate: 11–12	Low moderate: 8–9
Moderate: 9–10	Moderate: 10–11
Low moderate: 7–8	High moderate: 12–13
Low risk: 5–6	Most rescuable: 14–15

*The number after each item indicates the number of points scored.

† If there is undue delay in obtaining treatment, the final score should be reduced by one point.

*"After all I am alive only by accident.
I would have killed myself gladly that time any
possible way."*

Sylvia Plath, "A Birthday Present"

*"The woman is perfected,
Her dead
Body wears a smile of accomplishment."*

Sylvia Plath, "Edge"

References:

1. Boekelheide PD. Evaluation of suicide risk. Am Fam Physician 1978;*18*(6):109–113.
2. Golden KM. Suicide assessment: a clinical model. J Fam Pract 1978;*6*:1221–1227.
3. Murphy GE. Suicide and attempted suicide. Hosp Pract 1977;*12*(11):73–81.
4. Rockwell DA, Pepitone-Rockwell F. The suicidal patient. J Fam Pract 1978;*7*:1207–1213.
5. Sletten IW, Barton JL. Suicidal patients in the emergency room: a guide for evaluation and disposition. Hosp Community Psychiatry 1979;*30*(6):407–411. (Tables reproduced with permission.)

MANAGEMENT OF THE VIOLENT PATIENT

Signs of a Potentially Violent Patient

1. Drug intoxication or withdrawal.
2. Organic brain syndrome, acute psychosis, paranoia, borderline personality, or antisocial personality.
3. Tension in body posture.
4. Loud, forceful voice; threats of violence or boasts of violence.
5. Increased motor activity.

Tone of Interaction

1. Have one person in charge, dealing with the patient.
2. Show confidence, organization, and control—not anxiety or fear.
3. Don't bargain with the patient.
4. Don't argue with the patient.
5. Don't challenge the patient.
6. Don't console the patient.

Setting of Interaction

1. Use an area that is away from the stimuli of the ED, with no objects that could be dangerous.
2. Interview the patient alone.
3. Have someone nearby for back-up.
4. Stay between the patient and the door.
5. Stay at least an arm's length away from the patient.

Verbal Interaction

1. Use a soft voice.
2. Tell the patient what is expected of him, and that violent behavior will not be tolerated.
3. Tell the patient you want to help him.
4. Address the patient's feelings of violence.

Physical Restraint

1. A patient may not be responsive to verbal treatment.

2. Have a four- to five-person restraint team ready.

3. The restraint team should not have weapons, as the patient could take them.

4. The restraint team should initially stay about 20 feet from the patient.

5. Assign each team member to hold a particular limb or the head. Limbs should be held at the joint.

6. If necessary, use two mattresses and sandwich the patient between them.

7. Restrain the patient in a wheelchair or on a stretcher (prone or on his side).

Weapons

1. Ask the patient to place any weapons on the table or floor. Do not take weapons directly from the patient.

2. Once a patient has been restrained, remove all potentially dangerous items.

3. Wait for police to disarm the patient, if necessary.

Physical Examination

1. Explain the procedure to the patient. The familiar format may relieve the patient's tension.

2. Look for causes of violent behavior: drug intoxication or withdrawal; organic brain syndrome; infection; endocrinopathy (hypoglycemia, thyroid storm, uremia, adrenal crisis), hypoxia, trauma, brain tumor, and cerebrovascular accident (CVA).

Medication

1. Oral administration is preferred.

2. Haloperidol 5 mg (or 1–2 mg for elderly patients), every 30 minutes up to 10 doses or until the patient is calm. Do not use haloperidol if the patient is pregnant or breastfeeding, or if the cause of agitation is drug intoxication or withdrawal. If dystonia develops, give benztropine, 2 mg, or diphenhydramine, 50 mg IV.

3. For alcohol or barbiturate intoxication, keep the patient in a quiet environment.

4. For hallucinogens, give the patient diazepam and keep him in a quiet environment.

5. For life-threatening anticholinergic effects, administer bicarbonate, phenytoin, or physostigmine.

10

Patient Refuses Treatment or Tries to Leave

1. Treat the patient if there is a threat to his physical or mental health.

2. Establish that the patient is not competent to refuse treatment.

3. Meanwhile, obtain a court order to restrain the patient.

References:

1. Dubin WR. Evaluating and managing the violent patient. Ann Emerg Med 1981;*10*: 481–484.

2. Perry SW III, Gilmore MM. The disruptive patient or visitor. JAMA 1981;*245*:755–757.

3. Perry S. Effective management of the violent patient. ER Reports 1983;*4*(6):31–36.

> "Life was impossible, but it was endured.
> Whose life? Mine, but what does that mean?"
>
> CZESLAW MILOSZ

DEPRESSION

"Anxiety and hysteria are diagnoses of exclusion."
Marshall B. Segal, M.D., J.D.

Depression may be a sign of a serious underlying medical condition or it may be a primary disease entity itself, with the potential for a fatal outcome from suicide. The emergency physician must be able to recognize depressives who are an immediate suicide risk. They must also diagnose the medical cause when depression is the manifestation of an underlying medical illness. The medical causes of depression are summarized in the following table. "Evaluation of the Suicidal Patient" contains a suicide-risk score that can be used to identify patients who are at high risk of taking their own lives.

Medical Causes of Depression

DEFICIENCY STATES
Pellagra
Pernicious anemia
Wernicke's encephalopathy

DRUGS AND MEDICATION
Alcohol
Amphetamines
Antihypertensive agents
    clonidine
    diuretics—hypokalemia*
        or hyponatremia*
    guanethidine
    methyldopa
    propranolol
    reserpine
Birth control pills
Cimetidine
Digitalis
Disulfiram
Sedatives
    barbiturates
    benzodiazepines
Steroids/ACTH

ENDOCRINE DISORDERS
Acromegaly
Adrenal
    Addison's disease*
    Cushing's disease
Hyper- and hypoparathyroidism*
Hyper- and hypothyroidism*
Insulinoma
Pheochromocytoma
Pituitary

INFECTIONS
Encephalitis*
Fungal
Meningitis*
Neurosyphilis
Tuberculosis

MALIGNANT DISEASE
Metastases
    breast
    GI
    lung
    pancreas
    prostate
Remote effect: pancreas

METABOLIC DISORDERS
Electrolyte imbalance
    hypokalemia*
    hyponatremia*
Hepatic encephalopathy
Hypo-oxygenation*
    cerebral arteriosclerosis
    chronic bronchitis
    congestive heart failure*
    emphysema
    myocardial infarction*
    paroxysmal dysrhythmias
    pneumonia*
    severe anemia*
Uremia*

NEUROLOGIC DISORDERS
Alzheimer's disease
Amyotrophic lateral sclerosis
Creutzfeldt-Jakob disease
Huntington's chorea
Multiple sclerosis
Myasthenia gravis
Normal-pressure hydrocephalus
Parkinson's disease
Pick's disease
Wilson's disease

TRAUMA
Postconcussion

*Acute life-threatening disorders that must be diagnosed in the emergency room.

10

Reference:
    1. Jenike MA. Depressed in the ER. Emerg Med 1984;March:102–120. (With permission.)

11

PROCEDURES

EMERGENCY STETHOSCOPE 363

A SIMPLE TRICK TO ENSURE APPROPRIATE BP CUFF SIZE . 363

REMOVING CHEWING GUM FROM HAIR 364

REMOVING TAR FROM BURNS—A LITTLE PEARL 365

EMERGENCY RING REMOVAL 365

JUST A LITTLE STICK 366

ALLERGY TO LOCAL ANESTHETICS, OR IS BITING THE
BULLET EVER NECESSARY? 366

REGIONAL ANESTHESIA 368

ORAL ANESTHESIA 370

OUT, DAMNED SPOT! OUT, I SAY! (Macbeth V, i, 38) 374

EMERGENCY STETHOSCOPE

> *"If you tinker with something long enough you will break it."*
>
> Murphy

Dr. J. Edwin Seegmiller has suggested a simple method for improvising a stethoscope should you be involved in a medical emergency on an airplane. A headset for listening to recorded music is converted into a stethoscope by removing an earpiece from a second headset, everting it, and attaching it to the first headset's plug (Fig. 11-1).

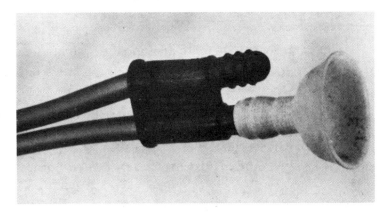

Fig. 11-1. Emergency stethoscope.

Reference:

   1. Seegmiller, J.E.: Stethoscopes on airplanes. N Engl J Med 1981;*305*:289. (Figure reprinted by permission of The New England Journal of Medicine.)

A SIMPLE TRICK TO ENSURE APPROPRIATE BP CUFF SIZE

If a small blood pressure cuff is used for a patient with a large arm, spurious systolic and diastolic pressures will be recorded with the potential for the inappropriate diagnosis and treatment of hypertension. The American Heart Association (AHA) now recommends that the inflatable bladder in the blood pressure cuff cover 75 per cent or more of the arm's circumference. Unfortunately, the range imprinted by the manufacturers on many standard size adult cuffs exceeds the acceptable limits recommended by the AHA.

"The problem can be remedied by re-marking, with an indelible marker, the right border of the range on a cuff at a point where 75 per cent of the arm's circumference is covered by the bladder. This is most easily done by multiplying the bladder length by 4/3, then marking the vertical line on the cuff at this distance from the left border of the cuff

11

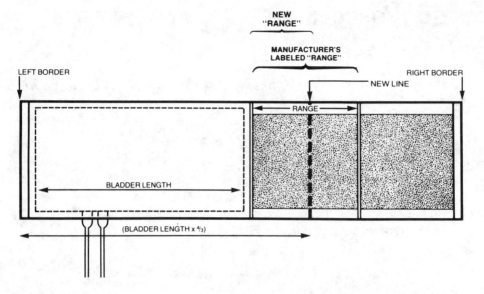

Fig. 11-2. Technique for re-marking the right border of the range on a blood-pressure cuff.

(Fig. 11–2). Thus, when the cuff is applied snugly to the arm, one will know (without measurement) whether the cuff size is appropriate: if on closure the left cuff border meets a point to the left of the new line, the cuff is adequate. If the left border meets a point to the right of the new line, a larger cuff is required.''

Reference:
1. Manning DM. Avoiding sphygmomanometer cuff "Hypertension." N Engl J Med 1981; *306*:109. (Quoted material and figure reprinted by permission of The New England Journal of Medicine.)

REMOVING CHEWING GUM FROM HAIR

Chewing gum can be easily removed from the hair by freezing the gum and crumbling it. Ice cubes or a topical refrigerant such as ethyl chloride are effective in freezing the gum, but care should be taken not to freeze the underlying skin since frostbite might result. About five seconds of spraying the refrigerant is usually adequate.

Reference:
1. Collure, DW. Removal of chewing gum from hair. Ann Emerg Med 1980;*9*:333.

REMOVING TAR FROM BURNS — A LITTLE PEARL

Tar burns can be extremely painful because the tar adheres to the injured tissue. Lard or margarine rubbed over the tar will dissolve it; the resulting gunk can then simply be rinsed off with water, and the underlying burn treated. Application of Neosporin cream is also effective.

EMERGENCY RING REMOVAL

Figure 11-3 illustrates a convenient technique for emergency removal of a ring from an edematous digit. If the swelling of the finger is likely to produce vascular compromise, it is best to employ a ring-cutting saw to facilitate immediate removal. When vascular obstruction is not imminent, the ring can be salvaged by the following method:

1. Apply soap liberally to a piece of string (or suture material) and pass the proximal end of the string beneath the ring with a curved hemostat.

2. Wrap the string tightly around the finger, proceeding distally toward the tip of the finger.

3. Unwrap the string, drawing the ring distally along the wrapped finger. You may have to repeat this procedure a few times to accomplish complete removal.

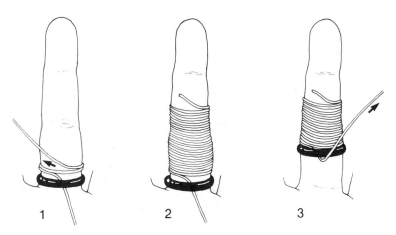

Fig. 11-3. A convenient technique for emergency removal of a ring.

1   2   3

11

JUST A LITTLE STICK

Intramuscular injections in children must be performed with caution and anatomic precision, since the margin for error is quite small in this age group. Complications shared by all intramuscular injections include muscle fibrosis and contracture, nerve injury, and abscess formation. Broken needles and accidental joint-space infiltration are always feared iatrogenic complications. The three major intramuscular injection sites used in children, along with salient features, are listed:

ANATOMIC AREA	FAVORABLE ASPECTS	POSSIBLE COMPLICATIONS
Lateral thigh (quadraceps femoris)	Absence of vital structures Largest muscle in body Useful in young infants	Fibrosis and muscle contracture Femoral artery thrombosis
Gluteal area	Shot unobserved by child	Muscle not well-developed until age 2 years Sciatic nerve injury in obese children, fatty infusion may occur
Deltoid region	Easily accessible area Reserved for single injections only	Contractures Radial and axillary nerve damage

Reference:
1. Bergeson PS, Singer SA, Kaplan AM. Intramuscular injections in children. Pediatrics 1982;70:944–947.

ALLERGY TO LOCAL ANESTHETICS, OR IS BITING THE BULLET EVER NECESSARY?

Many people report a history of allergy to local anesthetic agents and, as a result, either endure minor surgical procedures without anesthetic or are subjected to an otherwise unnecessary general anesthetic. Actually, very few of the adverse reactions to local anesthetics are allergic; they are due to sympathetic stimulation, vasovagal reactions, hyperventilation, and local responses to the trauma of the procedure. Toxic reactions can also occur if large amounts of the anesthetic are absorbed into the circulation.

An approach to the management of local anesthetic allergy is outlined here. Because there are two unrelated classes of local anesthetic agents, you can use an agent from the other class when the available information clearly identifies a particular anesthetic as producing the prior reaction. Local infiltration of 1 per cent diphenhydramine usually provides acceptable anesthesia for skin but not for dental procedures. Finally, skin testing and progressive challenge with lidocaine may be employed as outlined.

I. Management of Adverse Reactions to Local Anesthetic Agents

1. *Chemically unrelated agents:* Generic and proprietary names of some representative drugs:
   A. *Para-aminobenzoic acid esters*
      a. Procaine (Novocaine)
      b. Tetracaine (Pontocaine)
      c. Ethyl-p-aminobenzoate (Benzocaine)
      d. Bupivacaine (Marcaine)
   B. *Miscellaneous group*
      a. Lidocaine (Xylocaine)
      b. Mepivacaine (Carbocaine)
      c. Dibucaine (Nupercaine)

2. *Diphenhydramine (Benadryl) 1 per cent (10 mg/ml)*

3. *Skin testing and progressive challenge with lidocaine*
   a. Prick test with lidocaine 1 per cent, diluted 1:100.
   b. Prick test with lidocaine 1 per cent, full strength.
   c. Intradermal skin test with 0.02 ml lidocaine 1 per cent, diluted 1:100.
   d. Intradermal skin test with 0.02 ml lidocaine 1 per cent, full strength.
   e. Subcutaneous injection of 0.1 ml lidocaine 1 per cent.
   f. Subcutaneous injection of 0.5 ml lidocaine 1 per cent.

Injections are at 20-minute intervals unless the patient's history suggests a delayed reaction; in the latter case, there should be a delay of 24 hours between steps *d* and *e*, and a similar delay after step *f* before further administration of local anesthetic.

References:
   1. Gottlieb AJ, Zamkoff KW, Jastremski MS, et al. The Whole Internist Catalog. Philadelphia: WB Saunders, 1980:246.
   2. Nelson HS. Allergic reactions to drugs. Adv Asthma Allergy 1976; *3*:29.

11

REGIONAL ANESTHESIA

Median Nerve Block (Fig. 11-4)

The median nerve travels on the volar aspect of the wrist, passing deep to the flexor retinaculum. It lies deep to, or just radial to, the palmaris longus tendon. At the level of the ulnar styloid, a needle is passed between the palmaris longus and flexor carpi radialis tendons perpendicular to the skin to a depth of approximately 1 cm. If paresthesia is elicited, 1 to 2 ml of 2 percent xylocaine (lidocaine) is injected. If paresthesia is not elicited, another 2 ml is injected in the region. This method will anesthetize the radial half of the palm and the index and middle fingers.

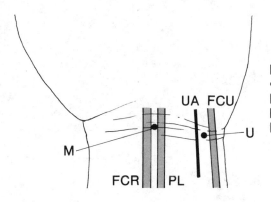

Fig. 11-4. Median and ulnar nerve block: Injection sites for median and ulnar nerves. •—Injection site. *M*—Median nerve. *FCR*—Flexor carpi radialis tendon. *PL*—Palmaris longus tendon. *UA*—Ulnar artery. *U*—Ulnar Nerve. *FCU*—Flexor carpi ulnaris tendon.

Ulnar Nerve Block (Fig. 11-4)

The ulnar nerve passes to the ulnar side of the ulnar artery and just to the radial side of the flexor carpi ulnaris tendon, on the volar aspect of the wrist. Injection is made between the ulnar artery and flexor carpi ulnaris tendon, using 2 ml of 2 percent lidocaine. This method will anesthetize the ulnar half of the palm and the dorsum of the hand, and the little finger and ulnar half of the ring finger.

Radial Nerve Block (Fig. 11-5)

The radial nerve leaves the radial artery, passes to the dorsal aspect of the forearm, and divides to supply the radial aspect of the dorsum of the hand. To block this nerve, the skin is penetrated just lateral to the radial artery, the needle is directed dorsally, and 2 ml of 2 percent lidocaine is injected subcutaneously in a "bracelet fashion".

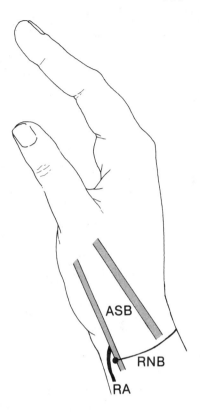

Fig. 11-5. Radial nerve block: Injection site for radial nerve. •—Injection site. *RA*—Radial artery. *ASB*—Anatomic snuff box. *RNB*—Path of infiltration for radial nerve block.

Digital Block (Fig. 11-6)

The fingers are supplied by a pair of nerves that course on either side of the digit, generally on the volar side. The needle is inserted perpendicularly to the palm on each side of the proximal phalanx at the fold between digit and palm, and 1 to 1.5 ml of lidocaine is injected. For proximal digital anesthesia, injection may be made from the dorsum of the hand at the level of the metacarpal head, or the base of the digit may be infiltrated circumferentially. Epinephrine should not be used; it might cause sufficient vasoconstriction to compromise circulation to the digit. Anesthesia of the toes is accomplished by a similar technique, injecting at the base of the toe.

Fig. 11-6. Digital Nerve Block: •—Injection site.

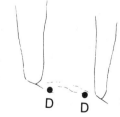

11

Ankle Block (Fig. 11-7)

Anesthesia of the sole of the foot is obtained by blocking the posterior tibial and sural nerves at the ankle. The tibial nerve runs deep to the posterior tibial artery as it courses behind the medial malleolus, and supplies the distal and medial sole of the foot. The sural nerve runs behind the lateral malleolus and supplies the heel and lateral sole of the foot. The needle is passed either medial or lateral to the Achilles tendon and advanced to the malleolus. From 2 to 4 ml of 1 per cent lidocaine with epinephrine 1:100,000 is injected for each nerve.

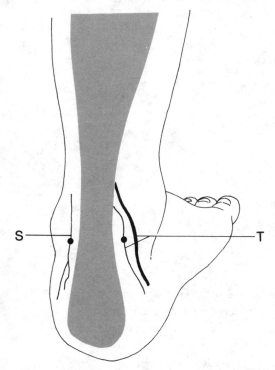

Fig. 11-7. Ankle Block: Injection sites for sural and tibial nerves. •—Injection site. S—Sural nerve. T—Posterior tibial artery and nerve.

"The feasibility of an operation is not the best indication for its performance."

Ward Cohen's Comment

ORAL ANESTHESIA

Local anesthesia can effectively break the pain cycle of a patient's toothache. It gives him comfort until definitive care can be provided by a dentist or oral surgeon. The sedation and abuse potential of narcotic analgesics are avoided.

Question the patient carefully regarding previous adverse reactions to anesthetics. If not contraindicated, use a long-acting anesthetic such as bupivacaine hydrochloride 0.25 per cent (Marcaine or Sensorcaine). Bupivacaine takes effect within two to ten minutes, and lasts up to seven hours. Epinephrine prolongs the anesthetic's effect and prevents bleeding at the injection site. The concentration of epinephrine should be 1:60,000 or less (Marcaine is available with epinephrine in the 1:200,000 concentration). Prepare a syringe with 1 to 2.5 ml of anesthetic solution and a small-gauge 1 5/8-inch needle.

Determine the site of pain by percussing the teeth. Correct placement of the anesthetic is important. Injections into muscle may result in soreness and trismus, but not anesthesia. Intravenous injection may produce systemic toxicity. Injection near a motor nerve will cause transient paralysis. If a hematoma forms, it should be treated with cold compresses for 24 hours, then hot compresses.

These directions are given for right-handed clinicians. Position the patient so that you can work comfortably. To inject the right side of the mouth stand on the patient's right facing him. To inject the left side stand slightly behind and to the right of the patient, so that you both face the same direction; bring your left arm around the patient's head and bend over to look into his mouth.

For each patient, clean the area to be injected with germicidal solution. You may also use a topical anesthetic prior to injection.

Inferior Alveolar Nerve Block

Inferior alveolar nerve block numbs the teeth on one side of the lower jaw, as well as the chin, tongue, and cheek on that side.

1. Using your index finger, locate the coronoid notch of the mandible. It is the deepest part of the anterior border of the mandibular ramus. Draw the skin over the notch toward the cheek (Fig. 11–8).

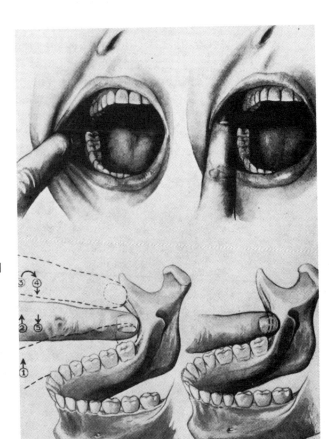

Fig. 11–8. Locating the coronoid notch of the mandible.

11

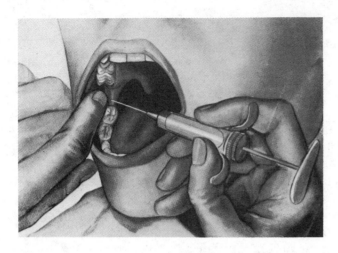

Fig. 11-9. Syringe parallel to the surface of the lower teeth. For inferior alveolar nerve block.

2. Hold the syringe parallel to the surface of the lower teeth. Direct it from the opposite bicuspids into the skin over the coronoid notch. Don't penetrate more than one-half inch (Fig. 11-9).

3. Aspirate for blood. If there is no return, inject the anesthetic slowly, taking at least two minutes for 2 ml. Withdraw the needle until about one-quarter of an inch remains in the tissue. Inject another 0.5 ml of anesthetic.

Posterior Superior Alveolar Nerve Block

This type of nerve block numbs the first, second, and third molars of the maxilla on one side.

1. Locate the posterior inferior surface of the malar prominence with your index finger. The prominence is palpable in the mucobuccal fold, opposite the tricuspids. Keeping the tip of the finger in place, form an angle with your finger to draw the lip and cheek away. Direct the syringe upward and medially, inserting the needle about three-quarters of an inch (Fig. 11-10 *A* and *B*).

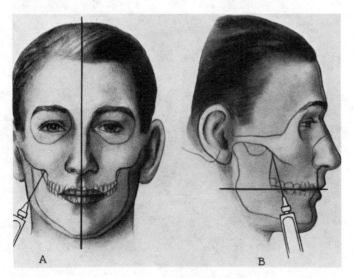

Fig. 11-10 *A* and *B*. Injection site for posterior superior alveolar nerve block.

A   B

2. Aspirate for blood. If there is none, slowly inject 2.5 ml of anesthetic. To fully anesthetize the first molar, inject an additional 0.25 ml over its apex (see Subperiosteal Infiltration Anesthesia).

Infra-orbital Nerve Block

An infra-orbital block numbs the maxillary incisors, cuspids, and bicuspids on one side.

1. Palpate the infra-orbital foramen with your thumb. It is at the junction of the middle and medial third of the infra-orbital ridge, and about 0.5 cm below it.

2. Keeping your thumb in place, lift the upper lip with your index finger (Fig. 11–11).

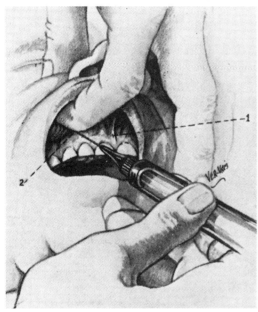

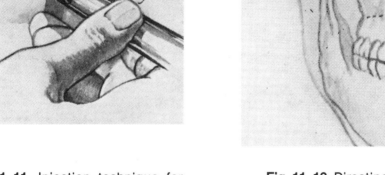

Fig. 11–11. Injection technique for infra-orbital nerve block.

Fig. 11–12. Directing the syringe into the infra-orbital foramen.

3. Insert the needle in the mucolabial fold, below the inner canthus of the eye. Direct the syringe upward and laterally into the infra-orbital foramen (just under your thumb). Don't insert the needle more than one-half of an inch (Fig. 11–12).

4. Withdraw the plunger. If you do not aspirate blood, inject 2 ml of anesthetic over one and half minutes. Massage the injected tissues with your thumb, to force the anesthetic into the infra-orbital canal.

11

Subperiosteal Infiltration Anesthesia

Subperiosteal infiltration anesthesia numbs the individual teeth of the maxilla.

1. Hold the syringe with the needle's bevel upward.

2. Insert the needle through the mucobuccal or mucolabial fold, over the affected tooth. Direct it toward the periapical region, until it touches bone. Slowly inject 1 ml of anesthetic.

Reference:

1. Archer WH. Anesthesia. *In:* Grossman LI (ed.). Lippincott's Handbook of Dental Practice. Philadelphia: J.B. Lippincott, Company, 1958;207–218. (Figures reproduced with permission.)

OUT, DAMNED SPOT! OUT, I SAY!
(MACBETH V, i, 38)

There are two approaches toward dress for the emergency room. You can wear scrubs that are cleaned by the hospital laundry or a private laundry; or you can wear your own clothing and learn to take out stains.

A word of caution: all solutions and solvents should be tested on a concealed part of the garment to determine if they affect the fabric or color. Isopropyl alcohol should be diluted with water (1:2) before it's used on acetate fabrics.

Stain and Treatment

Adhesive tape—Sponge the spot with cleaning fluid or hold an ice cube on the spot, then pick off the frozen adhesive.

Betadine—Rinse with cool water.

Blood—Soak washable fabric in cold water or in hydrogen peroxide (3%), then wash in warm water with detergent. Old stains may need to be soaked in an ammonia solution (1 tbsp per quart of water) before washing. Stubborn stains may respond to a paste of powdered starch and water that is applied, allowed to dry, and peeled off. An oxygen bleach (Snowy, Beads-o-Bleach) is another solution for difficult stains.

Nonwashable fabric should be sponged with cold water or peroxide. Stubborn stains may be sprinkled with sodium perborate crystals, then covered with a damp cotton pad. If this treatment yellows the fabric, sponge with white vinegar and rinse. Stubborn stains may also be treated with a chlorine bleach solution (e.g., 1 tsp Clorox per cup of water) applied in drops, and rinsed out after 5 to 15 minutes. If a stronger solution is used (1 part liquid chlorine bleach to 1 part water), it should be rinsed out immediately after application.

Carbon paper—If the material is washable, work liquid detergent into the stain, then rinse. For stubborn stains, drop ammonia directly on the spot before using detergent. Nonwashable material can be sponged with alcohol solution (1 part isopropyl alcohol to 2 parts water) then rinsed with cold water.

Charcoal—Any suggestions?

Coffee—If the fabric is washable, soak it in cool water, work detergent into the stain, then rinse. You may also soak the fabric in a solution of 1 part vinegar to 4 parts water, then hang the wet garment in the sun. Another method is to lay the stained fabric over a bowl, then pour boiling water through it from a height of 2 to 3 feet. Stubborn stains may respond to commercial coffee pot cleaner.

Nonwashable fabrics can be treated by squirting cool water through the stain with a syringe, catching extra water with a sponge held underneath the cloth. If a cream stain remains after using these methods, sponge the area with cleaning fluid.

Ink (Ballpoint)—Some inks can be washed out, whereas others are set by washing. Make a test mark of the same ink on similar material, and check the result of washing. Inks that do not wash out can be treated with various solvents, but test them on a concealed part of the material first. Some fabrics can be sponged with acetone. Isopropyl alcohol (1 part alcohol to 2 parts water) or amyl acetate (bought chemically pure from a drugstore) may be safer for other fabrics.

Iodine—Washable fabrics can be soaked in cool water, rubbed with a detergent, then washed. Another method is to moisten the stain, then hold it in the steam from a boiling teakettle.

Washable or nonwashable fabrics can be treated with isopropyl alcohol (for acetate fabrics, dilute 1 part alcohol to 2 parts water). Soak a cotton ball in alcohol and place it over the stain, then rinse or steam it. A sodium thiosulfate solution (1 tbsp per pint of water) may also work. Washable fabrics can be soaked in the solution. For nonwashable fabrics, a gauze pad soaked in the solution can be held over the stain for 15 minutes.

Mercurochrome or *Merthiolate*—If the fabric is washable, soak it in an ammonia solution (4 tbsp per quart of water), sponge with an alcohol solution (2 parts isopropyl alcohol to 1 part water), then rinse. If the fabric is nonwashable, sponge the area with isopropyl alcohol (dilute 1 part alcohol to 2 parts water for acetate fabric), or moisten the stain with a liquid detergent. Add one drop of ammonia and rinse.

Pencil—Pencil marks may be erased from cloth. If they remain, work detergent into the stain, then rinse. If the mark persists, place a few drops of ammonia on the stain, work in detergent, and rinse. Graphite pencil marks can be removed by rubbing mechanic's hand soap into the stain, then brushing it off.

Tea—Tea stains may respond to the methods described for coffee. Washable fabrics may also be soaked in borax solution (4 tsp per quart of water), then rinsed.

Urine—Urine stains may respond to soaking (washable fabrics) or sponging (nonwashable fabrics) with cool water, working in detergent, then rinsing with water (washable fabrics), or sponging with alcohol (nonwashable fabrics). Stubborn stains may respond to sponging with ammonia or with white vinegar.

Vomit—Soak washable fabrics (or sponge nonwashable fabrics) in a solution of ½ cup salt per 2 quarts water. Rinse, then wash with warm water and soap (or sponge nonwashable fabrics with alcohol).

11

References:
   1. Molle B, Charles I. Sincere's Home Cleaning Guide. Tucson: Sincere Auto Book Press, 1972.
   2. Moore AC. How To Clean Everything. New York: Simon & Schuster, 1968: 203–220.

12

POTPOURRI

DEVELOPMENT OF A SPECIALTY 377

WHAT TO DO WHEN YOU GROW UP 378

IS THERE A METHOD BEHIND THE MADNESS ? 380

ANSWERS TO COST CONSCIOUSNESS QUIZ 382

GAMES PHYSICIANS PLAY 383

A GUIDE TO PERCENTAGES 384

FUN WITH FIGURES 385

TO YOUR HEALTH! 389

ALL THOSE STRANGE THINGS WE DO TO OUR BODIES 392

15 TIPS TO HELP YOU SURVIVE A HOTEL FIRE 401

HOW TO SWIM WITH SHARKS 402

EMERGENCY MEDICINE LIBRARY 403

USEFUL REFERENCES 405

JUNK MAIL 405

PHONE DIRECTORY 406

DEVELOPMENT OF A SPECIALTY

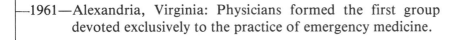

*"There is only one thing more foolish than to think
that one's own specialty can solve all problems,
and that is to think that another specialty can."*

Anonymous

—1961—Alexandria, Virginia: Physicians formed the first group
devoted exclusively to the practice of emergency medicine.

—1968—Falls Church, Virginia, and Lansing, Michigan: Through
conferences in these cities, the American College of
Emergency Physicians was founded.

—1970—University of Cincinnati: The first accredited residency
program in emergency medicine was founded.

—1973—American Medical Association Conference on the Education of Emergency Physicians discussed emergency
medicine as a possible specialty.

—1977—The American College of Emergency Physicians applied
for recognition to the American Board of Medical
Specialties.

—1979—Emergency Medicine was recognized by the American
Board of Medical Specialties.

—1980—First certifying examination in Emergency Medicine was
given by the American Board of Emergency Medicine.

References:
1. Riggs, LM Jr. A vigorous new specialty. N Engl J Med 1981;*304*:480–483.
2. ACEP News, September, 1982; 3–4.

12

WHAT TO DO WHEN YOU GROW UP

The accompanying table shows the projections of the Graduate Medical Education National Advisory Council for specialty shortages and surpluses by 1990. Many of the "popular specialties" will have a glut of physicians by 1990. The "best bets" look like Psychiatry (especially Child Psychiatry), Emergency Medicine, and Nuclear Medicine. There will probably never be too many *GOOD* physicians in any field.

The second table of data from the AMA's 1980 Physician Manpower Survey shows the current distribution of physicians in the United States and its territories. If you have picked one of the specialties with a surplus, you might want to consider locating in North or South Dakota. One can't help but wonder why there aren't more physicians in the Virgin Islands.

GMENAC Estimates of Physician Supply and Requirements for 1990

	PHYSICIANS	TOTAL RESIDENTS	TOTAL SUPPLY	REQUIRE-MENTS	SURPLUS (SHORTAGE)
All Physicians	504,750	88,500	535,750	466,000	69,750
General and Family Practice	84,800	9900	88,250	84,000	4250
General Pediatricians	35,300	7050	37,750	30,250	7500
Pediatric Allergy	750	450	900	900	—
Pediatric Cardiology	850	400	1000	1150	(150)
Pediatric Endocrinology	250	0	250	800	(550)
Pediatric Hematology-Oncology	500	200	550	1650	(1100)
Pediatric Nephrology	200	50	200	350	(150)
Neonatology	700	—	700	1300	(600)
General Internal Medicine	66,500	20,800	73,800	70,250	3550
Allergy and Immunology	3000	150	3050	2050	1000
Cardiology	14,250	1900	14,900	7750	7150
Endocrinology	3700	500	3850	2050	1800
Gastroenterology	6550	1000	6900	6500	400
Hematology-Oncology	7850	1300	8300	9000	(700)
Infectious Diseases	3050	500	3250	2250	1000
Nephrology	4600	700	4850	2750	2100
Pulmonary Diseases	6600	1050	6950	3600	3350
Rheumatology	2850	500	3000	1700	1300
Neurology*	8300	950	8650	5500	3150
Dermatology	7150	700	7350	6950	400
Psychiatry (General)	29,250	2550	30,500	38,500	(8000)
Child Psychiatry	4050	200	4100	9000	(4900)
Obstetrics-Gynecology	32,300	6200	34,450	24,000	10,450
General Surgery	32,100	9200	35,300	23,500	11,800
Neurosurgery	4850	700	5100	2650	2450
Ophthalmology	15,400	2600	16,300	11,600	4700
Orthopedic Surgery	19,000	3150	20,100	15,100	5000
Otolaryngology	8000	1400	8500	8000	500
Plastic Surgery	3700	600	3900	2700	1200
Thoracic Surgery	2700	450	2900	2050	850
Urology	8800	1600	9350	7700	1650
Emergency Medicine	8900	1000	9250	13,500	(4250)
Preventive Medicine	5550	0	5550	7300	(1750)
Anesthesiology*	18,750	2050	19,450	21,000	(1550)
Nuclear Medicine*	150	0	150	4000	(3850)
Pathology*	16,000	2450	16,850	13,500	3350
Physiatry*	2350	150	2400	3200	(800)
Radiology*	26,450	3800	27,800	18,000	9800
All other and unspecified	9200	1450	9700	—	N/A

*Full modeling methodology was not applied for practical reasons, so requirement in specialty is considered tentative.

Active Federal and Nonfederal Doctors (MDs) by State

	TOTAL	FEDERAL	NON-FEDERAL
Total physicians	467,679	17,901	449,778
Alabama	5229	190	5039
Alaska	627	118	509
Arizona	5859	324	5535
Arkansas	307C	131	2939
California	60,752	2384	58,368
Canal Zone	33	21	12
Colorado	6391	392	5999
Connecticut	8322	145	8177
Delaware	1047	46	1001
Washington, D.C.	4164	538	3626
Florida	21,131	757	20,374
Georgia	8549	489	8060
Hawaii	2265	245	2020
Idaho	1134	45	1089
Illinois	22,228	488	21,740
Indiana	7527	112	7415
Iowa	3917	70	3847
Kansas	4043	150	3893
Kentucky	5212	153	5059
Louisiana	6997	245	6752
Maine	1927	62	1865
Maryland	13,282	1537	11,745
Massachusetts	16,661	319	16,342
Michigan	15,571	224	15,347
Minnesota	8297	147	8150
Mississippi	3015	218	2797
Missouri	8508	177	8331
Montana	1153	53	1100
Nebraska	2509	67	2442
Nevada	1233	62	1171
New Hampshire	1701	46	1655
New Jersey	15,067	268	14,799
New Mexico	2292	149	2143
New York	49,978	873	49,105
North Carolina	9742	388	9354
North Dakota	956	37	919
Ohio	16,781	439	18,342
Oklahoma	4194	163	4031
Oregon	5232	113	5119
Pennsylvania	23,742	395	23,347
Puerto Rico	4145	133	4012
Rhode Island	2163	61	2102
South Carolina	4607	245	4362
South Dakota	884	75	809
Tennessee	7686	226	7460
Texas	24,058	1487	22,571
Utah	2570	78	2492
Vermont	1215	30	1185
Virginia	10,476	794	9682
Virgin Islands	92		92
Washington	8450	529	7921
West Virginia	2857	112	2745
Wisconsin	8005	146	7859
Wyoming	610	43	567
Pacific Islands	89	4	85
Outside U.S. Address	1044	1044	
unknown	6390	114	6276

Source: AMA Physician Masterfile, 1980. Special Tabulations. Division of Survey and Data Resources. American Medical Association. Chicago, 1981 (Dec. 31, 1980).

12

IS THERE A METHOD BEHIND THE MADNESS?

Many attempts have been made to find a pattern behind the variable activity of the emergency department. Some shifts are chaotically busy, while others are boringly quiet. Some days seem to be filled with psychiatric cases, while others are filled with heart cases. Here are descriptions of external forces that may be playing a role; try to predict your day from these trends.

Season

Blood pressures are mildly elevated on cold winter days compared with warm summer days among British men 55 to 64 years old. Cold weather, especially when combined with snowfall, is associated with an increased frequency of angina and coronary deaths. Polish patients with peptic ulcers have most epigastric pain in the early autumn and least in the spring and August. A New Hampshire poison center has no seasonal variability in the number of calls it receives. However, there is a predominance of calls about plants, insecticides, acetaminophen, and venom in summer, and a predominance of calls about vitamins, aspirin, cough and cold remedies, liniments, and food poisoning in winter.

In New South Wales (where the seasons are opposite to those in the northern hemisphere), manic bipolar disorders peak in September and October (spring), depressive bipolar disorders peak in August (late winter), and depressive psychoses peak in November (spring). The female suicide rate peaks in May and November (fall and spring), though there is no significant variation in the male suicide rate. Similar patterns occur in the US, where suicide rates are relatively high in spring and low in winter. Also, in Finland, suicide rates for females peak in June and October; rates for males peak in May. Homicide rates in the US have a sustained elevation from July through September, and another peak in December.

Day of the Week

In Manitoba, the highest incidence of sudden cardiac death in previously healthy men occurs on Monday. In Minnesota, the highest incidence of sudden cardiac death is on Saturday.

Weather

During the summer in Sacramento, ER visits for depression correlate with low barometric pressure; ER visits for schizophrenia correlate with high air pollution. Days characterized by high pollution in New Zealand show a negative association with ER visits and admissions for asthma! In clinical trials, high atmospheric concentrations of positive ions are related to inattention, decreased involvement, less sociability, less elation, more tension, greater fatigue, and more frequent organic symptoms.

Phase of the Moon

In India, the incidence of poisoning is significantly increased at the time of the full moon. In the US, the full moon as well as the new moon are associated with a high incidence of abnormal behavior.

References:

1. Beard CM, Fuster V, Elveback LR. Daily and seasonal variation in sudden cardiac death. Rochester, Minnesota 1950–1975. Mayo Clin Proc 1982;*57*:704–706.
2. Brennan PJ, Greenberg G, Miall WE, Thompson SG. Seasonal variation in arterial blood pressure. Br Med J 1982;*285*:919–923.
3. Briere J, Downs A, Spensley J. Summer in the city: urban weather conditions and psychiatric emergency-room visits. J Abnor Psychol 1983;*92*:77–80.
4. Bullock R, Hall R. The heart in winter. Practitioner 1982;*226*:465–466.
5. Charry JM, Frank BW, Hawkinshire V. Effects of atmospheric electricity on some substrates of disordered social behavior. J Pers Soc Psychol 1981;*41*:185–197.
6. Dawson KP, Allan J, Fergusson DM. Asthma, air pollution, and climate: a Christchurch study. NZ Med J 1983;*96*(727):165–167.
7. Gibinski K, Rybicka J, Nowak A, Czarnecka K. Seasonal occurrence of abdominal pain and endoscopic findings in patients with gastric and duodenal ulcer disease. Scand J Gastroenterol 1982;*17*:481–485.
8. Nayha S. Autumn incidence of suicides re-examined: data from Finland by sex, age, and occupation. Br J Psychiatry 1982;*141*:512–517.
9. Parker G, Walter S. Seasonal variation in depressive disorders and suicidal deaths in New South Wales. Br J Psychiatry 1982;*140*:626–632.
10. Paulozzi LJ. Seasonality of reported poison exposure. Pediatrics 1983;*71*:891–893.
11. Rabkin SW, Mathewson FAL, Tate RB. Chronobiology of cardiac sudden death in man. JAMA 1980;*244*:1357–1358.
12. Templer DI, Veleber DM. The moon and madness: a comprehensive perspective. J Clin Psychol 1980;*36*:865–868.
13. Thakur CP, Sharma RN, Akhtar, HSMQ. Full moon and poisoning. Br Med J 1980;*281* (6256):1684.
14. Warren CW, Smith JC, Tyler CW. Seasonal variation in suicide and homicide: a question of consistency. J Biosoc Sci 1983;*15*:349–356.

12

ANSWERS TO COST CONSCIOUSNESS QUIZ *

"When things go wrong, nobody ever thanks you for saving them money."

Marshall B. Segal, M.D., J.D.

Operating room use, 1 hour	$475–570	Complete blood count and differential	$ 13.00
25% albumin, 50 ml	31.00	Blood gases	36.00
Lactated Ringer's 1000 ml	4.30	Electrolytes, BUN and Glucose	25.00
Angiocath	5.00	Folic Acid	30.00
Ethilon Suture, 5–0	6.00	Magnesium serum	15.00
Transthoracic pacing kit	79.00	Theophylline level	27.00
Cockup splint	20.00	Culture sputum and smear	22.00
Adult electrodes	5.00	HCG pregnancy, slide	13.00
Kerlix	5.00	Urinalysis, regular	10.00
Cervical collar	33.00	Ankle x-ray	36.00
Endotracheal tube	7.00	Chest x-ray, PA single	41.00
O₂ by mask (daily charge)	50.00	X-ray, portable machine use	32.00
IPPB treatment	9.00	CT scan upper abdominal (pancreas, liver)	350.00
Long leg cast	27.00	Lung scan	150.00
CVP manometer	9.00		
Suture tray	15.00		
Skull series	67.00		
ECG	43.00		

*Quiz found on page 23.

GAMES PHYSICIANS PLAY

"Better to remain silent and be thought a fool than to speak up and remove all doubt."

Anonymous

Physicians have developed ways to deal with the uncertainty that frequently surrounds the cause of a patient's illness. The mechanisms are reflected in the phrases used when a case is discussed.

1. *Linguistic hedges:* "As far as I can tell", "I think...", "approximately", "at this time...."

2. *Use of probabilities:* "She probably just has...," "It's pretty unlikely that...,"

3. *Suggesting that a puzzling case be a lead-in for research:* "It would be interesting to see whether.... ."

4. *Consultation:* "Let's ask the infectious disease service what they think."

5. *Stalling.* This is glorified as "expectant management" or "a trial of watchful waiting."

6. *Gallows humor:* "I don't know what he has, but I know I'm glad I don't have it."

7. *Bypassing the issue:* "Either way, he has to be admitted." "I don't know what she's got, but it's obviously nothing serious."

Forming a diagnosis is important because a plan of treatment follows from it. A hypothesis is presented. In difficult cases, it is done by the highest-ranking physician, who quotes the literature and cites his own experience to support the hypothesis. If a diagnosis is suggested by someone of lower rank, it is used as a basis for therapy only if it is acceptable to the senior physician.

Diagnostic decisions are evaluated formally. Correct diagnoses (with their consequently correct treatments) are presented at grand rounds. They illustrate the skill and knowledge that were required to analyze complex cases.

Incorrect diagnoses are presented at morbidity and mortality conferences. The failure of diagnosis (and hence, treatment) is reflected in complications and death. In this ritual, the erring clinician is purged of his guilt and reaccepted by his peers. He shows his humility by publicly acknowledging his mistakes, and his magnanimity by accepting the responsibility for decisions that were, in reality, reinforced by the group. By demonstrating that he has learned what should have been done, the confessor provides the avenue for readmission to the group.

Reference:
1. Bosk CL. Occupational rituals in patient management. N Engl J Med 1980; *303:*71–76.

12

A GUIDE TO PERCENTAGES

"The expert is seldom in doubt but frequently in error."

Anonymous

In the context of medical communication, data are often presented as percentages. Usually they represent the results of a study published in the medical literature. Often, however, percentages are used rather loosely, to convey a meaning that is much less specific and less concrete than the original data. This practice can lead to some confusion as to just what is being communicated. To shed some light on this problem, the following list of terms and their meanings have been prepared.

Term	Meaning
100 per cent	This means always.
99 per cent	This also means always. The user of this term, however, is not sure if there is an exception and so leaves the door open for that possibility.
95 per cent	This means always, with one exception, and the user knows the exception.
90 per cent	This means almost always. The user knows there are exceptions, but can't remember them, hoping the precision implied by the use of this term will divert attention from what he doesn't know to what he knows.
70 per cent	This means most. This is one of the least accurate of the terms used. It is often used interchangeably with 60 per cent and 80 per cent, depending on the amount of emphasis required. Often used in series: "60..70..80 per cent."
50 per cent	This means about half.
30 per cent	This means some, used similarly to 70 per cent, along with 20 and 40 per cent.
10 per cent	This means rarely. See 90 per cent.
5 per cent	This means never. See 95 per cent.
1 per cent	This means never. See 99 per cent.

Rules for Using These Percentages

I.   *Rule of Decimals.* Any percentage with a decimal is correct. Do not use the table.

II. *Rule of Multiples.*
    A.   If the percentage is a multiple of ten, use the table.
    B.   If the percentage is a multiple of five, use the table only if the Qualifier Rule (see III) applies; otherwise, the table is correct.

Exceptions are 25 per cent and 75 per cent...see Fraction Rule (VI).

C. All other percentages are correct; do not use the table.

III. *Qualifier Rule.* If the percentage is qualified by such words as "about" or "around," use the table.

IV. *Round-off Rule.* Often when presenting data on slides, a lecturer will round off the percentages that are included on the slide. For example, 57.5 per cent will be rounded off to "about 60 per cent". When this happens, use the table.

V. *New Math Rule.* This rule is a corollary to the *Round-off Rule.* When presenting data from a slide that have not already been converted to percentages, the lecturer will do a quick estimate of the percentage. This estimate is usually grossly inaccurate, so round off to the nearest ten and use the table.

VI. *Fraction Rule.* Occasionally, data will be presented as rounded-off fractions, such as one-fourth or two-thirds. This procedure can be understood by using the table after rounding off the fraction to the nearest ten. For example, one-fourth is 25 per cent; rounded off to 30 per cent, it means "some."

FUN WITH FIGURES

Which of the following statements would you guess are true? Check your answers with the statistics provided in the tables.

_____ The safest means of travel is by railroad passenger train.

_____ Drownings occur most frequently in the summer months.

_____ The greatest number of fatal falls occur among infants.

_____ Violent deaths from motor vehicle accidents and firearms occur most frequently in the 15- to 24-year-old age group.

_____ The homicide rate is much higher than the suicide rate.

_____ Cardiovascular disease is the major cause of death in the U.S.

_____ The number of deaths caused by firearms has increased over the past 20 years.

_____ More Americans die from syphilis than from TB.

_____ Poisoning by gas occurs most frequently in the winter months.

_____ Ingestion of food, objects, and poison is the greatest cause of accidental death among children under 5 years of age.

_____ A girl born in 1980 can expect to live until she's 90 years old.

_____ Americans spend more for eyeglasses and medical appliances than they do for dental services.

_____ Ten per cent of the total expenditure for health goes toward administrative expenses.

Reference:
1. Lane, HU (ed.). The 1983 World Almanac & Book of Facts, New York: Newspaper Enterprise Association, 1982: 958, 964. (Tables reproduced with permission. The World Almanac & Book of Facts, 1983 edition, copyright Newspaper Enterprise Association, 1982, New York, New York 10166.)

12

Transportation Accident Passenger Death Rates, 1980

KIND OF TRANSPORTATION	PASSENGER MILES (billions)	PASSENGER DEATHS	RATE PER 100,000,000 PASSENGER MILES	1978-1980 AVERAGE DEATH RATE
Passenger automobiles and taxis*	2,200.0	29,050	1.32	1.30
Passenger automobiles on turnpikes	46.1	330	0.72	0.71
Buses	85.8	130	0.15	0.15
Intercity buses†	17.3	23	0.13	0.05
Railroad passenger trains	11.0	4	0.04	0.07
Scheduled air transport planes (domestic)	221.2	11	0.01	0.04

*Drivers of passenger automobiles are considered passengers.
†Class 1 only, representing 65 per cent of total intercity bus passenger mileage.

Accidental Deaths by Month and Type, 1978 and 1981

MONTH	1981 TOTALS	ALL TYPES*	MOTOR VEHICLE	FALLS	DROWN-ING†	FIRES, BURNS‡	INGEST. OF FOOD, OBJECT	FIRE-ARMS	POISON (SOLID, LIQUID)	POISON BY GAS
Total	*99,000*	*105,561*	*52,411*	*13,690*	*7026*	*6163*	*3063*	*1806*	*3035*	*1737*
January	8100	7836	2952	1388	190	868	299	154	314	254
February	7000	6892	2767	1092	166	793	244	128	238	229
March	7500	7791	3617	1080	320	640	260	143	313	177
April	7700	8129	4057	1135	460	520	237	127	237	134
May	8500	9115	4622	1083	930	357	243	107	248	107
June	8850	9434	4813	1057	1190	315	265	115	253	60
July	9500	10,484	5218	1160	1520	319	257	130	234	82
August	9300	9827	5185	1098	980	287	235	145	234	61
September	7800	9110	4941	1118	580	298	205	131	220	71
October	8350	9070	4972	1232	300	397	279	181	235	149
November	7850	8633	4622	1092	180	530	248	232	239	181
December	8550	9240	4645	1155	210	839	291	213	270	232
Average	*8250*	*8797*	*4368*	*1141*	*586*	*514*	*255*	*151*	*253*	*145*

Source: National Safety Council.
*Includes some deaths not shown separately.
†Includes drowning in water transport accidents. Some totals partly estimated.
‡Includes deaths resulting from conflagration regardless of nature of injury.

Accidental Deaths by Age, Sex, and Type, 1978

	ALL TYPES	MOTOR VEHICLE	FALLS	DROWN-ING	FIRES, BURNS	INGESTION OF FOOD, OBJECT	FIRE-ARMS	POISON (SOLID, LIQUID)	POISON BY GAS	% MALE ALL TYPES
All ages	*105,561*	*52,411*	*13,690*	*7026*	*6163*	*3063*	*1806*	*3035*	*1737*	*70*
Under 5	4766	1551	192	696	896	463	52	81	51	58
5 to 14	6118	3130	124	1010	586	91	297	37	76	69
15 to 24	26,622	19,164	538	2180	530	168	581	577	525	78
25 to 34	15,533	9648	502	1070	542	183	300	778	287	80
35 to 44	9491	4926	551	630	502	257	205	432	205	77
45 to 54	9174	4166	835	460	667	292	162	420	171	74
55 to 64	9600	3882	1266	450	733	410	112	305	185	70
65 to 74	9072	3217	1852	300	789	483	68	219	110	62
75 and over	15,185	2727	7830	230	918	716	29	186	127	47
Sex										
Male	73,881	38,139	7181	5875	3786	1765	1566	1800	1260	
Female	31,680	14,272	6509	1151	2377	1298	240	1235	477	
Percent										
male (%)	70	73	52	84	61	58	87	59	73	

Source: National Safety Council

Deaths and Death Rates for Selected Causes

1980 CAUSE OF DEATH (estimated)	NUMBER	RATE*	1980 CAUSE OF DEATH (estimated)	NUMBER	RATE*
All causes	*1,986,000*	*892.6*	Acute bronchitis and bronchiolitis	590	0.3
Viral hepatitis	790	0.4	Influenza and pneumonia	52,720	23.7
Tuberculosis, all forms	1770	0.8	Influenza	2590	1.2
Septicemia	9230	4.1	Pneumonia	50,130	22.5
Syphilis and its sequelae	180	0.1	Chronic obstructive pulmonary		
All other infective and			diseases	55,810	25.1
parasitic diseases	3730	1.7	Chronic and unqualified bronchitis	3940	1.8
Malignant neoplasms, including			Emphysema	14,130	6.4
neoplasms of lymphatic and			Asthma	2500	1.1
hematopoietic tissues	414,320	186.3	Ulcer of stomach and duodenum	5750	2.6
Diabetes mellitus	34,230	15.4	Hernia and intestinal obstruction	5430	2.4
Meningitis	1320	0.6	Cirrhosis of liver	31,330	14.1
Major cardiovascular diseases	989,690	444.9	Cholelithiasis, cholecystitis,		
Diseases of heart	763,060	343.0	and cholangitis	3110	1.4
Active rheumatic fever and			Nephritis, nephrosis, and nephrotic		
chronic rheumatic			syndrome	17,390	7.8
heart disease	7950	3.6	Infections of kidney	2640	1.2
Hypertensive heart disease	22,100	9.9	Hyperplasia of prostate	810	0.4
Ischemic heart disease	566,930	254.9	Congenital anomalies	13,730	6.2
Acute myocardial infarction	301,210	135.4	Certain causes of mortality in		
All other forms of heart			early infancy	22,570	10.1
disease	155,710	70.0	Symptoms and ill-defined conditions	29,130	13.1
Hypertension	7,140	3.2	All other diseases	112,510	50.6
Cerebrovascular diseases	170,420	76.6	Accidents	106,550	47.9
Arteriosclerosis	29,830	13.4	Motor vehicle accidents	54,200	24.4
Other diseases of arteries,			Suicide	28,290	12.7
arterioles, and capillaries	19,240	8.6	Homicide	25,090	11.3
			All other external causes	3510	1.6

Due to rounding estimates of death, figures may not add to total. Data based on a 10% sampling of all death certificates for a 12-month (Jan.-Dec.) period.

*Rates per 100,000 population.

Source: National Center for Health Statistics, US Department of Health and Human Services.

Principal Types of Accidental Deaths

YEAR	ALL TYPES	MOTOR VEHICLE	FALLS	BURNS	DROWNING	FIREARMS	MACHINERY	POISON GASES	OTHER POISONS
1960	93,806	38,137	19,023	7645	5232	2334	1951	1253	1679
1965	108,004	49,163	19,984	7347	5485	2344	2054	1526	2110
1970	114,638	54,633	16,926	6718	6391	2406	–	1620	3679
1975	103,030	45,853	14,896	6071	6640	2380	–	1577	4694
1980	–	52,600	12,300	5500	7000	1800	–	1500	2800
1981	–	50,800	11,700	4900	6000	1900	–	1700	2600
DEATH RATES PER 100,000 POPULATION									
1960	52.1	21.2	10.6	4.3	2.9	1.3	1.1	0.7	0.9
1965	55.8	25.4	10.3	3.8	2.8	1.2	1.1	0.8	1.1
1970	56.4	26.9	8.3	3.3	3.1	1.2	–	0.8	1.8
1975	48.4	21.5	7.0	2.8	3.1	1.1	–	0.7	2.2
1980	–	23.2	5.4	2.4	3.1	0.8	–	0.7	1.2
1981	–	22.2	5.1	2.1	2.6	0.8	–	0.8	1.1

12

Source: National Center for Health Statistics, US Department of Health and Human Services.

Years of Life Expected at Birth

YEAR	TOTAL POPULATION	MALE	FEMALE
1980*‡	73.8	70.0	77.7
1979*‡	73.8	69.9	77.8
1975	72.5	68.7	76.5
1970	70.8	67.1	74.7
1965	70.2	66.8	73.8
1960	69.7	66.6	73.1
1950	68.2	65.6	71.1
1940	62.9	60.8	65.2
1930	59.7	58.1	61.6
1920†	54.1	53.6	54.6
1910†	50.0	48.4	51.8
1900†	47.3	46.3	48.3

*Provisional
†Based on data for death registration states only.
‡Based on estimate of the population.

Average Lifetime in the US

1980‡ AGE INTERVAL	NUMBER LIVING*	AVERAGE LIFE EXPECTANCY†	1980‡ AGE INTERVAL	NUMBER LIVING*	AVERAGE LIFE EXPECTANCY†
0–1	100,000	73.6	45–50	93,469	32.1
1–5	98,743	73.6	50–55	91,380	27.8
5–10	98,486	69.8	55–60	88,126	23.7
10–15	98,323	64.9	60–65	83,324	19.9
15–20	98,174	60.0	65–70	76,545	16.4
20–25	97,676	55.3	70–75	67,640	13.3
25–30	97,011	50.6	75–80	56,355	10.4
30–35	96,353	45.9	80–85	41,431	8.2
35–40	95,649	41.3	85 and over	26,395	6.5
40–45	94,797	36.6			

*Of 100,000 born alive, number living at beginning of age interval.
†Average number of years of life remaining at beginning of age interval.

US Health Expenditures

	1950	1960	1965	1970	1975	1979	1980	1981
Total (billions)	$12.7	$26.9	$41.7	$74.7	$132.7	$215.0	$249.0	$286.6
Type of Expenditure								
Health services and supplies	11.7	25.2	38.2	69.3	124.3	204.5	237.1	273.5
Hospital care	3.9	9.1	13.9	27.8	52.1	86.1	100.4	118.0
Physician services	2.7	5.7	8.5	14.3	24.9	40.2	46.8	54.8
Dentist services	1.0	2.0	2.8	4.7	8.2	13.3	15.4	17.3
Nursing home care	.2	.5	2.1	4.7	10.1	17.6	20.6	24.2
Other professional services	.4	.9	1.0	1.6	2.6	4.7	5.6	6.4
Drugs and drug sundries	1.7	3.7	5.2	8.0	11.9	17.2	19.3	21.4
Eyeglasses and appliances	.5	.8	1.2	1.9	3.2	4.6	5.1	5.7
Expenses for prepayment and administration	.5	1.1	1.7	2.7	4.4	9.3	10.7	11.2
Gov't public health activities	.4	.4	.8	1.4	3.2	6.2	7.0	7.3
Other health services	.5	1.1	1.1	2.1	3.7	5.1	6.0	7.2
Research and medical facilities construction	1.0	1.7	3.5	5.4	8.4	10.5	11.8	13.1
Research	.1	.7	1.5	2.0	3.3	4.8	5.3	5.7
Construction	.8	1.0	2.0	3.4	5.1	5.7	6.5	7.5

Source: Health Care Financing Administration, US Department of Health and Human Services.

TO YOUR HEALTH!

Alcohol slows reaction time, decreases coordination, releases inhibitions, and produces personality changes ranging from euphoria to belligerence to drowsiness. Its influence in accidental injury and death is described in several studies. The results are compiled in the next table.

The laws in your state that concern drunk driving are presented in a subsequent table. You may be interested in working with some of the organizations listed.

The sensible, controlled use of alcohol may make you lose business— the kind of business you don't want.

Presence of Alcohol in Victims of Accidental Injury or Death

TYPE OF ACCIDENT	SEVERITY OF INJURY	LOCATION AND DATE OF STUDY	BLOOD ALCOHOL LEVEL IN gm/100 ml	PER CENT WITH BLOOD ALCOHOL LEVEL GREATER THAN SPECIFIED
Fall	External	Finland, 1975	0.105	46
	Fatal	California, 1965–1966	0.100	60
	Fatal	NYC, 1974–1975	0.100	41
Head Injury	Amnestic for	Sweden, 1980	Positive	52
	period of accident	Sweden, 1980	0.250	36
Drowning	Fatal	Baltimore, 1968–1971	0.030	47
	Fatal	Baltimore, 1968–1971	0.100	38
	Fatal	NYC, 1974–1975	0.100	53
Burns	Fatal	California, 1965–1967	0.100	64
	Fatal	NYC, 1974–1975	0.100	40
Motor Vehicle	Fatal	USA, 1981	0.010	
		(16–19 year olds)		21
		(16–19 year old males, single vehicle, weekend night)		35
		(20–24 year old males, single vehicle, weekend night)		40
	Fatal	London, 1971–1980	0.080	32
		(pedestrian)	Positive	25
		(car driver)	Positive	55
		(car passenger)	Positive	77
		(motorcyclist)	Positive	45
		(bicyclist)	Positive	14

12

State Laws Pertaining to Drunk Driving*

STATE	DRINKING AGE	FIRST OFFENSE LICENSE SUSPENSION	STATE TASK FORCE	BLOOD ALCOHOL CONCENTRATION (BAC) DEFINING DRIVING WHILE INTOXICATED (DWI) (gm/100 ml)	MADD, SADD, AND RID CHAPTERS†	PENDING LEGISLATION	EXISTING MEASURES
Alabama	19	90 days	Yes	0.10	MAD, SADD, RID		Dram shop liability (retail server of alcohol responsible for consequences)
Alaska	21 (1/84)	90 days (10/83)	No	0.10	MADD, SADD, RID		
Arizona	19	30 days	Report issued	0.10	MADD, SADD, RID	Mandatory rehabilitation· Simplified legislation to clarify laws	
Arkansas	21	90 days–1 yr	Report issued	0.10	MADD, SADD		
California	21	None	Report issued	0.10	MADD, SADD		Toll-free number to report DWI suspects
Colorado	21;18,3.2 beer	1 yr (.15 BAC)	Yes	0.15‡	MADD, SADD, RID	(Drinking age 21; revocation 0.10 BAC	REDDI § line: license revocation; dram shop liability
Connecticut	20 (10/83)	6 mo. (10/83)	Yes	0.10	SADD, RID		Dram shop liability
Delaware	21 (1/84)	3 mo.	Yes	0.10‡	MADD, SADD		
District of Columbia	21; 18, beer and wine	6 mo.	No	0.10‡	SADD		
Florida	19	6 mo.	Yes	0.10	MADD, SADD, RID		Statewide rehabilitation program
Georgia	19	1 yr	Report issued	0.12‡	MADD, SADD, RID	Drinking age 21; dram shop liability	
Hawaii	18	90 days	Report issued	0.10	SADD		
Idaho	19	180 days	No	0.10‡	SADD, RID		Toll-free REDDI hot line
Illinois	21	1 yr maximum	No	0.10	SADD, RID		Dram shop liability
Indiana	21	60 days–1 yr.	Yes	0.10	MADD, SADD, RID		
Iowa	19	120 days	Report issued	0.13‡	MADD, SADD, RID	Drinking age 21; REDDI program	Toll-free line; CB radio watch; dram shop liability
Kansas	21;18,3.2 beer	Limited use	Report issued	0.10	MADD, SADD, RID	Driving while impaired 0.05-0.10 BAC	REDDI hot line
Kentucky	21	None	Yes	0.10	MADD, SADD		
Louisiana	18	60 days	Yes	0.10	MADD, SADD		Mandatory education and community service
Maine	20	45–90 days	Yes	0.10	SADD		
Maryland	21	60 days maximum	Report issued	0.13	MADD, SADD		
Massachusetts	20	30 days–1 yr	Report issued	0.10	MADD, SADD, RID	Drinking age 21	Dram shop liability
Michigan	21	6 mo.–1 yr	Yes	0.10	MADD, SADD, RID		Dram shop liability
Minnesota	19	30 days	Yes	0.10	MADD, SADD		Dram shop liability
Mississippi	21;18,3.2 beer	90 days–1 yr	Report issued	0.10	MADD, SADD, RID		
Missouri	21	90 days	Yes	0.13‡	MADD, SADD, RID		REDDI program; administrative license revocation
Montana	19	6 mo	No	0.10	SADD		Montanans Against Drunk Drivers
Nebraska	20	6 mo	Yes	0.10	MADD, SADD	Age 21; open container; license revocation	REDDI program; trooper incentive program
Nevada	21	90 days	No	0.10	MADD, SADD		New law: 2 days in jail or 48 hours of public service
New Hampshire	20	90 days	Report issued	0.10	MADD, SADD, RID		

State	Drinking age	License suspension	Accident report	BAC	Organizations†	Other laws	Programs§
New Jersey	21	6 mo	No	0.10	MADD, SADD, RID		$1000 license surcharge for convicted drivers
New Mexico	21	None	Report issued	0.10	MADD, SADD		
New York	19	6 mo	Report issued	0.10	MADD, SADD	Blood test for drivers in serious accidents	"STOP DWI" education program; dram shop liability; Limited dram shop liability
North Carolina	21;19, beer and wine	1 yr	Report issued	0.10	MADD, SADD, RID		Dram shop liability
North Dakota	21	91 days	Yes	0.10	MADD, SADD		
Ohio	21; 19, beer	60 days	Yes	0.10	MADD, SADD, RID	Education program for first offenders	REDDI program; dram shop liability
Oklahoma	21	1 yr	No	0.10	MADD, SADD, RID	BAC to .05; breath tests for serious accidents	
Oregon	21	1 yr	Yes	0.08 (10/83)	MADD, SADD		Dram shop; REDDI program; CB reporting system
Pennsylvania	21	1 yr	Report issued	0.10	MADD, SADD, RID		Dram shop liability
Rhode Island	20	3-6 mo	No	0.10	MADD, SADD		Toll-free hot line; dram shop liability
South Carolina	21;18, beer and wine	6 mo	Yes	0.10	MADD, SADD, RID	Drinking age 20 (beer and wine); open-container law	
South Dakota	21;18, 3.2 beer	30 days	No	0.10	SADD		
Tennessee	19	1 yr	No	0.10	MADD, SADD, RID		Mandatory education requirement; Hot line program; Dram shop liability
Texas	19	1 yr maximum	Report issued	0.10‡	MADD, SADD, RID		
Utah	21	90 days	Report issued	0.08	SADD, RID		
Vermont	18	1 yr	No	0.10	MADD, SADD, RID		Drinking age 19 vetoed by governor; dram shop liability
Virginia	21;19, beer	6 mo	Report issued	0.10	MADD, SADD		Toll-free hot line; CB radio reporting system
Washington	21	90 days	Report issued	0.10	MADD, SADD		
West Virginia	19	6 mo	Report issued	0.10	MADD, SADD		Administrative license suspension
Wisconsin	18	3 mo	No	0.10	MADD, SADD, RID		Dram shop liability
Wyoming	19	90 days	No	0.10	SADD	Drinking age 21; BAC .08; no plea bargaining at .10	Toll-free REDDI hot line; cram shop liability

*Data as of August 1, 1983

†MADD—Mothers Against Drunk Drivers.
SADD—Students Against Driving Drunk.
RID—Remove Intoxicated Drivers.

‡"Presumed intoxicated" or "defined as intoxicated" BAC number, whichever is greater.

§REDDI—Report Every Drunken Driver Immediately.

References:
1. Brismar B, Engstrom A, Rydberg U. Head injury and intoxication: a diagnostic and therapeutic dilemma. Acta Chir Scand 1983;149:11-14.
2. Centers for Disease Control. Alcohol as a risk factor for injuries—United States. MMWR 1983;32:61-62.
3. Centers for Disease Control. Patterns of alcohol use among teenage drivers in fatal motor vehicle accidents—United States 1977-1981. MMWR 1983;32:344-347.
4. Crompton MR. Alcohol and fatal road traffic accidents. Med Sci Law 1982;22:189-194.
5. Honkanen R, Ertama L, Kuosmanen P, et al. The role of alcohol in accidental falls. J Stud Alcohol 1983;44:231-245.
6. Insurance Information Institute. Drunk Driving in America. Newsweek 1983; November, 14, 113. (Table reproduced with permission.)

12

ALL THOSE STRANGE THINGS WE DO TO OUR BODIES

"If the mind that rules the body, ever so far forgets itself as to trample on its slave, the slave is never generous enough to forgive the injury, but will rise and smite the oppressor."

Henry Wadsworth Longfellow

In recent years there has been an increased interest in and concern for personal fitness with an associated mushrooming participation in sports, such as jogging and bicycling. In addition to the usual sorts of orthopedic injuries one expects from athletic endeavors, the new surge in participatory sports has resulted in the recognition of a diverse array of unusual syndromes. We have been collecting reports of these syndromes with great interest, primarily from *Letters to the Editor* in the *New England Journal of Medicine,* which are summarized in the next section. We are sure that this collection is neither all inclusive of the syndromes that have been so far described nor static. We eagerly await each issue of the New England Journal to see what new and unusual syndrome will be described. When you see patients who have strange complaints and findings, remember to take a careful history of their vocations and avocations. Who knows, perhaps you can even have a syndrome named after yourself (ideally as the describer and not the victim).

Health Problems Related to Jogging

In the last ten years a steady, sustained increase in jogging has taken place. Reasons often cited for engaging in this pastime include weight loss, general conditioning, and sheer enjoyment. Although the health benefits are substantial, there are a variety of health risks involved, some trivial and some serious. A selection of them are presented here in detail.

Sudden death from jogging is the most serious risk. It may be the result of ischemic heart disease or other cardiac disease, but it is usually caused by an automobile or truck. Sudden death is not limited to the older runner.[24] Most physicians recommend a physical examination for persons over the age of 35 years who begin an exercise program and gradually progressive levels of exercise for individuals of any age group. Other cardiac problems include bradyarrhythmias and left ventricular enlargement. Proteinuria and hematuria are also common. They both resolve spontaneously and are of little consequence for the runner.

Gastrointestinal symptoms include cramping abdominal pain and loose bowel movements or diarrhea.[6] In an informal survey of members of a running club in London,[30] 25 per cent had symptoms of abdominal cramps or diarrhea during or after competitive running. Only 6 per cent had severe nausea or retching. Most ran on an empty stomach, with an average of 3.5 hours after eating when training and 6 hours after eating when racing. In addition, 30 per cent reported an urge to defecate while running.

Several unique problems occur in joggers. Jogger's nipple[15] is one example. Irritation of the nipples caused by friction against the shirt leads to pain and bleeding. It occurs in both male and female runners. Twenty such cases occurred during the Mayor Daley Marathon in 1977.[20] Taping the nipples or using petrolatum jelly has been recommended to avoid this problem.

A case of nephroptosis in a 28-year old male runner has been reported.[8] He began to experience right subcostal pain within the first quarter-mile of his daily run. After the run the pain would give way to a residual ache which lasted 20 to 30 minutes. Diagnosis was made after the patient noted a mass in the right upper quadrant. During abdominal ultrasonography the kidney could be seen to move from the retroperitoneum to within 1.5 cm of the anterior abdominal wall.

Another unusual affliction, radial nerve palsy,[25] has been reported in a runner. The patient presented with numbness and tingling in the left arm. The symptoms would appear after running four miles or more and would resolve with rest. On examination, there was sensory loss over the dorsum of the left hand and forearm. Apparently, the runner ran with his elbows tightly flexed, compressing the radial nerve between the humerus and triceps. Symptoms resolved when he held his arms with less flexion while running.

The Vicious Cycle[21]

This urologic syndrome occurs in males who have recently begun an exercise program involving cycling or use of a cycling type of exercise machine. They present with symptoms of urinary obstruction, frequent urination, urinary retention, decrease in the force of the urinary stream, dribbling, and nocturia. There is no history of discharge or dysuria. Physical examination and urinalysis are normal. Avoidance of direct pressure on the perineum while riding results in relief of symptoms. We are also aware of an unpublished case of vulvar edema.

Unicyclist's Sciatica[7]

After riding a unicycle in excess of 3 km, a man experienced bilateral pain, radiating from the buttocks down the posterior area of the thighs, into the posteromedial calves, and the medial halves of the feet. The pain increased with thigh flexion and was associated with paresthesias and hyperesthesias with a similar distribution. Burning dysuria with normal urinalysis lasted two days after the incident.

12

Cyclist's Palsy[2]

A male patient was forced to discontinue a bicycle tour after two weeks. He had developed numbness, weakness, and loss of coordination in both hands. Over the next two weeks, he noted muscle wasting in the hands, continued numbness in the ring and little fingers, and difficulty with fine motor control and pincer grasp. This syndrome is caused by compression of the ulnar nerve at the point of emergence of that nerve from the bony pisohamate tunnel at the base of the palm. It also occurs in construction workers from pneumatic drills, in carpenters from wood planes, and in secretaries from staplers and carriage returns. Symptoms gradually improve with physical therapy.

Pudendal Neuritis from Cycling[9]

A 46-year-old man reported penile insensitivity. It developed after a 2-day, 180-mile bicycle trip, riding on a narrow, hard-leather seat. While he was able to achieve and maintain erection during intercourse, there was loss of sensation to light touch along the penile shaft. Symptoms resolved over 4 weeks after switching to a padded seat.

A "New Wave" of Subconjunctival Hemorrhage[1]

A 20-year-old man presented with bilateral red eyes. Physical examination revealed bilateral subconjunctival hemorrhage. The night before it developed, the patient had been dancing the "pogo," which is performed to "new wave" music. This dance involves repeated bouncing movements for long periods of time.

Disco Felon[32]

A 17-year-old girl presented with a classic felon of the left middle finger. She had originally noted a small crack on her finger that had later become infected. She thought that the crack had developed from snapping her fingers while disco dancing, a frequent pastime. The felon was drained with an ulnar incision and packed. Her recovery was uneventful.

Space Invaders' Wrist[17]

This syndrome results from frequent playing of the Space Invaders video game, using a standard paddle and push-button device over a period of approximately one month. Pain and stiffness in the right wrist (use of the device by the left hand is nearly impossible) were exacerbated by repeated playing of the game and resolved after about ten days of abstinence.

Cuber's Thumb[33]

The cause of this syndrome was the use of an inexpensive "Rubik's Cube," which had a tendency to stick during rotations. The user held the cube in the left hand with one of the corners braced against the left thumb. The patient experienced localized, exquisitely tender swelling on the volar surface of the left metacarpophalangeal joint. The condition was originally diagnosed as gout, but several days later, the cube jammed on a rotation, thrusting the corner against the painful metacarpal, establishing the diagnosis. While treatment of cuber's thumb is accomplished by buying a more expensive model, no cure for cube addiction has been described, and only the passage of time has led to recovery.

Slot Machine Tendonitis[19]

This syndrome develops after a weekend of playing slot machines. Patients complain of pain in the right shoulder. Physical examination reveals classic bicipital tendonitis, with point tenderness over the long head of the biceps. The pain is reproduced by the motion required to work the slot machines. Rest or an early jackpot is helpful. Nonsteroidal anti-inflammatory agents will also alleviate the pain in the shoulder, but not the odds. Cases of this syndrome are usually limited to regions within driving distance of casinos.

Pachinko Thumb

Pachinko, oriental pinball, involves manipulating a lever with the thumb. Excessive playing can cause pain and swelling at the metacarpophalangeal joint of the playing hand. As with Space Invaders' wrist, abstinence is the best treatment. Intractable addicts who must continue playing can be given some relief with splinting, although this often causes their scores to fall.

Gamba Leg[12]

Gamba leg syndrome developed in a patient who had begun, two months prior to presentation, to play the treble viola de gamba, an early string instrument that is gripped between the knees while playing. She complained of numbness and paresthesias on the medial aspect of the left leg in the distribution of the cutaneous branch of the saphenous nerve. Symptoms resolved after placing a cloth pad between the instrument and the knee.

Cymbal Player's Shoulder[13]

A 19-year-old woman presented with bilateral anterior shoulder pain, made worse by flexion of the elbow and shoulder. It had

12

progressed over the last seven days, during which time she had participated in 22 hours of band rehearsals, playing the cymbals. At the time of presentation she was unable to pick up the cymbals because of the pain. Physical examination revealed tenderness along the biceps tendon, with pain elicited by active flexion of the elbow against resistance. This case represents another instance of bicipital tenosynovitis. After rest and nonsteroidal anti-inflammatory medication, she was able to perform again.

Frisbee Finger[5]

This malady occurs as a result of prolonged play with a Frisbee. An abrasion appears on the middle finger on the dominant hand, with or without concomitant clear vesicles distal to the abrasion, and vesicles on the thumb of the same hand. It is more likely to occur in an urban setting, where the sliding of the Frisbee over hard surfaces produces jagged edges on the Frisbee. The syndrome can occur with smooth-edged Frisbees, however. Abstinence is the only effective preventive and curative procedure; bandages are easily worn away or become entangled on the Frisbee, making play difficult.

Waterslide Injuries[16]

The records of 61 patients injured on waterslides were reviewed. Riders sit on a mat and slide down an inclined plane constructed of fiberglass or concrete over which water is circulated. Alternatively, they may ride down head first in a prone position. Injuries occur when riders hit the waterslide or other riders on the slide. Injuries most commonly affect the head and face; types and frequency are listed.

Lacerations	53%
Contusions and abrasions	25%
Fractured bones	7%
Sprains	7%
Fractured teeth	6%
Concussions	3%

Alpine Slide Anaphylaxis[29]

Alpine slides are recently introduced devices that allow skiers to fulfill their desires to go down mountains in the summertime and to give mountain owners a source of revenue in the summer. They are curving cement tracks going down a mountain that one traverses on a wheeled sled. A cluster of anaphylactic reactions has recently been linked to an alpine slide in Vermont. A careful study has shown that individuals at risk for anaphylaxis who sustain abrasions while riding the slide during grass-pollen season apparently introduce enough pollen through the abrasions to trigger an allergic reaction. The reactions primarily occur in late June to early August, which is the grass-pollen season in the mountains. Individuals with an atopic history or history of allergic rhinoconjunctivitis are at increased risk for this problem and should be warned about the danger. If there is an alpine slide in your area, it would seem fitting to bring this problem to the attention of personnel there so appropriate measures could be taken to warn patrons and treat those who have reactions.

Wrist Injuries in Rollerskating[31]

In a letter to the *New England Journal of Medicine,* Ullis presents statistics on injuries from rollerskating during the first nine months of 1979. The region from the distal radius and ulna to the fingertips accounts for 47 per cent of all such injuries. Fractures of the wrist were present in 12 per cent. Ten per cent had sprains of the wrist, and fracture of the distal radius or ulna occurred in 6 per cent.

Water Skiing Injuries[14]

Water skiing is the cause of a variety of injuries. Injuries result from falling into the water, colliding with solid objects, becoming entangled in the rope, being struck with the skis, or being run down by a boat. A unique mechanism of injury is the "water ski douche," caused by forceful entry of water through a body orifice after a fall at high speed or after a tow through the water in a sitting position. Potential injuries are listed below.

Water Skiing Injuries and Sequelae

ENT Injuries
  Ruptured eardrums
  Otitis media
  Sinusitis
  Disruption of middle ear articulations
  Round or oval window rupture

Gynecologic Injuries
  Vaginal laceration—may tear the posterior
    cul-de-sac with subsequent peritonitis
  Tears of the cervix, uterus, or fallopian tubes
  Salpingitis and tubo-ovarian abscess
  Spontaneous abortion

GI Injuries
  Rectal laceration
  Rectal perforation

12

Mechanical Bull Injuries

"I'm so lonely in the saddle since my horse died..." (from a folk song.)

Fads come and go, leaving behind a mini-epidemic of injuries related to the activity. One of the most striking of these epidemics has been the injuries associated with the mechanical bull. It is a machine that simulates a bull ride with movement up and down, side to side, and an undulation front to back. Most injuries occur when falling from the mechanical bull, striking the bull, landing on the floor, or injuring the hand and wrist in the handle. Thus, the "empty saddle syndrome"[4] has been applied to these injuries. The mechanical bull was popularized by its role in a movie, leading to another name, the "urban cowboy syndrome."[28]

Most injuries occur in patients who have had no prior bull-riding experience, and all of whom have consumed alcohol prior to the injury. The majority of injuries are minor—sprains and contusions. More serious injuries include fractures of the hand and wrist and compression fractures of the cervical and lumbar vertebrae.[34] In addition, a case of rhabdomyolysis has been reported.[26]

Dog Walker's Elbow[18]

This syndrome was reported in a male patient who frequently walked his dog on a leash. It seems the dog had been to obedience school but was not a star pupil. As a result, he would usually walk to the left of the patient, but was wont to tug on the leash frequently to investigate bushes, poles, and the like as well as to chase after other animals, especially squirrels and cats. The patient usually carried the leash in the left hand with the forearm supinated and the elbow extended to 150 degrees. When his left arm became tired, he held the leash in his right hand, with the forearm pronated and with the elbow extended to 150 degrees. A lateral epicondylitis of the left elbow and a medial epicondylitis of the right elbow resulted.

OPEC Otitis[27]

A 35-year old man presented with bilateral burning ear pain. He had been siphoning gasoline from a car when he "got a mouthful". He choked, felt gasoline go up into his nose, and then felt severe burning in the mouth, nose, and especially the ears. On examination, both tympanic membranes were reddened, with distinct air-fluid levels bilaterally. He was treated with phenylephrine nasal spray and beclomethasone, two puffs intranasally every four hours. That night, the right ear "popped," followed by a taste of gasoline. Tympanocentesis of the left ear was performed the next day. Recovery was uneventful. Talk about getting an ear full!

The Sunglass Syndrome[10]

This syndrome is a compression neuropathy of the infra-orbital nerve caused by wearing large sunglasses for long periods. Symptoms begin as a sensation of numbness, paresthesia, and dysesthesia in the area beneath the eyes and over the cheeks. It progresses to include the nose, with numbness and dysesthesia, in which the air moving in and out of the nasal passages produces an uncomfortable sensation. After approximately three to four weeks, the numbness also affects the upper incisors. Symptoms resolve over two to three weeks after discontinuation of sunglasses use.

Tobacco Primer's Wrist[22]

This syndrome is common in the tobacco belt. Tobacco priming requires frequent movement of the arm with pronation in association with extension and abduction of the thumb. It is followed by forceful and rapid flexion and adduction of the thumb to prune the tobacco leaves manually from the stalk. These patients present with pain and swelling over the origin of the tendons of the abductor pollicis longus and extensor pollicis brevis. Crepitation may be noted with direct pressure and with thumb abduction and extension. Treatment with infiltration of a depot steroid and splinting leads to recovery in several days.

Penile Frostbite[11]

A 59-year-old physician was jogging while wearing polyester, double-knit trousers and Dacron and cotton boxer style undershorts for a period of approximately 25 minutes in windy weather at $-8^{\circ}C$. At this time, he began to note a painful, burning sensation at the penile tip. Symptoms progressed during the remaining five minutes of the run. On physical examination ten minutes later, the glans was noted to be frigid, red, tender on manipulation, and anesthetic to light touch. Rapid rewarming over the next 15 minutes was accomplished with return of the affected part to normal. Rewarming techniques that cause friction to the affected area should be avoided.

French Vanilla Frostbite[23]

An 18-month-old girl was treated to her first French vanilla ice cream cone, which she ate enthusiastically for 30 minutes, never removing her mouth from the delightful treat. When she returned home, her lips were noted to be swollen, dusky, and warm. Over the next two days they blistered; then they crusted over and healed without event over the next seven days. A classic example of "cold sores"?

12

Popsicle Panniculitis[3]

Once the popsicle was invented, could popsicle panniculitis be far behind? This form of panniculitis is produced by sucking on cold objects, such as popsicles and ice cubes. It is characterized by the presence of a reddish purple discoloration of the cheeks. On occasion the cheek may feel indurated. Tenderness and warmth are unusual.

The lesions are most obvious 24 to 48 hours after the cold injury. They are most commonly confused with cellulitis. The patients with popsicle panniculitis are afebrile and feel well. The lesions subside without treatment, leaving no permanent injury.

The next time you see a red-faced child, inquire about prolonged sucking on popsicles or ice cubes. Misdiagnosis may leave you red-faced.

"Take care of your health; you have no right to neglect it, and thus become a burden to yourself, and perhaps to others."

William Hall

Peanuts

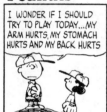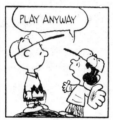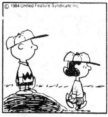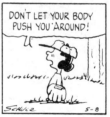

With permission of United Feature Syndication, Inc., 1984.

References:
1. Caspari RF. A "new wave" of subconjunctival hemorrhage? N Engl J Med 1980;*303:*1420.
2. Converse TA. Cyclist's palsy. N Engl J Med 1979;*301:*1397–1398.
3. Epstein EH Jr, Oren ME. Popsicle panniculitis. N Engl J Med 1970;*282:*966.
4. Eyck RPT, Longmire AW. Mechanical bull injuries: the empty saddle syndrome. Ann Emerg Med 1981;*10:*582–584.
5. Faust HS. Frisbee finger. N Engl J Med 1975;*293:*304.
6. Fogoros RN. "Runner's Trots." Gastrointestinal disorders in runners. JAMA 1980;*243:*1743–1744.
7. Gold S. Unicyclist's sciatica—A case report. N Engl J Med 1981;*305:*231–232.
8. Goldberg J. Jogger's kidney: a case of acquired nephroptosis. N Engl J Med 1981;*305:*590.
9. Goodson JD. Pudendal neuritis from biking. N Engl J Med 1981;*304:*365.
10. Gwinup GR. The sunglass syndrome. N Engl J Med 1983;*308:*1168.
11. Hershkowitz M. Penile frostbite, an unforeseen hazard of jogging. N Engl J Med 1977;*296:*178.
12. Howard PL. Gamba leg. N Engl J Med 1982;*306:*1115.
13. Huddleston CB, Pratt SM. Cymbal-player's shoulder. N Engl J Med 1983;*309:*1462.
14. Kizer KW. Medical hazards of the water skiing douche. Ann Emerg Med 1980;*9:*268–269.
15. Levit F. Jogger's nipples. N Engl J Med 1977;*297:*1127.
16. Malpass CA Jr, Schuman SH, Sobczyk R. Waterslide injuries. Ann Emerg Med 1981;*10:*360–363.
17. McCowan TC. Space invaders wrist. N Engl J Med 1981;*304:*1368.
18. Mebane WN III. Dog walker's elbow. N Engl J Med 1981;*304:*613–614.
19. Neiman R, Ushiroda S. Slot machine tendonitis. N Engl J Med 1981;*304:*1368.
20. Nequin ND. More on jogger's ailments. N Engl J Med 1978;*208:*405–406.
21. O'Brien KP. Sports urology: the vicious cycle. N Engl J Med 1981;*304:*1367–1368.
22. Parsons JS. Tobacco primer's wrist. N Engl J Med 1981;*305:*768.
23. Peterson LR, Peterson LC. French vanilla frostbite. N Engl J Med 1982;*307:*1028.
24. Pfeiffer RJ. Cardiac arrest and jogging. Ann Emerg Med 1982;*11:*678–679.
25. Pickering TG. Runner's radial palsy. N Engl J Med 1981;*305:*768.

26. Powers RD, Lamb GC, Matyasz RC, et al. Urban cowboy rhabdomyolysis. N Engl J Med 1981;*403:*427.

27. Reynolds S, Tanberg D, Flynn J. OPEC otitis. N Engl J Med 1982;*306:*114.

28. Seager SB, Jui-Aenlle L, Faux L. The urban cowboy syndrome. Ann Emerg Med 1981; *10:*252–253.

29. Spitalny KC, Farnham JE, Witherell LE, et al. Alpine slide anaphylaxis. New Engl J Med 1984;*310:*1034–1036.

30. Sullivan SN. The gastrointestinal symptoms of running. N Engl J Med 1981;*304:*915.

31. Ullis K. Wrist injuries in rollerskating. N Engl J Med 1979;*301:*1350.

32. Walker FW, Lillemoe KD, Farquharson RR. Disco felon. N Engl J Med 1979;*301:* 166–167.

33. Waugh D. Cuber's thumb. N Engl J Med 1981;*305:*768.

34. Williamson JE, Allison EJ Jr, Williams RM. Fractures of the hand associated with riding the mechanical bull. Ann Emerg Med 1982;*11:*452–454.

15 TIPS TO HELP YOU SURVIVE A HOTEL FIRE

1. *DON'T PANIC.*

2. *Locate the exits* as soon as you check in. Find out what is behind the exit door. Count the doors between the exit and your room; you may have to find it by touch in a fire. It wouldn't hurt to take a flashlight with you to keep in the night stand.

3. *Familiarize yourself with the hotel room.* Do the windows open? How high from the ground floor are you? Does the bathroom have an exhaust fan that could be used to remove smoke?

4. *Leave the hotel at the first sign of smoke.* If you make the mistake of ignoring the real thing, it may well be your last mistake. If your door is too hot to touch, stay in your room and fight the fire (see no. 14).

5. *Take your key when you leave.* If the escape routes are blocked by smoke or fire, your room may still provide a safe haven (see no. 14). Keep the key where you can find it, i.e., in the night stand next to the flashlight.

6. *Shut the door when you leave.* Doors will retard the entry of smoke and fire into your room and give you a better place to retreat to if you can't get out.

7. *Stay on your hands and knees.* Smoke and heat rise.

8. *Cover your head and back with a wet towel.*

9. *Crawl to the exit.* Stay on the wall that is on the same side as the exit. Count doors as you pass them so you will know when you reach the exit.

10. *DO NOT USE THE ELEVATOR.*

11. *Go down the exit stairwell first.* Hold on to the handrail. Be prepared to encounter smoke and fire on the way down. If you do, don't go through it. Go back.

12. *Go to the roof if you can't go down.* Leave the roof door open to vent the stairwell. (This is the only door you should leave open. Any other you go through should be shut). Wait on the side of the building where the wind is blowing the smoke away from you. If you can't open the roof door, stay behind it until the fire fighters arrive.

12

13. *Look before you leap.* Ground floor—obviously the best escape route is out the window. Above the third floor—unlikely you'll survive the jump. In between—your choice. Stop and fight the fire. If you jump, jump out away from the building.

14. *Fight the fire.* Open the window to vent any smoke in the room. Don't break it, as you may need to close it at some point to keep smoke out. Call the fire department. Don't call the hotel. The staff may delay calling the fire department until an employee has confirmed the fire.

> Turn on the bathroom fan.
> Cover your face with a wet towel.
> Fill the tub and sink with water.
> Stuff wet towels, sheets, or blankets in the cracks around the door.
> Keep everything wet.
> Remove combustible material from near the door and windows.
> Use the ice bucket or wastebasket to throw water on the doors and walls to keep them cool.
> Swing a wet towel around the room to help clear the smoke.
> If there is a fire outside the window, keep the window shut, close the draperies, and keep the area wet.

15. *DO NOT PANIC.*

"By medicine life may be prolonged, yet death will seize the doctor too."

Shakespeare

Adapted from a lecture by William Clark, M.D.

HOW TO SWIM WITH SHARKS

Actually, no one wants to swim with sharks. The best way to avoid injury from sharks is, of course, to avoid shark-infested waters. However, sometimes you will be caught unaware. If you are unskilled in swimming with sharks when this happens, you are probably beyond help. The following rules, if mastered beforehand by diligent practice, may allow you to survive.

1. Assume unidentified fish are sharks. Just because a fish is docile in the absence of blood does not mean it is not a shark.

2. Do not bleed. Bleeding will cause a more aggressive attack and will often provoke other sharks in the vicinity to attack. In addition, it tends to confuse sharks, which may know they have injured you but are unable to understand why you don't bleed. They may begin to doubt their powers or to think the swimmer has supernatural powers.

3. Counter any aggression promptly. Sharks rarely attack without warning. Usually there is a preliminary exploratory action. This should be countered immediately to avoid an attack. The best countermove is a sharp blow to the nose.

4. Get out if someone else is bleeding. This provokes aggressive behavior in the most docile of sharks.

5. Use anticipatory retaliation. Sharks have poor memories and often will forget that the swimmer is skilled. They will need repeated anticipatory retaliation. It will serve to remind the shark that you are both alert and unafraid. The procedure is the same as in Rule 3—a sharp blow to the nose. It is important, however, that you do not injure the shark and draw blood, for two reasons. First, you may provoke uninvolved sharks to attack. Second, it may become difficult to distinguish swimmers from sharks. Indeed, aggressive swimmers can be worse than sharks, for none of these rules will check their behavior.

6. Disorganize an organized shark. This is done by diversion. Sharks, as a group, are prone to internal dissension; by introducing something minor or trivial, the swimmer can often get them to fight among themselves. It is, of course, unethical for a swimmer under attack to divert the sharks to another swimmer.

Reference:
1. Cousteau V, John RJ (trans.). How to swim with sharks: a primer. Persp Biol Med 1973; *16:*525.

EMERGENCY MEDICINE LIBRARY

The 27 books listed here have been recommended to provide a core reference libary for the hospital Emergency Department. This list is from a careful review by the Emergency Medicine faculty of Wright State University of 703 texts in 40 categories. Although one might disagree with certain selections, the list is well researched and a handy guide for starting your library.

We chain our references to the wall so that they are immediately available but not able to "walk away".

Emergency Medicine. Concepts and Clinical Practice. Edited by Peter Rosen, Frank J. Baker II, G. Richard Braen, Robert H. Dailey, and Richard Levy. St. Louis, C.V. Mosby Co., 1983. 1626 pages. $100.00 (two volumes).

Office Practice of Medicine. William T. Branch. Philadelphia, WB Saunders, 1982. 1318 pages. $75.00.

Illustrated Handbook in Local Anesthesia, 2nd edition. Ejnar Eriksson. Philadelphia, WB Saunders, 1980. 159 pages. $45.00. (currently out of print).

Clinical Interpretation of Laboratory Tests, 9th edition. Frances K. Widmann. Philadelphia, FD Davis Publishing Co. 1983. 601 pages. $18.95.

AMA Drug Evaluations, 5th edition. Chicago, AMA Drug Division, 1983. 2000 pages. $64.00.

Cecil Textbook of Medicine, 16th edition. Edited by James Wyngaarden and Lloyd H. Smith. Philadelphia, WB Saunders, 1982. 2600 pages. $75.00.

Current Therapy. Edited by Robert E. Rakel. Philadelphia, WB Saunders, 1984. 1104 pages. $42.00.

Treatment of Cardiac Emergencies, 3rd edition. Emanuel Goldberger and Myron Wheet. St. Louis, C.V. Mosby Co., 1982. 422 pages. $26.95.

12

Manual of Dermatology, 2nd edition. Edited by Donald Pillsbury and Charles Heaton. Philadelphia, WB Saunders Co., 1980. 360 pages. $27.50.

Electrocardiography in Clinical Practice. Te-Chuan Chou. New York, Grune & Stratton, 1979. 624 pages. $46.50.

Manual of Neurologic Therapeutics, 2nd edition. Martin A. Samuels. Boston; Little, Brown and Co., 1982. 461 pages. $15.95.

Orthopedic Neurology: A Diagnostic Guide to Neurological Levels. Stanley A. Hoppenfeld. Philadelphia, JB Lippincott, 1977. 131 pages. $25.00.

Manual of Gynecologic and Obstetric Emergencies. Ben-Zion Taber. Philadelphia, WB Saunders, 1984. 528 pages. $25.95.

Handbook for Prescribing Medications During Pregnancy. Richard L. Berkowitz, et al. Boston: Little, Brown and Co., 1981. 257 pages. $12.95.

Pediatrics, 17th edition. Abraham Rudolph, et al, eds. E. Norwalk, CT, Appleton-Century-Crofts, 1982. 2240 pages. $75.00.

Emergency Psychiatry for the House Officer. Beverly Fauman and Michael Fauman. Baltimore, Williams & Wilkins, Company 1981. 184 pages. $9.95.

Radiology of Emergency Medicine, 2nd edition. John H. Harris, Jr. and William H. Harris. Baltimore, Williams & Wilkins, Company 1981. 720 pages. $68.95.

Emergency Radiology of the Acutely Ill or Injured Child. Leonard Swischuk. Baltimore, Williams & Wilkins, Company 1979. 496 pages. $48.95.

Davis-Christopher Textbook of Surgery, 12th edition. David C. Sabiston, Jr. Philadelphia, WB Saunders, 1981. 2481 pages. $75.00.

Synopsis of Ophthalmology, 5th edition. William H. Havener. St. Louis, C.V. Mosby Co., 1979. 675 pages. $28.50.

DePalma's The Management of Fractures and Dislocations: An Atlas, 3rd edition. John F. Connolly. Philadelphia, WB Saunders, 1981. 2153 pages. $120.00 (two volumes).

The Management of Trauma, 3rd edition. Edited by George D. Zuidema, Robert B. Rutherford, and Walter F. Ballinger. Philadelphia, WB Saunders, 1979. 849 pages. $65.00.

Clinical Management of Poisoning and Drug Overdose. Lester Haddad and James Winchester. Philadelphia, WB Saunders, 1982. 1040 pages. $77.50.

Differential Diagnosis: The Interpretation of Clinical Evidence, 3rd edition. Edited by A. McGehee Harvey, James Bordley III, Jeremiah A. Barondess. Philadelpia WB Saunders, 1979. 738 pages. $42.50.

Bedside Diagnostic Examination, 4th edition. Edited by Elmer DeGowin and Richard L. DeGowin. New York, Macmillan, 1981. 952 pages. $22.95.

Atlas of Bedside Procedures. Edited by Thomas Vander Salm, Bruce S. Cutler, and H. Brownell Wheeler. Boston; Little, Brown & Co., 1979. 408 pages. $22.50.

Grant's Atlas of Anatomy, 8th edition. Edited by James E. Anderson. Baltimore, Williams & Wilkins Company 1983. 640 pages. $37.50.

Reference:
1. Hamilton GC, Epstein FB, Jagger J, et al. A new library for emergency medicine. Ann Emerg Med 1983;*12:*687–696.

USEFUL REFERENCES

We have found it handy to keep the following compendium of important, but impossible to remember data, in a loose leaf binder in the ED.

Drug Dosage in Renal Failure
Bennett W, Aronoff G, Morrison G, et al. Drug prescribing in renal failure: dosing guidelines for adults. Am J Kidney Dis 1983;*3:*155–193. Reprints can be purchased for $3.00 from the National Kidney Foundation, 2 Park Avenue, New York, NY 10016.

Drug Interactions
The Medical Letter Handbook of Drug Interactions. Rizack MA, Hillman CD (eds.). New Rochelle, New York: The Medical Letter, 1983. Copies may be purchased from the Medical Letter, 56 Harrison St., New Rochelle, NY 10801 for $7.50.

Treatment of Sexually Transmitted Diseases
The Medical Letter 1984;*26*:5–10 and updated recommendations published regularly.

The Choice of Antimicrobial Drugs
The Medical Letter 1984;*26*:19–26.

Health Information for International Travel
Morbidity Mortality Weekly Reports, vol. 32, August 1983.

Physicians' Desk Reference for Nonprescription Drugs
Available from Medical Economics Company Inc., Box 2019, Mahopac, NY 10541 for $14.95 each (prepaid).

Physical Growth Charts for Children
Physical growth: national center for health statistics percentiles. Am J Clin Nutr 1979;*32:*607–629.

JUNK MAIL

An internist saved all the unsolicited mail he received from the pharmaceutical industry and a variety of other sources for the calendar year 1982. Statistics related to this junk mail are listed.

Total weight	502.75 lb
Most pieces from one source	89
Number of pharmaceutical companies sending literature	55
Number of mailings for courses or seminars	281
Number of "throwaway" journals	41
Cost of subscription to these journals	$1099.55

12

Reference:
Breslow RA. Junk mail. N Engl J Med 1983;*308:*1168.

PHONE DIRECTORY

Antivenin Index	405-271-5454	Oklahoma City Poison Control (Assists in locating antivenin for snakebite.)
Radiation	615-482-2441	Methodist Hospital, Oak Ridge, Tenn.
	215-243-2990	Radiation Management Corporation (Provides services for Commonwealth Edison nuclear power plants.)
Organ Donation	713-799-6126 Ext. 5238	Eye Bank Association of America
	1-800-24-Donor	Organ Donation Information and Referral Hotline
Air Evacuation	202-697-9560	Pentagon
Centers for Disease Control	404-329-3311	Special Immunobiologics Drugs for Parasitic Diseases
Diving Injuries	512-536-3281	Hyperbaric Oxygen Facility Information
Health Information for International Travel	518-474-3186	New York State Bureau of Communicable Disease Control
Product Problem Reporting	800-638-6725	Hotline operated by US Pharmacopeia for reporting any problem with drugs, medical devices, or laboratory products that may pose a health hazard.
Pet Poison Hotline	217-333-3611	Animal Poison Control (Advice around the clock from veterinary toxicologist at the University of Illinois.) *Note*—call is not toll free; advice is.
Chemtree	800-424-9300	Information about chemical emergencies
National Pesticide Network	800-858-7378	Expert advice about pesticide poisoning
National Institute of Occupational Safety and Health	513-684-4382 or 513-684-3784.	For answers to questions about occupational hazards

INDEX

Note: Page numbers in *italics* refer to illustrations; page numbers followed by t refer to tables.

Abdomen, acute, in children, 313, 313t
    in differential diagnosis of child abuse, 333t
    peritoneal lavage in diagnosis of, in trauma patient, 108 110, 109t
    examination of, in trauma patient, 99t
    stab wound of, 111
Abortion, 219t
Abrasions, periorbital, vs. swollen eye, in children, 295t
Abruptio placentae, 220
Abscess, peritonsillar, in children, 300t
    retropharyngeal, 300t
Accident(s), presence of alcohol in victims of, 389t
Acetaminophen poisoning, *140*, 140–141, 141t
    antidote for, 136t
Acetaminophen products, over-the-counter, 142, 142t
Acid poisoning, antidote for, 136t
Acid(s), ingestion of, management of, 148–149, 149t, *150*, *151*
    injury of eye due to, 233
Acid-base balance, calculation of, 345–346
Acid-base status, altered, in newborns, 291
    anion gap and, 349–352
Acid-fast stain, procedure for, 342
Acidosis, hyperchloremic, 352
    lactic, causes of, 350t
    metabolic, anion gap and, 352
ACLS (Advanced Cardiac Life Support) instructions for mega-code station, 87–88
Activated charcoal, in treatment of poisoning, 135t
Air, dry, in air transport of critically ill patient, 11t
Air ambulance, in air transport of critically ill patient, 12
Air temperature, rise in, dangers of, 170–171, 171t
Air transport, of critically ill patient, 6–12
    and PO₂ saturation, at different altitudes, 6, 6t
    pressure changes with altitude during, 6, 6t
    problems during, 9t–11t
        remedial actions for, 9t–11t
    requirements of oxygen during, 7, *7*, 7t
    volume expansion of gases during, 8, 8t
Airsplint, air transport of patient with, 10t
Airway, establishment of, in trauma patient, 91
    obstruction of, cardiopulmonary resuscitation for, in conscious victim, 44t–45t
        in unconscious victim, 46t–47t

Airway (*Continued*)
    obstruction of, management of, *72,* 72–73, *73*
        retrograde stylet in, 74, *74*
Albumin, concentration of, decrease in, calcium for, 348 349
Alcohol, levels of, calculation of, 349
    presence of, in accidental injury or death, 389t
Alkali poisoning, antidote for, 136t
Alkaline substance(s), ingestion of, management of, 148–149, 149t, *150*, *151*
    injury of eye due to, 232–233
Alkaloid poisoning, antidote for, 136t
Allergy, to local anesthetics, 366–367
    vs. swollen eye, in children, 295t
AMA standards of conduct, 4–5
Aminophylline, dosage of, in bronchospasm, 244–245, 244t, 245t
Ammonium chloride, in bromide poisoning, 136t
Amphetamine poisoning, antidote for, 136t
Amyl nitrite, in cyanide poisoning, 137t
Analgesics, ingestion of during pregnancy, congenital malformations and, 222t
Anaphylaxis, alpine slides and, 396–397
    in children, drugs for, 71t
Anemia, air transport of patient with, 9t
    red blood cell indices in, 341t
Anesthesia, ankle block, 370, *370*
    digital nerve block, 369, *369*
    inferior alveolar nerve block, *371*, 371–372, *372*
    infra-orbital nerve block, 373, *373*
    local, allergy to, 366–367
    median nerve block, 368, *368*
    oral, 370–374, *371*, *372*, *373*
    posterior superior alveolar nerve block, *372*, 372–373, *373*
    radial nerve block, 368, *369*
    regional, *368*, 368–370, *369*, *370*
    subperiosteal infiltration, 374
    ulnar nerve block, 368, *368*
Angel dust, 146
Angioedema, in children, 300t
Anion gap, and metabolic acidosis, 352
    calculation of, 349–352
    decreased, 351t
    increased, 350t
Ankle(s), eversion injuries of, *194*, 194–195
    fractures of, *192*, 192–195, *193*, *194*
    injuries of, compartment syndromes in, symptoms of, 195
    inversion injuries of, *192*, 192–193. *193*
    reflexes in, 195

Antacids, comparison of, 274–275, 274t–275t
Anti-infectives, ingestion of during pregnancy, congenital malformations and, 221t–222t
Antiarrhythmics, 254t–255t
  and postural hypotension, 239
Antibiotics, for bite wounds, 130, 130t
  for pneumonia, in children, 311t
  in wound closure, 201
Anticholinergic poisoning, antidote for, 136t
Anticholinesterase poisoning, antidote for, 136t
Anticoagulants, ingestion of during pregnancy, congenital malformations and, 222t
Anticonvulsants, ingestion of during pregnancy, congenital malformations and, 222t–223t
Antidotes, to poisons, 135, 136t–139t
Antihistamine poisoning, antidote for, 136t
Antihistamines, ingestion of during pregnancy, congenital malformations and, 221t
Antishock trousers, 107–108, 108t
Antivenins, 139t
Anuria, pulmonary edema in patient with, 258
Anus, fissure of, and rectal bleeding in children, 314t
Arrhythmia(s), identification of, 251, 251t, 252, 253
Arsenic poisoning, antidote for, 136t
Aspiration, of foreign body, in children, 300t
Aspirin poisoning, 142–144, 143, 143t
  acid-base disturbances in, 143, 143t
  determination of severity of, Done nomogram in, 142, 143
  symptoms of, 142
  treatment of, 144
Asthma, acute attacks of, admission criteria for, 242–243
  in children, 302, 303t
    theophylline for, 306–307, 307t
Asystole, algorithm for management of, 58–59
Atropine, in anticholinesterase poisoning, 136t
  in organophosphate poisoning, 148
Atropine poisoning, antidote for, 136t
Autopsy, request for, in children, 334–335

Back, examination of, in trauma patient, 99t
Barium salt poisoning, antidote for, 136t
Belladonna alkaloid poisoning, antidote for, 136t
Benztropine, in phenothiazine poisoning, 139t
Bite(s), animal, infected, treatment of, 129
  management of, 128–130
  poisoning due to, 139t
  rabies prophylaxis in, 129–130
  tetanus prophylaxis in, 129–130
  antibiotic prophylaxis for, 130, 130t
  human, hepatitis and, 129
  insect, vs. swollen eye, in children, 295t
Bladder, effects of organophosphate poisoning on, 147t
Bladder control, loss of, air transport of patient with, 10t
Blast injury(ies), trauma resulting from, 114, 115t
Bleeding, rectal, in children, 314, 314t–315t
  vaginal, during pregnancy, 217–218, 218t, 219t, 220

Blood, in feces, detection of, 343–344
  loss of, due to fractures, 178, 178t
  uncrossmatched, use of in trauma patient, 102–104
Blood pressure, normal ranges of, in children, 283
Blood pressure cuff, size of, 363–364, 364
Blood products, volume for intravenous administration of, in pediatric trauma patient, 106t
Blood urea nitrogen (BUN), in shock, 53, 53
Bloodletting, 19
Botulism, 264–265
Boutonniere deformity, 185, 185t, 186
Bowel(s), obstruction of, 208, 208t
Bradycardia, algorithm for management of, 60
Breast-feeding, ingestion of drugs during, 220–221, 221t–224t
Bromide poisoning, antidote for, 136t
Bronchial tree, effects of organophosphate poisoning on, 147t
Bronchospasm, aminophylline dosage in, 244–245, 244t, 245t
Burn(s), air transport of patient with, 11t
  estimate of extent of, in children, 286
  flash, of eyes, 233
  removal of tar from, 365

Cadmium poisoning, antidote for, 136t
Caffeine, ingestion of during pregnancy, congenital malformations and, 223t
  overdose of, 152
Calcium, levels of, calculation of, 348–349
Calcium blockers, and postural hypotension, 239
Calcium gluconate, in detergent poisoning, 137t
  in oxalate poisoning, 138t
Carbon monoxide poisoning, antidote for, 136t
Cardiac failure, air transport of patient with, 9t
Cardiopulmonary resuscitation, drug concentrations during, 78, 78
  equipment for, checklist of, 67–68
  for complete airway obstruction, in conscious victim, 44t–45t
    in unconscious victim, 46t–47t
  in infants and children, 42t–43t, 48t, 49, 284, 284t
  one and two rescuer, 38t–41t
  one rescuer, 36t–37t
  precautions in administration of, 65–67
  review of, 35, 36t–48t
  steps in administration of, 63–65
Cardiovascular system, effects of organophosphate poisoning on, 147t
Cathartics, saline, in treatment of poisoning, 135t
Catheter(s), arterial pulmonary, algorithm for management of patient without, 52
  balloon-tipped, temporary placement of, 82, 82, 83, 84
  Foley, in bladder injuries following pelvic fracture, 117
    in intestinal obstruction, 208
    in urethral injuries following pelvic fracture, 117
  placement of, in trauma patient, 92

Catheter(s) (*Continued*)
　intravenous, flow rates of, 78–79, 79t
　suction, selection of, in children, 284t
　Swan–Ganz, 86
　transtracheal, insertion of, *72*, 72–73, *73*
Caustic substance(s), ingestion of, management of, 148–149, 149t, *150*, *151*
Cell counts, calculation of, *338*, 338–339
Cellulitis, orbital, 232t
　　in children, classification of, 296t
　　periorbital, vs. swollen eye, in children, 295t
　　preseptal, 295t
Centers for Disease Control, antiparasitic drugs available from, 268–269, 269t
　immunobiologic agents available from, 268–269, 269t
Cerebrospinal fluid, cell count in, 340
Cervical spine, injuries of, 179t
Charcoal, activated, in treatment of poisoning, 135t
Chemical injury(ies), of eye, 232–233, *233*
Chest, examination of, in trauma patient, 98t, 98t–99t
　pain in, in children, 312, 312t, 313t
Chest tube(s), stabilization of, 113, *113*
Chewing gum, removal of, from hair, 364
Child abuse, differential diagnosis of, 332, 332t–333t
Child(ren), abuse of, differential diagnosis of, 332, 332t–333t
　acute abdomen in, 313, 313t
　administration of drugs to, weight of child and, 285, 285t
　angioedema in, 300t
　aspiration of foreign body in, 300t
　asthma in, 302, 303t
　　theophylline for, 306–307, 307t
　autopsy request for, 334–335
　burns in, estimate of extent of, 286
　cardiopulmonary resuscitation in, 284, 284t
　cardiovascular resuscitation drugs for, 70t
　chest pain in, 312, 312t, 313t
　closure of wounds in, 322–323
　comatose, 324–327, 325t, 326t, 327t
　　due to poisoning, 327, 327t
　　intracranial causes of, 325
　　metabolic causes of, 326, 326t
　　traumatic causes of, 324–325, 325t
　congestive heart failure in, 297–298, 297t, *298*
　croup in, 300t
　diabetic ketoacidosis in, 287
　diarrhea in, oral rehydration solutions in, 317–318, 317t
　digitalization in, 298, *298*
　emergency care of, 280–281, 281t
　emergency drugs for, 69, 70t, 71t
　epiglottitis in, 300t
　intracranial pressure in, increased, 323–324, 324t
　intramuscular injections in, 366, 366t
　Kawasaki syndrome in, 329–330
　maintenance fluids in, 285, 286t
　neurologic dysfunction in, Reyes syndrome and, 288
　normal values in, blood pressure, *283*
　　heart rate, 282t
　　respiratory rate, 282t
　nursemaid's elbow in, 321

Child(ren) (*Continued*)
　orbital cellulitis in, classification of, 296t
　otalgia in, 293
　peritonsillar abscess in, 300t
　pertussis in, 309
　pneumonia in, 310–311, 310t, 311t
　pulmonary testing in, *304*, 304–305, *305*
　rectal bleeding in, 314, 314t–315t
　resuscitation of, intravenous equipment for, 69
　　medications for, 68
　　ventilatory equipment for, 69
　retropharyngeal abscess in, 300t
　Reyes syndrome in, 288–289
　scabies in, 331
　sexual abuse in, 318–319
　sickle cell anemia in, 298, 299t
　sinusitis in, 294–295
　status epilepticus in, 328, 328t–329t
　stiff neck in, 320t, 321
　stridor in, 299, 299t, 300t
　suprapubic urine specimen from, 319
　swelling of eye in, 295–296, 295t, 296t
　tonsillitis in, 300t
　trauma in, 105–106, 105t, 106t
　uvulitis in, 296–297
　wheezing in, 301–302
　whooping cough in, 309
"Chinese Restaurant Syndrome," vs. myocardial infarction, 247–248
Chlamydia, infections due to, in infants, 307–308
Chlorpromazine, in amphetamine poisoning, 136t
Cholecystitis, acute, 209–210
　differential diagnosis of, 210
Cholecystography, in cholecystitis, 209–210
Cholinergic compound poisoning, antidote for, 136t
Ciliary body, effects of organophosphate poisoning on, 147t
Circulation, assessment of, in trauma patient, 91
Clostridium botulinum, botulism due to, 264–265
Colitis, acute, and rectal bleeding in children, 314t
　antibody-associated, 315t
　chronic ulcerative, 315t
Colon, obstruction of, 208, 208t
Colostomy, air transport of patient with, 9t
Coma, in children, 324–327, 325t, 326t, 327t
　due to poisoning, 327, 327t
　intracranial causes of, 325
　metabolic causes of, 326, 326t
　traumatic causes of, 324–325, 325t
Compartment syndromes, in ankle injuries, symptoms of, 195
Congenital malformations, ingestion of drugs during pregnancy and, 221t–224t
Congestive heart failure, in children, 297–298, 297t, *298*
　drugs for, 71t
Conjunctivitis, acute, 232t
　chlamydial, in infants, 308
　vs. swollen eye, in children, 295t
Copper poisoning, antidote for, 136t
Cornea, trauma to, 232t
　ulcer of, 232t

Cost-consciousness quiz, 23
answers to, 382
CPR. See *Cardiopulmonary resuscitation.*
Crohn's disease, and rectal bleeding in children, 315t
Croup, in children, 300t
Crutches, sizes of, 322, 322t
Cryptitis, and rectal bleeding in children, 314t
Cutaneous lesions, in differential diagnosis of child abuse, 332t
Cyanide poisoning, antidote for, 137t
Cycling, exercise program involving, urologic syndrome in, 393

Dacryocystitis, vs. swollen eye, in children, 295t
Death rates, accidental, by age, sex, and type, 386t
by month and type, 386t
principal types of, 387t
selected causes of, 387t
in transportation accidents, 386t
Decontamination, in organophosphate poisoning, 148
Deferoxamine, in iron poisoning, 138t, 145
Depression, medical causes of, 360, 361t
Dermatitis, vs. swollen eye, in children, 295t
Detergent poisoning, antidote for, 137t
Diabetes, ketoacidosis and, and coma in children, 326t
in children, 287
Diagnosis(es), decision-making process in, 383
Diarrhea, in children, oral rehydration solutions in, 317–318, 317t
infectious, and rectal bleeding in children, 314t
Digitalization, in children, 298, *298*
Digoxin, dosage of, in children, *298*
nomogram for, 258–259, *259*
Dimercaprol (BAL), in heavy metal poisoning, 137t
Diphenhydramine, in phenothiazine poisoning, 139t
Disaster management, evacuation procedures in, 170
Dissection, thoracic aortic, 206, 207t
Dissociation, electromechanical, algorithm for management of, 59
Diuretics, and postural hypotension, 239
ingestion of during pregnancy, congenital malformations and, 223t
Drug(s), administration of, by endotracheal intubation, 76–77
weight of child and, 285, 285t
and coma in children, 327, 327t
and postural hypotension, 239
anti-asthma, ingestion of during pregnancy, congenital malformations and, 223t
antiarrhythmic, 254t–255t
antiparasitic, available from Centers for Disease Control, 268–269, 269t
associated with hyperthermia, 172t, 174t
asthmatic patient's response to, 303t
cardiovascular, ingestion of during pregnancy, congenital malformations and, 223t
concentration of, during cardiopulmonary resuscitation, 78, *78*

Drug(s) (*Continued*)
dosages of, emergency, in newborns, 291t
dosing schedules for, 32
during breast-feeding, 220–221, 221t–224t
during pregnancy, 220–221, 221t–224t
for cardiovascular resuscitation in children, 70t
for relief of esophageal obstruction, 230
for treatment of urinary tract infections, 270
in management of tonic-clonic status epilepticus, 276
in management of violent patient, 359
in pediatric resuscitation cart, 69
in prevention of bacterial endocarditis, 256t
in prevention of meningitis, 264, 264t
in treatment of acute pulmonary edema, *257*
over-the-counter, abuse of, 152, 152t
pediatric emergency, 69, 70t, 71t
prescription, top ten selling, 33
psychotherapeutic, ingestion of during pregnancy, congenital malformations and, 223t
Drunk driving, state laws regarding, 390t–391t
Duplications, and rectal bleeding in children, 315t
Dysrhythmias, cardiac, algorithms for management of, 54–62

Ear, pain in, in children, 293
Ectopic pregnancy, 219t
Ectopy, ventricular, vs. ventricular aberration, 251, 251t, *252*, *253*
Edema, pulmonary, acute, treatment of, *257*
in anuric patient, 258
EDTA, in arsenic poisoning, 137t
Elbow(s), injuries of, dog walking and, 398
Electrocardiogram, in diagnosis of right ventricular infarction, 248, *249*
in identification of arrhythmias, 251, 251t, *252*, *253*
Embolism, pulmonary, 246, 246t, 247t
Emergency, definition of, 3–4
Emergency department, activity of, factors influencing, 380–381
Emergency medicine, core reference library for, 403–404
development of, as a specialty, 377
Encephalitis, and coma in children, 326t
Endocarditis, bacterial, prevention of, drugs in, 256t
Endotracheal tube, air transport of patient with, 11t
selection of, in children, 284t
Epiglottitis, acute, in adults, 231
in children, 300t
Epiphyseal plate, fractures of, 180, 181t
Epistaxis, causes of, 225–226
location of bleeding in, anterior, 226
posterior, 226–228, *227*
superior, 226
management of, 225–228, *227*
Erythrocyte sedimentation rate, calculation of, 341
Erythromycin, in chlamydial infections, in infants, 308
in pertussis, in children, 309
Esophagitis, and rectal bleeding in children, 315t

Esophagus, obstruction of, due to food, 229–230

varices of, and rectal bleeding in children, 315t

Ethanol, in methanol poisoning, 138t

Ethylene glycol poisoning, antidote for, 137t

Euvolemia, 273

Evacuation procedures, in disaster management, 170

Extensor tendon(s), injuries to, 185, 185t, *186*

Eye(s), chemical injury of, 232–233, *233*

flash burns of, 233

red, causes of, 232, 232t

swelling of, in children, 295–296, 295t, 296t

Eye of Horus, 29–30

Fabric, removal of stains from, 374–375

Face, injuries of, evaluation of, 224, *225*

Fainting, 238, 238t

Feces, blood in, detection of, 343–344

Felon, of finger, dancing and, 394

Fibrillation, ventricular, monitored, algorithm for management of, 55

unmonitored, 56–57

Finger(s), felon of, dancing and, 394

injury to, 185, 185t, *186*

Frisbee and, 396

removal of ring from, 365, *365*

Fires, in hotels, tips for surviving, 401–402

Fissure, of anus, and rectal bleeding in children, 314t

Fluid(s), maintenance, in children, 285, 286t

Fluid volume, requirements for, in pediatric trauma patient, 105t

Fluoride poisoning, antidote for, 137t

Foot, glass fragments in, x-rays of, 182

Foreign body, and rectal bleeding in children, 315t

aspiration of, in children, 300t

Formaldehyde poisoning, antidote for, 137t

Fracture(s), blood loss due to, 178, 178t

complications of, 177, 177t–178t

of ankle, *192*, 192–195, *193*, *194*

of epiphyseal plate, 180, 181t

of pelvis, bladder injuries in, 116–117

in trauma patient, 116

urethral injuries in, 116–117

Frostbite, 175

of the lips, due to ice cream, 399

penile, 399

Gallbladder, visualization of, 209–210

Ganglionic blockers, and postural hypotension, 239

Gas, in soft tissues, causes of, 22t

Gas gangrene, air transport of patient with, 10t

Gasoline, siphoning of, injuries due to, 398

Gastroenteritis, acute infectious, features of, 316t, 317

Gastrointestinal tract, decontamination of, following poisoning, 135t

effects of organophosphate poisoning on, 147t

problems of, jogging and, 392–393

Genitalia, examination of, in trauma patient, 99t

Glasgow Coma Scale, in assessment of comatose trauma patient, 95, 95t, 97t

Glass fragments, x-rays of, 182

Glaucoma, acute, 232t

Gold poisoning, antidote for, 137t

Gram stain, procedure for, 341

Guaiac slide test, for detection of fecal blood, 343–344

Hair, removal of chewing gum from, 364

Hand(s), glass fragments in, x-rays of, 182

injuries of, assessment of, 182–186, 183t, 184t, 185t, *186*, *187*

types of, 184, 184t

sensation in, 183

vascular supply to, 182–183

Head, examination of, in trauma patient, 98t

Headache, 239, 240t–241t

Headgear, protective, removal of from trauma patient, 119, *119*

Health expenditures, 388t

Heart disease, air transport of patient with, 9t

Heart rate, in children, 282t

Heat, injuries due to, in long-distance running, 171–172

Heat stroke. See *Hyperthermia.*

Heavy metal poisoning, antidote for, 137t

Hemangioma, and rectal bleeding in children, 315t

Hematocrit, calculation of, 338

in shock, 49–52

Hematuria, algorithm for workup for, 271

in differential diagnosis of child abuse, 333t

Hemodynamic manipulation, techniques of, 84–85, *85*

Hemolytic-uremic syndrome, and rectal bleeding in children, 315t

Hemorrhage, acute, classes of, 101t

control of, in trauma patient, 91

pneumatic antishock trousers in, 107–108, 108t

epidural, in children, 325t

subconjunctival, dancing and, 394

subdural, in children, 325t

Hemorrhoids, and rectal bleeding in children, 315t

Hemostasis, in wound closure, 199

Henoch-Schonlein purpura, and rectal bleeding in children, 315t

Hepatitis, due to human bites, 129

prevention of, 260–261, 260t, 261t

in needle-stick injuries, 262–263

viral, serologic findings in, 260t

Hepatitis B immune globulin, in prevention of hepatitis B, 261t

HIDA scan, in acute cholecystitis, 209

Hormones, ingestion of during pregnancy, congenital malformations and, 223t

Hydatidiform mole, 219t

Hyperglycemia, sodium for, 348

Hypernatremia, and coma in children, 326t

Hyperplasia, nodular lymphoid, and rectal bleeding in children, 315t

Hypertensive crisis, in children, drugs for, 71t

Hyperthermia, 172, 172t, *173*, 174, 174t
  drugs associated with, 174t
  initial treatment of, 174
Hypervolemia, 272
Hypochlorite poisoning, antidote for, 137t
Hypoglycemia, and coma in children, 326t
  in children, drugs for, 71t
  in newborns, 290–291
Hyponatremia, 272–273
  and coma in children, 326t
Hypotension, in children, drugs for, 70t
  in newborns, 290
  postural, drugs and, 239
Hypothermia, in newborns, 289–290
Hypovolemia, 273
Hypoxia, in children, drugs for, 71t

Ileus, postoperative, air transport of patient
    with, 9t
Immobilized patient, air transport of, 11t
Immunobiologic agents, available from Centers
    for Disease Control, 268–269, 269t
Infant(s). See also *Newborn(s)*.
  chlamydial infections in, 307–308
  irritable, 292
  sudden death of, in differential diagnosis of
    child abuse, 333t
Infarction, myocardial, vs. "Chinese Restau-
    rant Syndrome", 247–248
  pulmonary, vs. pneumonia, in children, 299t
  right ventricular, 248, *249*
  vs. osteomyelitis, in children, 299t
Infection(s), air transport of patient with, 11t
  chlamydial, in infants, 307–308
  nasal vestibular, vs. swollen eye, in children,
    295t
  of urinary tract, single-dose treatment of,
    270
Injections, intramuscular, in children, 366,
    366t
Intestine(s), obstruction of, 208, 208t
  parasites of, and rectal bleeding in children,
    314t
Intracranial air, air transport of patient with,
    9t
Intramuscular injections, in children, 366, 366t
Intravenous catheters, flow rates of, 78–79, 79t
Intravenous fluids, air transport of patient
    with, 11t
Intravenous infusion, improvisation of, 80
Intubation, endotracheal, administration of
    drugs via, 76–77
  retrograde stylet in, 74, *74*
  nasotracheal, complications of, 75
    contraindications for, 75
    indications for, 75
    procedure for, 75–76
Intussusception, and rectal bleeding in chil-
    dren, 314t
Iodine poisoning, antidote for, 137t
Ipecac, syrup of, in iron poisoning, 145
  in treatment of poisoning, 135t
Iridocyclitis, 232t
Iritis, 232t
Iron poisoning, 144–145
  antidote for, 138t

Irradiation, vs. radioactive contamination,
    164–165, 164t
Irrigation, in chemical injuries of eye, 232–233
Isoniazid poisoning, antidote for, 138t

Jaw wires, air transport of patient with, 10t
Jogging, health problems related to, 392–393

Kawasaki syndrome, in children, 329–330
Ketoacidosis, diabetic, and coma in children,
    326t
  in children, 287
Knee(s), injuries of, in adolescents, 187–190,
    188, 189t, 190t, 191t
  due to overuse, 190t–191t
Kwell, in treatment of pediculosis, 127

Labor, premature, air transport of patient
    with, 11t
Laboratory test(s), 336–353. See also specific
    tests.
  reasons for ordering, 337
Lacerations, periorbital, vs. swollen eye, in
    children, 295t
Lacrimal glands, effects of organophosphate
    poisoning on, 147t
Law(s), state, regarding drunk driving, 390t–
    391t
Lead poisoning, antidote for, 138t
Leg(s), injury to, musical instruments and, 395
Les torsades des pointes, 250, *250*, 250t
Lice, and pediculosis, 127–128
Life expectancy, average, 388t
Ligament(s), anterior cruciate, injury to, 189t
  medial collateral, 189t
Lighting, air transport of patient requiring, 11t
Limb(s), edematous, cast on, air transport of
    patient with, 10t
  replantation of, 118, *118*
Lumbar spine, x-rays of, 180

Magnesium sulfate, in barium salt poisoning,
    136t
Malformations, congenital, ingestion of drugs
    during pregnancy and, 221t–224t
Mallet finger, 185t, *186*
Marine life, poisoning due to, 122–125
Mean arterial pressure (MAP), in shock, 49–
    52, *50*, *52*
Mechanical bulls, injuries due to, 398
Meckel's diverticulum, and rectal bleeding in
    children, 314t
Medication(s). See *Drug(s)*.
Medicine, Oriental, 18–19
  bloodletting, 19
  cupping, 19
  skin scrape, 18–19
Meningitis, and coma in children, 326t
  prevention of, 263–264, 264t
Meniscus, injuries to, 190t
Mercury poisoning, antidote for, 138t

Methanol poisoning, antidote for, 138t

Methemoglobinemic agent poisoning, antidote for, 138t

Methenamine, in phosgene poisoning, 139t

Methylene blue, in methemoglobinemic agent poisoning, 138t

Midgut, volvulus of, and rectal bleeding in children, 314t

Migraine headache, 240t

Milk, intolerance to, and rectal bleeding in children, 314t

Monosodium glutamate, sensitivity to, 247–248

Mucomyst, in acetaminophen poisoning, 136t, 141, 141t

Musculoskeletal system, examination of, in trauma patient, 99t

Mushrooms, poisoning due to, 125–127, 126t

Myocardial infarction, vs. "Chinese Restaurant Syndrome", 247–248

N-acetylcysteine, in acetaminophen poisoning, 136t, 141, 141t

Nail bed, injuries to, 185

Naloxone, in narcotic poisoning, 138t

Narcotic poisoning, antidote for, 138t

Narcotics, use of, 26, 27t

Neck, examination of, in trauma patient, 98t
stiff, in children, 320t, 321

Needle-stick injury(ies), management of, 262–263

Neonate, air transport of, 11t

Nerve(s), peripheral, testing of, 196, 196t

Neuritis, pudendal, cyclist's, 394

Neurologic dysfunction, in children, Reyes syndrome and, 288

Neuropathy, compression, due to sunglasses, 399

Newborn(s), altered acid-base status in, 291
drug dosages for, emergency, 291t
hypoglycemia in, 290–291
hypotension in, 290
hypothermia in, 289–290
positive pressure ventilation in, 291
stabilization of, 289–291, 291t

Nitrite poisoning, antidote for, 138t

Nitrogen saturation, air transport of patient with, 10t

Nitroglycerin, topical, hazards of, 80

Nose, bleeding from, causes of, 225–226
management of, 225–228, 227

Nursemaid's elbow, in children, 321

Obstruction, intestinal, 208, 208t
of esophagus, due to food, 229–230
of upper airway, in children, 299t, 300t
x-rays of, 300

Occupational hazards, 154, 154t, 155, 156t–162t

Ocular findings, in differential diagnosis of child abuse, 332t

Odor(s), recognition of, 16–17

Oliguria, sudden acute, algorithm for management of, 53

Orbital cellulitis, 232t

Organ donation, intercenter criteria for, 14
role of emergency physician in, 13–15, 15

Organophosphate poisoning, 147–148, 147t

Orotracheal tube, pediatric, specifications for, 105t

Orthopedic injury(ies), 177, 177t

Osgood-Schlatter disease, 191t

Osmolal gap, calculation of, 352–353

Osseous lesions, in differential diagnosis of child abuse, 333t

Osteochondritis dissecans, 191t

Osteomyelitis, vs. infarction, in children, 299t

Otalgia, in children, 293

Otitis, due to siphoning gasoline, 398

Oxalate poisoning, antidote for, 138t

Oxygen, air transport of patient receiving, 11t
in carbon dioxide poisoning, 136t

Pacemaker, balloon-tipped, temporary placement of, 82, 82, 83, 84
electronic, air transport of patient with, 9t

Palsy, cyclist's, 394

Pancreatitis, acute, 210–213
differential diagnosis of, 211
early signs of, morbidity and mortality and, 212
etiologic factors in, 212
major complications of, early signs of, 212
symptoms of, 210–211
treatment of, 211

Panniculitis, popsicles and, 400

Parasites, diseases due to, drugs in treatment of, 269t
intestinal, and rectal bleeding in children, 314t

Patella, dislocation of, 190t

Patient(s), immobilized, air transport of, 11t
psychiatric, air transport of, 11t
walk-out, 28–29

Pediculosis, 127–128

Pelvis, fracture of, bladder injuries in, 116–117
in trauma patient, 116
urethral injuries in, 116–117

Penicillamine, in heavy metal poisoning, 137t

Penis, frostbite of, jogging and, 399
zipper injuries of, 120, 120

Percentages, in results of medical studies, 384–385

Pericardiocentesis, 80–82, 81

Perineum, examination of, in trauma patient, 99t

Peritoneal lavage, in diagnosis of acute abdomen, in trauma patient, 108–110, 109t
in evaluation of stab wounds, 111

Pertussis, in children, 309

Phencyclidine (PCP), 146

Phenol poisoning, antidote for, 138t

Phenothiazine poisoning, antidote for, 139t

Phenothiazines, and postural hypotension, 239

Phenylpropanolamine, overdose of, 152

Phosgene poisoning, antidote for, 139t

Physician(s), number of active, 379t
projected supply of, 378, 378t

Physostigmine, in anticholinergic poisoning, 136t

Placenta previa, 218, 220

Pneumatic antishock trousers, 107–108, 108t
air transport of patient with, 10t
Pneumomediastinum, air transport of patient with, 9t
Pneumonia, in children, 310–311, 310t, 311t
vs. infarction, in children, 299t
Pneumonitis, chlamydial, in infants, 308
Pneumoperitoneum, air transport of patient with, 9t
Pneumothorax, air transport of patient with, 9t
Poisoning, and coma in children, 327, 327t
by marine life, 122–125
catfish, 124
coral, 123
jellyfish, 122–123
sea urchins, 123–124
stingrays, 124–125
due to Christmas decorations, 153–154
due to mushrooms, 125–127, 126t
treatment algorithm for, 126
gastrointestinal decontamination following, 135t
management of, 134, 135t
Poisons, antidotes for, 135, 136t–139t
Pollutants, environmental, 154, 154t, *155*, 156t–162t
Polyps, and rectal bleeding in children, 314t
Postictal states, and coma in children, 326t
Potassium, concentration of, disorders of, 344–345, 344t
Pralidoxime, in organophosphate poisoning, 148
Pralidoxime chloride, in anticholinesterase poisoning, 136t
Pregnancy, ectopic, 219t
ingestion of drugs during, 220–221, 221t–224t
tests of, *215*, 215–216, 216t, 217t
vaginal bleeding during, 217–218, 218t, 219t, 220
Prescriptions, abbreviations used in, 31
checklist for, 30–31
for liquids, 32
Pressure, intracranial, increased, in children, 323–324, 324t
Proctitis, and rectal bleeding in children, 314t
Protein, intolerance to, and rectal bleeding in children, 314t
Pseudosyncope, 238, 238t
Psychiatry, 354–361. See also specific disorders.
Pulmonary edema, acute, treatment of, *257*
in anuric patient, 258
Pulmonary embolism, 246, 246t, 247t
Pulmonary testing, in children, *304*, 304–305, *305*
Pulmonary vascular pressures, respiratory variation of, 86, *86*
Pupils, of eyes, effects of organophosphate poisoning on, 147t
Pyridoxine, in isoniazid poisoning, 138t

Quaternary ammonium compound poisoning, antidote for, 139t

Rabies, prevention of, 131–132, 132t–133t
in animal bite wounds, 129–130
Radiation, dosage of, effects of, 163, 163t
injury due to, antidotes for, 167
decontamination procedures for, 165–167
management of, 164–167, 164t, 165t, 168t–169t
Radioactive contamination, treatment of, 165–167
vs. irradiation, 164–165, 164t
Radioactive packages, labeling of, 165, 165t
Radioassays, in pregnancy diagnosis, 217t
Rectum, bleeding from, in children, 314, 314t–315t
Reflexes, testing of, in ankle, 195
Refractometer, in measurement of specific gravity of urine, 343
Replantation, of limbs, 118, *118*
Respiratory manipulation, clinical formulas for, 346–348
Respiratory rate, in children, 282t
Resuscitation, artificial methods of, 35
cardiovascular, in children, drugs for, 70t
of trauma patient, 92
Resuscitation cart, pediatric, 68–69
Retractor, eyelid, improvisation of, *233*
Retrograde stylet, in management of upper airway obstruction, 74, *74*
Reyes syndrome, 288–289
and coma in children, 326t
Rhythm, supraventricular, with pulse, algorithm for management of, 62
RID, in treatment of pediculosis, 127
Rifampin, in prevention of meningitis, 264, 264t
Ring, removal of, from finger, 365, *365*
Running, long-distance, heat injuries in, 171–172

Salicylate poisoning. See *Aspirin poisoning.*
Saline cathartics, in treatment of poisoning, 135t
Salivary glands, effects of organophosphate poisoning on, 147t
Scabies, in children, 331
Sciatica, unicyclist's, 393
Septic shock, in children, drugs for, 70t
Serum immune globulin, in prevention of hepatitis A, 261t
in prevention of non-A, non-B hepatitis, 261t
Sexual abuse, in children, 318–319
Sharks, rules for swimming with, 402–403
Shingles, 277
Shock, classification of, 49
definition of, 49
management of, 49–53, *50*, *52*, *53*
treatment of, in trauma patient, 101–102, 101t
Shoulder(s), injury to, musical instruments and, 395–396
Sickle cell anemia, in children, 298, 299t
Silver poisoning, antidote for, 139t
Sinusitis, in children, 294–295
Skin disease(s), inflammatory, topical steroids in treatment of, 24–25, 24t, 25t

Smell, sense of, in identification of medical
   conditions, 16–17
   in identification of toxins, 16–17
Snake bites, antivenin for, 139t
Sodium, levels of, calculation of, 348
Sodium chloride, in bromide poisoning, 136t
Sodium nitrite, in cyanide poisoning, 137t
Sodium sulfate, in barium salt poisoning, 136t
Sodium thiosulfate, in cyanide poisoning, 137t
Soft tissues, causes of gas in, 22t
Spider bites, antivenin for, 139t
Spinal cord, segments of, testing of, 196, 196t
Spine, cervical, injuries of, 179t
   lumbar, x-rays of, 180
Stab wound, of abdomen, 111
Stain(s), acid-fast, procedure for, 342
   Gram, 341
   removal of, from fabric, 374–375
Starling curve, of ventricular function, 84–85,
   85
Statistics, miscellaneous, 385, 386t–388t
Status asthmaticus, in children, drugs for, 71t
Status epilepticus, in children, 328, 328t–329t
   drugs for, 71t
   tonic-clonic, management of, 276
Steroids, topical, in treatment of inflammatory
   skin diseases, 24–25, 24t, 25t
Stethoscope, improvisation of, 363, *363*
Striated muscle, effects of organophosphate
   poisoning on, 147t
Stridor, in children, 299, 299t, 300t
Stryker frame, air transport of patient with,
   10t
Suction, air transport of patient receiving, 11t
Sudden infant death, in differential diagnosis
   of child abuse, 333t
Suicidal patient, evaluation of, 355–356
   high risk factors in, 356t
   risk score and death rate in, 356t
   risk-rescue rating in, 357t
Sulfadiazine, in prevention of meningitis, 264,
   264t
Surgery, cataract, air transport of patient fol-
   lowing, 9t
   retinal, 9t
Sutures, 202–203, 203t
   techniques of use of, 203t
   types of, 202
Sweat glands, effects of organophosphate poisoning on, 147t
Swimming, with sharks, rules for, 402–403
Sympathetic ganglia, effects of organophosphate poisoning on, 147t
Syncope, 238, 238t
Syndrome of inappropriate ADH secretion
   (SIADH), 273
Syrup of ipecac, in iron poisoning, 145
   in treatment of poisoning, 135t

Tachycardia, ventricular, algorithm for management of, 60–61
   recurrent, algorithm for management of,
   62
Tar, removal of from burns, 365
Tattoos, 20–21
   resulting from trauma, 204
   significance of, 21

Teeth, avulsion of, due to trauma, 230
Telangiectasia, and rectal bleeding in children,
   315t
Temperature, of air, rise in, dangers of, 170–
   171, 170t
Temporal arteritis, 241t
Tendonitis, of patellar tendon, 191t
Tendons, extensor, injuries to, 185, 185t, *186*
Testis(es), torsion of, 214–215
Tetanus, prevention of, 204, 205t
   in animal bite wounds, 129–130
   in open wounds, 205t
   primary immunization against, 205t
   risk of, in open wounds, 205t
Tetralogy of Fallot, in children, drugs for, 71t
Thallium poisoning, antidote for, 139t
Theophylline, in asthmatic child, 306–307,
   307t
Thoracic aortic dissection, 206, 207t
Thoracic aortic transection, 112
Thumb(s), injury to, 185, 185t, *186*
   Pachinko and, 395
   Rubik's Cube and, 395
   motion of, *187*
Tinnitus, 228, 228t–229t
Tonometry, *234*, 234–236, *235*
   false readings in, causes of, 236
   uses of, 234–235
   contraindications to, 236
Tonsillitis, in children, 300t
Toxic shock syndrome, criteria for diagnosis
   of, 266–268, *267*
   differential diagnosis of, 268
   management of, 268
   risk of recurrence of, 267–268
Toxin(s), in osmolality, 353t
   occupational, 154, 154t, *155*, 156t–162t
Tracheostomy, air transport of patient with,
   10t
Traction, balanced, air transport of patient
   with, 10t
Transection, thoracic aortic, 112
Trauma. See also *Trauma patient.*
   avulsion of teeth due to, 230
   coma due to, in children, 324–325, 325t
   corneal, 232t
   facial, evaluation of, 224, *225*
   penetrating, air transport of patient following, 9t
   tattoos resulting from, 204
Trauma patient, acute abdomen in, peritoneal
   lavage in diagnosis of, 108–110, 109t
   blast injuries in, 114, 115t
   comatose, assessment of, Glasgow Coma
   Scale in, 95, 95t, 97t
   initial assessment of, 90–92
   primary survey in, 90–91, 96t
   resuscitation phase in, 92
   secondary survey in, 92
   pediatric, 105–106, 105t, 106t
   pelvic fractures in, 116
   removal of protective headgear from, 119,
   119
   replantation of limbs in, 118, *118*
   severity of injury in, assessment of, 93, 93t,
   94, *94*
   treatment of shock in, 101–102, 101t
   use of uncrossmatched blood in, 102–104

Trauma patient (*Continued*)
  with multiple injuries, assessment of, secondary survey in, 98t–99t
    diagnostic work-up for, 100t
    examination of, 96t–100t
    overlooked injuries in, 106
Trauma Score (TS), in assessment of injury, 93, 93t, 94, *94*, 96t
Tricyclic antidepressant poisoning, antidote for, 139t
Tubes, endotracheal, selection of, in children, 284t

Ulcer, corneal, 232t
  peptic, and rectal bleeding in children, 315t
Ultrasonography, Doppler, in diagnosis of torsion of testis, 214
  in acute cholecystitis, 209
  in placenta previa, 218, 219t
Unconscious patient, air transport of, 9t
Upper airway, obstruction of, by foreign objects, 300–301, 301t
  in children, 299, 299t, 300t
    management of, 72, *72–73*, *73*
      retrograde stylet in, 74, *74*
Urinary tract, infections of, single-dose treatment of, 270
  injuries of, following pelvic fracture, 116–117
Urine, slide tests of, in pregnancy diagnosis, 215–216, 216t
  specific gravity of, calculation of, 342–343
  specimen of, suprapubic, in children, 319
Urine sediment, sampling of, 342
Urinometer, in measurement of specific gravity of urine, 342
Uveitis, 232t
Uvulitis, in children, 296–297

Varices, esophageal, and rectal bleeding in children, 315t
Vasodilators, and postural hypotension, 239

Ventilation, positive pressure, in newborns, 291
  transtracheal catheter, *72*, *72–73*, *73*
Ventricular aberration, vs. ventricular ectopy, 251, 251t, *252*, *253*
Ventricular ectopy, vs. ventricular aberration, 251, 251t, *252*, *253*
Violent patient, management of, 358–360
Vitamin K, in warfarin poisoning, 139t
Volvulus, of midgut, and rectal bleeding in children, 314t

Warfarin poisoning, antidote for, 139t
Water skiing, injuries due to, 397
Waterslides, injuries due to, 396
Wheezing, in children, 301–302
Whooping cough, in children, 309
Wound(s), botulism in, 265
  closure of, 198–201
    antibiotics in, 210
    debridement in, 199
    hemostasis in, 199
    in children, 322–323
    irrigation in, 198–199
    local anesthetic in, 198
    tetanus prophylaxis in, 201
  prevention of tetanus in, 204, 205t
Wrist(s), injury of, rollerskating and, 397
  tobacco priming and, 399
  video games and, 394

X-ray(s), chest, in thoracic aortic transection, 112
  in intestinal obstruction, 208
  of foreign object, 300
  of fractures of epiphyseal plate, 180, 181t
  of glass fragments, 182
  of lumbar spine, 180

Zipper injuries, of penis, 120, *121*